Geographies of Women's Health

Around the globe, environmental and social transformations are reshaping women's mental and physical health experiences, their access to health care services, and their roles in care giving.

This international collection explores the relationships between society, place, gender, and health, and how these play out in different parts of the world. The chapters work together in examining the complex layering of social, economic, and political relations that frame women's health. The authors demonstrate that women's health needs to be understood "in place" if gains are to be made in improving women's health and health care. Policy implications are woven throughout as contributors explore the close connections between policy structures, access to health and health care resources, and modes of service delivery. What happens in the offices of government can have profound influences on women's ability to create and sustain healthy lives.

The contributors use both qualitative and quantitative methodologies, representing the many lenses now being employed in understanding the health of women. Many chapters use women-centered research strategies and draw on feminist theory in explicating the links between health and place. What is significant in these accounts is that women are rarely best viewed as "victims" but as women exploring and using active strategies in managing health and illness and accessing both formal and informal health care systems.

Isabel Dyck is a social geographer and Associate Professor in the School of Rehabilitation Sciences, University of British Columbia. Her research interests include feminist analyses of the work experiences of women with chronic illness and health care access for immigrant and minority group women.

Nancy Davis Lewis is Associate Dean of Social Sciences and Professor of Geography at the University of Hawaii. Her research explores a wide range of health issues from human ecology to the health transition.

Sara McLafferty is Professor of Geography at Hunter College of the City University of New York. Her research has explored geographic inequalities in health and access to health care in cities and the use of spatial analysis methods in examining these issues.

Routledge international studies of women and place
Series editors: Janet Henshall Momsen and Janice Monk

Geographies of Women's Health

Edited by Isabel Dyck,
Nancy Davis Lewis,
and Sara McLafferty

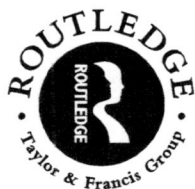

ROUTLEDGE

London and New York

First published 2001
by Routledge
11 New Fetter Lane, London EC4P 4EE

Simultaneously published in the USA and Canada
by Routledge
29 West 35th Street, New York, NY 10001

Routledge is an imprint of the Taylor & Francis Group

Typeset in Sabon by Keystroke, Jacaranda Lodge, Wolverhampton
Printed and bound in Great Britain by Biddles Ltd, Guildford and King's Lynn

British Library Cataloguing in Publication Data
A catalogue record for this book is available from the British Library

Library of Congress Cataloging in Publication Data
Geographies of women's health/edited by Isabel Dyck, Nancy Davis
Lewis, and Sara McLafferty.
     p. cm.
     Includes bibliographical references and index.
1. Women—Health and hygiene—Cross-cultural studies.
2. Women—Medical care—Cross-cultural studies.
3. Medical geography. 4. World health—Case studies.
I. Dyck, Isabel. II. Lewis, Nancy, 1946– III. McLafferty, Sara, 1951–

RA564.85 .G47 2000
614.4′2′082—dc21   00–045838

ISBN 0–415–23607–X

Contents

Illustrations

Figures

Tables

Contributors

Adrian J. Bailey is currently a Senior Lecturer in the School of Geography at the University of Leeds and Adjunct Associate Professor of Geography at Dartmouth College. His interests in the health of international migrants have focused on the experiences of Puerto Ricans and Salvadorans in New York, and among immigrant children, Latinos, and Asians in New England.

Susan Craddock is Assistant Professor of Women's Studies and Geography at the University of Arizona. Her research interests focus on disease as both an outcome and a producer of social difference and inequity. Her publications include *Dis/Placing Disease: Poverty, Deviance, and Public Health Policy*.

Joyce Davidson is currently undertaking postdoctoral research at the Institute of Health Research, University of Lancaster. Her research focuses on women with agoraphobia, and seeks to make gendered links between place, embodiment, and mental health. Her current research draws on her background in philosophy, where she worked with feminist theories of identity. She has published in *Hypatia*, a journal of feminist philosophy.

Isabel Dyck is a social geographer and Associate Professor in the School of Rehabilitation Sciences, University of British Columbia. Her research interests include feminist analyses of the home and work experiences of women with chronic illness, health care access for immigrant, minority group women, and integration issues for immigrant families. Current research includes examination of the home as a site for long-term care.

Anne Ellaway is a researcher working with Sally Macintyre exploring the processes by which place of residence might influence health and the ability to lead healthy lives. Published work includes the role of housing and neighborhood conditions in producing health outcomes.

Jim Glassman is a Killam Postdoctoral Fellow in the Department of Geography at the University of British Columbia and Assistant Professor in the Department of Geography at Syracuse University. His current research is on state policies promoting manufacturing development in Thailand and on the role of the gendering of assembly work in Thailand's industrial transformation.

Patricia Gober is Professor of Geography at Arizona State University, where she has taught since 1975. She has been President of the Association of American Geographers, and has served on boards and committees for the National Science Foundation, the Population Reference Bureau, and the National Oceanographic and Atmospheric Administration. Dr. Gober is author of numerous works focusing on urban geography, population geography, and migration.

Elizabeth Hoban is a public health worker with a background in Primary Health Care education, program development, and public health research. She has been working in Australian Indigenous health and international public health in Africa and Southeast Asia for the past fifteen years. Her research has examined barriers to cervical cancer screening in Indigenous communities and the development of appropriate service delivery systems. She is currently working towards a PhD at the Key Centre for Women's Health in Society at Melbourne University.

Caroline Kerner is currently a research associate at Boston University. Her research interests include women's health and Latino/a immigration.

Maureen Kirk is a Gunggalida Aborigine from Burketown. She was the cancer support officer for Indigenous women at the Royal Women's Hospital, Brisbane, prior to her secondment to The University of Queensland to undertake research. She is a member of several national and regional committees related to breast and cervical cancer and serves on the National Advisory Committee for Health Promotion for Indigenous Health Workers. She is currently project director for state-wide efforts to increase Indigenous women's access to cancer screening and treatment.

Nancy Davis Lewis is Associate Dean of Social Sciences and Professor of Geography at the University of Hawaii. Her research explores a wide range of health issues, including the health of women. Her current research is on the relationship between climate change and infectious disease in the Pacific Islands. This is set within a context of gender, social vulnerability, and the human dimensions of global change. She serves as the Secretary General of the Pacific Science Association and on the editorial boards of *The Contemporary Pacific, Ethics, Place and Environment* and *Pacific Science*.

Andrea Litva is currently a lecturer in Medical Sociology in the Department of Primary Care, University of Liverpool. Her teaching and research interests center on lay perceptions of health, illness, and health care, public involvement in health care decision making, and using social theory and qualitative methods in health services research.

Sally Macintyre is Director of the Medical Research Council's Social and Public Health Sciences Unit at the University of Glasgow. Following on from a general interest in the social patterning of health, her recent research interests are in the patterning of health by social class, area of residence, and gender.

Sara McLafferty is Professor of Geography at Hunter College of the City University of New York. Her research and publications have explored geographic inequalities in health and access to health care in cities and the use of spatial analysis methods in examining these issues. She has also investigated the impacts of economic restructuring and policy transformations on women's access to employment and health care services.

Lenore Manderson is a medical anthropologist and social historian. She is Professor of Women's Health and Director of the Key Centre for Women's Health in Society, The University of Melbourne. Her primary research interests on which she has published widely are related to infectious disease in poor resource communities, and to gender, sexuality, and women's health. She is a Fellow of the Academy of Social Sciences of Australia.

Ines Miyares is Associate Professor of Geography at Hunter College at the City University of New York. Her research addresses the formation and function of urban immigrant, refugee, and transnational communities, and Latin America. Her publications have focused on the Hmong, Cubans, Russians, and the Latin American community in the New York metropolitan area.

Graham Moon is Professor of Health Services Research at the Institute for the Geography of Health, University of Portsmouth. He is editor of *Health and Place* and a former Chair of the Royal Geographical Society–Institute of British Geographers' Geography of Health Research Group. He has published extensively on health geography and social perspectives on health and health policy. His current research interests focus on conceptions of place in health policy, health-related behavior, and the genealogy of post-1945 medical geography.

Pamela Moss is an Associate Professor in the Faculty of Human and Social Development at the University of Victoria, British Columbia. She teaches as a socialist, poststructuralist, and feminist, and she is active in feminist community politics around issues in women's housing and women's health advocacy. Her writing considers the themes of body, self, and identity in numerous contexts. Publications include an edited collection of essays on the geographical uses of autobiography, and a feminist methodology text for students in geography.

Alison Mountz is a doctoral student in geography at the University of British Columbia. Her research interests include transnational migration, urban geographies, and feminist methodology.

Kay Peggs is lecturer in sociology in the School of Social and Historical Studies, University of Portsmouth. She has published in such journals as the *British Journal of Sociology*. Her present research lies in the field of gender, aging, and consumption.

Cynthia Pope is a PhD candidate in the Department of Geography and Regional Development at the University of Arizona with concentrations in medical and feminist geography. Her MA research focused on women crossing the border from Mexico into the United States for prenatal care. For the PhD, she is exploring issues related to women and health in Latin America, in particular how women perceive and respond to HIV risk in Havana, Cuba.

Jan Rigby is a teaching fellow at the School of Geographical Studies, University of Bristol. Her research interests include applications of GIS and spatial analysis to the geographies of ill-health, and the role of early environment and life-course events in health outcomes, and she has recently completed a study of breast cancer.

Mark W. Rosenberg is Professor of Geography at Queen's University in Kingston, Ontario. His research interests focus on women's health, the elderly population, persons with disabilities, and access to health and social services. He is currently working on a three-year study of the geographies of women's health and is co-author of the book *Growing Old in Canada*. He serves as Secretary of the International Geographical Union Commission on Health, Environment and Development and Chairperson of the Association of American Geographers' Medical Geography Specialty Group.

Carol Thomas is a Senior Lecturer in Applied Social Science at Lancaster University, and works closely with the university's Institute for Health Research. Her research interests include disability studies, especially disabled women's social experiences, the psycho-social needs of cancer patients, and understanding health inequalities. She is the author of *Female Forms: Understanding and Experiencing Disability*, together with a wide range of articles and book chapters on disability and health-related topics.

Sue Tripathi received her PhD in medical geography from Kent State University. She is currently a research analyst in the Department of Health, Adams County, Colorado. Her research interests focus on gender and health-related topics, including HIV/AIDS, STDs, substance abuse, and related areas.

Yvonne Underhill-Sem is a Lecturer at the University of Waikato/Te Whare Wanaga o Waikato. A Cook Islands New Zealander with close family ties to Papua New Guinea, she has taught at the University of Papua New Guinea and University of Waikato and has also worked as a strategic health planner. Her research interests include population mobility and ethnic identities among Pacific Islanders in New Zealand. More recently she has critiqued demographically driven population policies in the third world and worked on the Pacific Island contribution to the Cairo population meeting.

Allison Williams is an Assistant Professor in the Department of Geography, University of Saskatchewan and a research faculty with the Saskatchewan Population Health and Evaluation Research Unit (SPHERU). Her research examines how environments operate as determinants of and pathways to health, particularly for First Nations Peoples, the elderly, home care practitioners, and specifically women. A major focus is women's paid and unpaid caring work that takes place in the home. She is active in research partnerships with public health departments, community groups, and various health care organizations.

Richard A. Wright is Professor of Geography and Chair of the Geography Department at Dartmouth College, New Hampshire. His research explores the social and spatial construction of labor markets in US metropolitan areas, and the transnational social and economic lives of Salvadoran immigrants.

Acknowledgments

This edited collection had its beginnings in conversations with Jan Monk and Janet Momsen who encouraged us to contribute to their series on the geographical aspects of women's lives. Their support and helpful comments were invaluable during the long process of producing the volume. We would like to thank them for their support for women geographers and leadership in the development of feminist geography more generally; this has been an inspiration to us, as for many, and we are indebted to their interest and energy in fostering the publication of research in many fields of relevance to the geographies of women's lives.

Thanks and appreciation are due to our contributors, whose patience with delays and ready willingness to make changes helped us though the process. We would also like to acknowledge our health geography colleagues who have supported our endeavor, especially Mark Rosenberg who organized a panel featuring book authors at the Association of American Geographers' 96th Annual Meeting in Pittsburgh, 2000. The diligent and cheerful assistance of Elisa Lin during the detailed final editing and compilation of the book at UBC was much appreciated.

Our appreciations would be incomplete without a final note on the pleasure of our long-distance collaboration in producing the collection. Our enthusiasm for the project overcame the initial challenges of working in virtual space, and electronic communication allowed us to continue discussion emanating from various countries and three continents during the book's production. Thanks go to Eric Rowe at UBC for his patient untangling of computer glitches along the way.

1 Why geographies of women's health?

Isabel Dyck, Nancy Davis Lewis,
and Sara McLafferty

Introduction

The last decade has seen an escalating interest in understanding the health of women. As women's health has been explored, the limits of biomedical approaches in understanding health and illness have become evident. Reliance on biological and physiological explanation of women's health and illness is challenged by documentation of the ways in which women's location in complex social, political, and economic relations affects the content and meaning of their lives, including their experience of health and sense of well-being. Gender is shown to be a major axis of difference that affects health status, while class, "race," and nationality are also interrelated in complex ways with health inequalities. Social science is now commonly, but not universally, acknowledged as an essential ingredient in understanding women's health, one that must take into account the various dimensions of "context" in which women live.

Although social science scholarship concerned with women's health has not always employed feminist theory, feminist inquiry has made important contributions in two main ways. First, through centering women's experiences and locating these experiences in wider social relations and political economies, conventional ways of conceptualizing women's health issues have been extended. The organization of gender relations and the gendering of activities situate women in conditions conducive to health and ill-health. Women's working conditions in and outside the home, their position in the household, their reproductive roles and associated sexual practices all contribute to their experience of health. Second, feminist scholarship has been influential in prescribing research methods that are appropriate for investigating gendered social relations and their impact on where and how women live. Research based in the successive waves of feminism has challenged woman as a unitary concept. In addition, the inadequacy of Western feminism's concepts in explaining women's lives in developing countries has been exposed, and ways in which research can be ethically conducted along feminist principles with emancipatory aims has been debated. Together, these contributions have opened up ways of exploring women's health that emphasize the importance of the *interconnections* between the biological, psychological, social, cultural, economic, and political dimensions of health and illness.

Social science scholarship on women's health also grows out of pragmatic concerns about the impacts for women of global and regional transformations. What women *do* and the environments in which they live are changing. The opportunities and resources for improving health are being transformed in the context of social, economic, and technological processes which affect the types of work women and men engage in and the organization of reproduction. In the developing world, economic recession, structural adjustment, environmental deterioration, and ethnic strife have had special ramifications for the health – or ill-health – of women. Similar concerns are emerging in Eastern Europe and the former Soviet Union, where the health impacts of decades of environmental degradation are only now being revealed. Around the globe, women's increasing participation in the paid labor force, widening class divisions, and restructuring of health and social services are reshaping women's health and access to health care. In addition, the international financial community's belated recognition of women's role in economic development has increased the burdens on women, responsible now not only for their own health, but for that of their families, the environment – and the economy.

Until recently the contribution of geography has been largely absent in these investigations of women's health. With this volume, in which many but not all authors are geographers, we begin to fill that lacuna. We explore a wide range of issues concerning women's health, and suggest ways in which geographic inquiry can further our understanding of the health of women. As in other social science disciplines, we move away from a medical focus to a broader understanding of health, locating the discussion within political and economic processes and social change. How such processes play out in particular places brings a distinct geography to women's health issues and to their health care, whether as consumers or providers. How women's health is defined and responded to, what conditions produce health or ill-health, and what resources are available to women as they manage their own or their families' health and illness are all shaped within particular polities, economies, and cultural discourses about gender.

The authors of the chapters employ both qualitative and quantitative methodologies in their inquiries and the approaches taken are diverse and representative of the many lenses now being employed in understanding the health of women. Running through many of the contributions is the inclusion of women's own perspectives of health and illness and ways of managing health. These bring further nuances to the depiction and understanding of the complex interactions between place, gender, and health. The chapters suggest the importance of both traditional research approaches and women-centered methods in understanding women's health. What is significant in these accounts is that women are rarely best viewed as "victims," but should be seen as women exploring and using active strategies in managing health and illness and accessing both formal and informal health care systems. Together the chapters begin to tease out relationships between society, place, gender, and health, and how these play out in different parts of the world. They reflect the changing concerns of inquiry in the field of women's health; chapter topics take us beyond the confines of medical definitions, medical sites, and biomedical provinces of knowledge to other areas, both conceptually and spatially beyond the clinic.

Research on women's health

In the biomedical research arena, until a decade and a half ago, the health of women had been largely ignored. A reason given was that white males were a convenient research norm. Kreiger and Fee (1994), however, argued that the lack of research on white women, and men and women in non-white racial and ethnic groups was not for convenience, but rather that these omissions must be read as evidence of a logic of difference. From a global perspective, we do not know to what extent the majority of research findings, which influence health strategies around the world, include the 90 percent of the global population not represented in these studies (Feacham *et al.* 1989). Greater research focus on lung cancer, perceived to be a male cancer, than on breast cancer was often cited as an example of this gender bias. Ironically, recent research findings suggest that a gene linked to the abnormal growth of lung cells is much more active in women than in men, and that nonsmoking females are three times more likely to develop lung cancer than nonsmoking males (Arnold and Eckstein 2000).

In the latter half of the 1980s, women's health appeared on the political – and research – agenda. It was a decade in which groups, including many feminist organizations, exerted increasing pressure on policy makers to address women's health. This resulted, on the biomedical front, in the creation of the Office for Research on Women's Health and the Women's Health Initiative in the United States. Federal, provincial, and territorial working groups were set up in Canada and a number of research centers for women's health were set up in Australia and elsewhere. Thomas and Rigby in this volume discuss the EU's European Women's Health Project, an example of this heightened interest, and highlight the dissonance, attributed in large part to political pressures, between the survey as designed and the final product.

In the international arena, women's health also took center stage. Women's health was central to the debates at the International Conference on Population and Development in Cairo, September 1994. It was also a major component of the Platform for Action at the Fourth World Conference on Women in Beijing and a major theme at the concurrent NGO Forum on Women in Huairou, in September 1995. It continues to be central in follow-up activities. An important message from Beijing was that health is a human right and women's rights are human rights. The understandable focus on maternal and child health and "safe motherhood" was expanded to include all aspects and stages of women's lives and to encompass physical, mental, social, and economic health, or "safe womanhood" (Lewis *et al.* 1994). This increased interest in women's health resulted in a plethora of meetings, publications, initiatives, and research agendas (Lewis 1998). Narrow, biomedically based models of women's health are being replaced with broader socio-ecological models of health. These increasingly recognize the value of social science research (Caldwell 1993; Caldwell *et al.* 1990; Chen *et al.* 1993) and the contribution of transdisciplinary approaches (Bird and Rieker 1999; Rosenfield 1992; *Social Science and Medicine* 1992, 1996). Gender, however, had not always been explicitly incorporated into these frameworks (Caldwell and Caldwell 1994). Ruzek (1993) called for a social model of health that puts women's health needs at the center of the analysis and focuses attention on the diversity of women's health over the life-cycle.

Conceptualizing women's health

A social model of health situates women's and men's health in particular social, economic, and political circumstances – varying over time and space. It emphasizes that the biological, although the site of acute and chronic disease symptoms or traumatic injury, must be closely related to social relations and processes in understanding why and how people are sick. Feminist analyses emphasize the influence of structured inequalities based on gender – but also those pertaining to class, "race," sexual orientation, and age – on women's health. Health status and experience are understood as gendered phenomena. Gender is not equated with "sex difference" in this framework of understanding. Rather it refers to the socially and culturally constructed meanings around biological sex which inform notions of femininity and masculinity and associated norms of behavior. Such meanings and related gender identities and performance are not fixed. They shift over time and vary across space, so that what constitutes being a woman or a man in a particular society is a negotiated position. Feminist scholarship has documented and theorized the subordination of women within webs of meaning about masculinity and femininity that are translated into the organization of polities and economies and attendant social life and health. Doyal (1995), for example, suggests that women experience both material discrimination and cultural devaluation that, respectively, affect their access to the resources necessary to maintaining a healthy life and threaten their emotional health. This holds, Doyal points out, despite the wide variation in women's situations within their own societies and between countries. Drawing on international research, she shows that what women do as mothers, daughters, or wives, whether in domestic, waged, or unpaid community work, affects their health and how they manage health problems, sometimes detrimentally. Furthermore, attention to gender signals the importance of investigating the role played by women in care-giving, whether as professionals or family caregivers, and the further impact such care-giving may have on a woman's own health. Health cannot be compartmentalized as a separate issue in women's lives; rather it is integral to everyday life, its absence or presence closely linked to the organization of social relations at different geographical scales and an individual's positioning in society.

Whether emphasis is placed on political economy, cultural and social change, or women's agency in seeking to improve their health, *where* in the world women pursue their lives also matters to how they experience and manage health and illness. Cross-cultural variations are shown, for example, in life-cycle concerns, disease incidence, and dealing with threats to health (Whelehan *et al.* 1988). Health status and access to health care statistics also show inequalities between women throughout the world and within particular polities and economies. Yet gender, represented through a depiction of "the inseparability and co-mingling of their various tasks that tends to differentiate women's lives from those of men" (Doyal 1995: 21), remains an important social determinant of health. In short, being a woman is associated with particular hazards to health. Following from this, Doyal advocates analyses of how the activities of women's day-to-day lives impact on their health, taking into account material context, cultural constraints, and women's lived experience. Being healthy, she suggests, goes beyond subjective well-being to being free from sustained constraints on achieving one's potential and enjoying a satisfying life.

This conceptualization of health is similar to the approach of the World Health Organization (1986) and other holistic frameworks (e.g. Epp 1986) informing health promotion activities. These view health not merely as the absence of disease but as a resource for living – enabling people to cope with and change their physical, social, and economic environments in realizing their aspirations. Since the mid-1980s, increasing emphasis has been placed on the socio-environmental factors affecting health, culminating in a population health perspective which, however, has not gone without critique (see Hayes and Dunn 1998 for a review). The attendant politics of broader definitions of health also differ. Health promotion frameworks still tend to focus on individual change, despite recognizing the large part played by social determinants of health. Additionally, feminists, noting the inadequate articulation of gender in these frameworks of health, claim improvement of women's health must be based on analyses that promote understanding of how intersections of gender with other axes of social difference construct and maintain health inequalities.

Geographers have been well positioned to explore the complex links between "environments" and health in this shift to holistic models of health, whether at the scale of geopolitical positioning or the local level of everyday life. In the midst of the process of reconceptualizing health, Canadian geographers noted the potential contribution of their discipline to the project of "achieving health for all" (Rosenberg *et al.* 1990). Since then, medical, social, and cultural geographers have explored the contribution of social theory to understanding health, health care, and disability issues, and in so doing created a "new" medical geography or "health geography." Engaging with concepts of space and place in new and varied ways and working with a "cultural turn" throughout human geography, geographers have analyzed health, illness, and health care access as phenomena with intricate links between the "personal," the local, and global processes. Calls to reinsert space and place in medical geography were accompanied with a reworking of these concepts. Place, rather than being seen simply as location with the concomitant understanding of space as a "container" of action, is theorized as a relational and dynamic concept (Jones and Moon 1993; Kearns 1993).

Incorporation of social theory in analyses also brought health geography closer to work in cognate areas. An emphasis on narrative and a focus on the body, as both corporeal and discursively inscribed, forged new spaces for inquiry (see for example, Dorn and Laws 1994; Kearns 1995, 1997). Experiential accounts, the interrogation of medical categories, and the spatial and discursive constitution of the "deviant" bodies of the physically or mentally ill are areas commanding recent attention. A special issue of *Environment and Planning D: Society and Space* (1997) and collected volumes concerned with illness and disability (Butler and Parr 1999; Kearns and Gesler 1998) signal an emerging concentration of work in the spirit of the "new" health geography. These collections included analyses of the specificities of women's health and disability, although women's health was slow to attract attention in geography.

Geography and women's health

Somewhat later than other social scientists (Matthews 1995) geographers are adding their multiple voices to the exploration of women's health concerns, employing both quantitative and qualitative methods and contributing from a number of different theoretical perspectives. In 1989 Pearson had claimed that medical geography was genderless and colorblind, and later Litva and Eyles (1995) suggested that while there were feminists doing medical geography, there was no feminist medical geography. In the past decade, however, geographers have made important contributions to understanding women's health and developing feminist approaches. A special issue of *Geoforum* (1995) was the first collection in a journal explicitly addressing "geographies of women's health" and Moss and Dyck (1996) put forward a feminist materialist framework for analyzing the links between environment, illness experience, and the formation of (dis)abled identities (see also Moss and Dyck this volume). Focusing on concepts of place and space, and working closer with social theory, geographical inquiry has delved further into understandings of the contextual nature of women's health status and experience. Directions of inquiry also have become more inclusive in capturing the wide range of health issues pertinent to women (Lewis *et al.* 1994).

Core topics of investigation have been those surrounding reproductive health (Abel and Kearns 1991; Gober 1994; McLafferty and Templaski 1995;

Rosenberg 1988) and access to health care (Dyck 1995a; Flad 1995; Iyun and Oke 2000; Ross *et al.* 1994a, 1994b; Senior and Williamson 1990; von Reichert *et al.* 1995), but other aspects of women's emotional and physical health have been added, including issues related to the commercial sex industry, experiential accounts of living with chronic illness, and health over the life course (Asthana 1996a; Dorn 1998; Dyck 1995b, 1998, 1999; Elliot 1995; Lewis and Kieffer 1994; Macintyre *et al.* 1996; Moss 1997; Moss and Dyck 1999). Immigrant women's health and health care experiences are beginning to be noted (Dyck 1995a; Elliott and Gillie 1998), as are issues of empowerment for women in relation to their health (Asthana 1996b; Garvin 1995). On the other side of the coin women as health care providers are being given some attention (Harrison 1995). Throughout these studies, gender is shown to be an important dimension of health – in its construction, in its experience, in health care access – with women negotiating their health in the context of gendered relations and processes operating at different scales.

In these forays into various aspects of women's health, geographers have revisited conventional methodological approaches in attempts to understand the links between place, space, gender, and health. A tradition of quantitative approaches has been augmented by qualitative approaches as newly framed questions prescribe different methods within shifting areas of concern (see, for example, *The Professional Geographer* 1999). Bringing women's experiences and perspectives into the construction of knowledge about women's health through qualitative strategies shows both the diversity of women's experiences and the common threads of their health concerns. Yet, while qualitative methods have been privileged in much feminist research (Reinharz 1992), "counting women" is also important if we are to gain a full perspective on the many dimensions of women's positioning in societies throughout the world (see *The Professional Geographer* 1996). Quantitative methods can be used to document the broad contours of difference in women's health and well-being and their access to resources and services. Focusing on measurable dimensions of women's lives, the methods reveal how place-based differences in indicators of women's well-being are connected to social, economic, and environmental processes that operate locally, nationally, and globally (Macintyre *et al.* 1996). Women's positions in the social and service networks that are so critical for promoting health and preventing ill-health can also be described quantitatively (Gober 1994). The chapters in this book demonstrate the need to be flexible in thinking about methodology, employing ethically sound methods that fit the purposes of inquiry and reflect the voices and concerns of study participants. The chapters show a wide range of different ways of using both quantitative and qualitative approaches.

From political economy to the personal: interweaving scales and concerns

Not all chapters in this volume draw specifically on feminist theory, but their approaches are consistent in employing theoretical perspectives and methodologies which reveal something of the complex links between global economies, local experiences of place, and women's experiences of health and "self." As the chapters show, a variety of methods and theoretical approaches bring different perspectives to how we might study and understand women's health, and include gender – as it intersects with other social divisions such as age, "race," and class – as an important determinant of health. They bring a rich, textured analysis to how global and local changes intertwine in affecting the lives and health of women and work together in uncovering the layers of social, economic, and political relations and discourses that frame women's health. As the chapters move from national and international scales to "the geography closest in" – the body (cf. Rich 1986) – and engage a wide range of theoretical perspectives, they demonstrate that women's health needs to be understood "in place" if gains are to be made in improving women's well-being and access to health care. Policy implications are woven through the chapters as some authors take up the close connections between policy structures, access to health and health care resources, and modes of service delivery. What happens in the offices of government can have profound influences on women's ability to create and sustain healthy lives.

Part I: Globalization, structural change, and political realignment: implications for women's health

None of the contributions in this volume is global in scope. This is not surprising given the difficulty of attempting to develop valid and meaningful indices of women's status, including health status, even conventionally defined, at the global scale (United Nations 1991) and the considerable difficulties even at the regional level, e.g. the European Union (Thomas and Rigby this volume). The contributions in Part I address women's health from different theoretical and methodological perspectives, at different scales and for places at different points on the continuum of development. The lives of the women represented by these studies are variously affected by globalization, structural adjustment, the fluidity of capital and labor, national and international health policies, and political shifts within nations and regions.

Based on their involvement with the European Women's Health Project, Thomas and Rigby critique the final report, *The State of Women's Health in the European Community* (CEC 1997). They argue that the project started out with a clear commitment to a broad socio-structural and socio-cultural perspective but ended up as a traditional epidemiological study. There were several reasons for this, including problems of data availability, quality and comparability. However, the two primary forces were administrative imperatives of diplomacy and the general dominance of the positivistic epidemiological paradigm in health research. The dissonance between the project as designed and the final project highlights both political and practical challenges to be faced as the health, and ill-health, of women across the globe is explored. The authors ask how seriously member countries take the health needs of women.

Shifting the focus to Africa, Craddock explores the tensions existing between the non-industrialized and the industrialized countries in the HIV/ AIDS arena. She employs a social and political ecological framework to explore risk for women in East Africa. In suggesting that poverty as a category is too vague to be useful and must be broken into investigations of empowerment and entitlement, she makes explicit a consideration in a number of the other contributions to this volume. While she challenges geographers to contribute to an expanded scale of inquiry that encompasses the local, regional, and international scales, she argues that the most effective way to examine the effects of international institutional practices is increased attention to localized studies.

In a study in Northern Thailand, Glassman explores a topic ignored by most geographers, especially in the industrializing world, that of health in the workplace. The issues he explores are salient for women factory workers throughout Thailand and the industrializing world. The author argues that this is but one example of a gendered capitalist industrialization project that creates similar constraints and pressures for labor in disparate places, and reproduces similar patterns of work and workplace injury across the globe. This gendered and geographical class analysis highlights the relative disadvantage of workers in the north of Thailand. As in Craddock's contribution, empowerment, or lack thereof, is central to Glassman's analysis. Connection with workers across national and international spaces is problematic but may offer possibilities in a new global era.

In the concluding chapter in Part I, Gober and Rosenberg revisit earlier research and explore changes in the geography of access to abortion services for North American women over time. As in all the chapters in this part, but more explicitly than some, it addresses the role of the state, in this case in supporting or restricting women's right to abortion. It is the only chapter in this part directly focusing on access to care, a central theme in much research by health geographers (Rosenberg 1998). The chapter explores how differences in political systems and societal values nuance the debate about a woman's right to choose in the United States and Canada. As a historical analysis it differs from the chapter by Pope in Part II that calls into question some myths concerning women from Mexico who cross the US–Mexico border for obstetrical services. Together they focus our gaze on borders and the changing nature of borders in a global era. The authors conclude that North American women's ability to exercise their legal rights to have an abortion will depend increasingly on where they live.

Part II: *Providing and gaining access to health care: local areas and networks*

The local scale of inquiry, including the spaces and places of everyday life, occupies a central location in geographical studies of women's health. Positioned between the global and the personal, it considers the connections between wider social processes and women's health and access to health care in local areas. Several themes run through much of the literature on women's health at this geographical scale. The first is the need to understand how women's lives intersect with locally based social networks and networks of services, resources, and opportunities in affecting health and access to health care. For women, access to health care means much more than just distance and location; it includes the extent to which services are appropriate, affordable, and culturally "safe" (Dyck and Kearns 1995; Timyan *et al.* 1993). Time geographic factors constrain access (Young 1999). Not only are these constraints increasing in many areas with women's "double" and "triple" days, but they vary by class, ethnicity, and "race." Another theme is the local imprint of general social and economic processes on women's health inequalities, health care access, and mobilization (Asthana 1996b; McLafferty and Templaski 1995). How general processes play out in local areas is an important topic of investigation. Finally, as illustrated in several chapters in Part II, the mixing of qualitative and quantitative methodologies offers useful insights in local-scale investigations.

The chapters in Part II explore the links between the global and the local as expressed in women's changing roles in health care provision and their access to essential health services. Williams examines the impacts of economic restructuring and cutbacks in health care programs on women home health care workers in northern Ontario, Canada. An innovative mixed methodology that combines quantitative survey analysis and qualitative depth interviews reveals how home care workers' experiences are being transformed by health care cutbacks and privatization. They describe mounting pressures to increase productivity, changing definitions of tasks and responsibilities, and the resulting compression of their daily work lives in time and space. Given the predominance of women in the health care workforce, these patterns are likely to be repeated in many other parts of the industrialized world where health care privatization is in full swing.

An analysis of access to health care among Salvadoran immigrant women in New Jersey by Kerner, Bailey, Mountz, Miyares, and Wright also explores the local imprints of political and social processes. Women's narratives show how socially constructed immigration policies intersect with poverty and geographical constraints to limit access to essential preventive health care services. For these women, access is critically related to immigration status – the fear of violating current immigration status, misunderstandings about their health care rights as immigrants, and efforts to create an identity that will help them improve their immigration status. Issues of identity, power, marginalization, and citizenship are interwoven as women negotiate an unfamiliar and often unsupportive care landscape.

Pope's careful analysis of why women cross the US–Mexican border for prenatal care points out the complexity of women's health care choices in a politically charged border region. Rarely are women's decisions motivated by a desire for US citizenship, as commonly depicted in the media; rather, they reflect consideration of service opportunities in relation to the resources and constraints of everyday life. Social networks are important in directing women to affordable, quality prenatal care services across the border. Service providers often support border crossing, framing health care access in community, as opposed to political, terms. Social networks are also central in Tripathi's chapter which explores Indian women's efforts to gain treatment for sexually transmitted diseases. Using depth interviews along with the quantitative methodology of Q analysis, Tripathi finds that poverty, social stigma, and limited geographical availability of services constrain access to treatment; however, some women overcome these barriers by creating and drawing upon supportive, locally based social networks. Defined on the basis of religion, culture, caste, and gender, these networks represent an important informal resource that compensates in part for inadequacies in the formal medical care system.

Research partnerships are a central theme in Manderson, Kirk, and Hoban's chapter on barriers to the diagnosis and management of cervical cancer among Indigenous women in Australia. Prepared in partnership with Indigenous women, this chapter draws attention to the ethics of field research and how feminist participatory research can contribute to health policy by exploring issues of cultural safety, power, and reciprocity. Continuous consultation throughout the project gives voice to women's concerns while highlighting place-based geographical, social, and cultural barriers to treatment. More importantly, the authors argue that research partnerships can be seen as part of a process of reconciliation that acknowledges the historical production of health and illness in Indigenous communities, and recognizes and responds to community concerns.

Part III: Embodied health and illness, perceptions, and place

The chapters of this part bring the focus of inquiry to the embodiment of health and illness, and to the formations of ideas about health and its management. The spaces of everyday life are those through which the body is experienced and perceptions of health and illness constituted and negotiated. These dimensions of geographical inquiry emphasize the social construction of categories concerning the body, health, and illness. Within this general framework, the chapters demonstrate different ways of tracing connections between holistic conceptions of health, experiential accounts of health and illness, and the interrogation of medical categories as powerful, cultural constructions at the level of the "personal" and the local. An interest in theories of the body and the "self" is prominent in four of the chapters, reflecting a current preoccupation with how we can understand the healthy or ill body outside medical discourse and picking up on general questions concerning gender, place, body, and subjectivity (McDowell 1999). The situatedness of lay perceptions of health and illness in people's experience and perceptions of place, with recognition of their recursive constitution, is a theme tying together the last two chapters of Part III. How people interpret health and illness and respond to health problems has been shown to be profoundly social, open to change, and linked to the constitution of place and its social and cultural transformations and continuities (for early important contributions see Cornwell 1984; Donovan 1986). While qualitative inquiry has been prominent in this field, the quantitative methodology of Ellaway and Macintyre's study shows an alternative way of pursuing the theme of the interconnections between perceptions of place and health.

The importance of cultural comparison is highlighted in this set of chapters. The inclusion of Underhill-Sem's work in Papua New Guinea in contrast to others from Canada and Britain illuminates how culture as lived in particular places mediates health experience. The chapters show how culture and place interact in how health is talked about and understood, whether by professionals, women themselves, or through the categories used in research. They also indicate how health and illness are negotiated on a day-to-day basis in particular, local contexts. Theory and method are closely intertwined in these explorations, as authors trace various ways in which the specificities of place, with the social and the spatial recursively interconnected, are involved in how women experience and perceive health and illness. It is at this level of the everyday that the embeddedness of lay perceptions of health and illness in local networks of knowledge and experiences of place is observed, and that the body as the locus of experience *and* a "surface of inscription" emerges as one deemed healthy or ill.

Davidson, in her chapter, works with insights from the psychological works of Kierkegaard, particularly his understanding of anxiety, as she analyzes material from interviews with women suffering from agoraphobia, a medically defined disorder describing fear of public spaces. The women experience this as a crisis of body boundaries as they try to accomplish day-to-day tasks, especially in the mall – a place of practical and symbolic significance to women's household work. In interviews women talked of the spatial and temporal phenomenology of their experiences, and the spatial strategies they developed in coping with their difficulties in negotiating the self in an environment predicated on a masculine economy. Davidson, while emphasizing the women's everyday struggles, brings a note of optimism in that women can improve and come to experience public spaces positively.

Moss and Dyck also work closely with theory as they analyze the embodied experience of chronic illness. Empirical examples of women's employment experiences as they struggle with invisible disability are used to demonstrate the interconnections between body, environment, and illness. Understanding the body as both corporeal and constructed through discourse, the authors trace the material practices and lived spaces through which women's bodies are inscribed and associated meanings are reproduced. The authority of medical discourse in designating the body as diseased is discussed in relation to women's own experiences of their body and "ableness" in the context of processes of marginalization. The body and how it is theorized are central to Underhill-Sem's chapter on counting and accounting for fertility. She draws on traditional fertility analysis and its policy implications as well as field work in Papua New Guinea to explore the disjuncture between the meaning of fertility in the disembodied numbers of standard demographic analysis and the birthing experiences as related by women. This chapter suggests how culture and place situate the ways in which birth and fertility are talked about and measured, casting doubt on the generalizability of social science and medical categories to other cultural contexts.

Litva, Peggs, and Moon use qualitative methods to hear the accounts of young women defining health and describing their concerns about maintaining health on leaving home to attend university. Again a focus on the body provides an entry point to understanding the relationship between place, perceptions of health, and women's feelings of control over their health. For the young women of this study, fitness and food are arenas of concern in relation to health. They describe controlling the body as a strategy in coping with the uncertain "worlds and locales" of their changed environment. However, the management of the body and its health was closely related to appearance, in that having an attractive, "healthy" looking body was seen as an important resource in making the transition from home to university life.

Just as perceptions of health may be place-related, perceptions of place may be related to health. Ellaway and Macintyre use traditional survey methods and measures of mental and physical health to examine links between gender differences in perceptions of local residential environments and men's and women's health. Collecting data in four contrasting neighborhoods in the West of Scotland, the authors conclude that perceptions of area are associated with health, with some measures showing a stronger gender association than others. Their analysis indicated a stronger association for men on one mental health measure, with women showing a stronger association with physical symptoms, but they caution that associations between assessments of area and health cannot be assumed. The authors of these last two chapters show how different methodologies can be useful in unraveling the complex relationships between perceptions of health and place and health outcomes.

Women's health on the agenda: consolidation and future directions

This book provides a range of theoretical and methodological approaches that are being used in research concerned with understanding women's health. The topics indicate some of the current interests of authors whose work has pertinence to understanding women's health, as this unfolds in different political economies, cultures, and neighborhoods. The chapters indicate commonalities in health and health care access linked to gender – seen through the prism of the daily activities of women's paid and unpaid labor, significant life events such as pregnancy and giving birth, diseases of unsafe sexual practices, and the association of these with geopolitical positioning. They suggest the vast diversity in women's experiences as they attempt to maintain their health and that of their families, manage mental and physical illness, and create effective help-seeking pathways. The chapters also show the importance of the interactions of lay perceptions, professional discourse, and medical categories in shaping how women think about health, illness, and their bodies as they negotiate their everyday activities. A focus on place and the spatiality of everyday life suggests that there will be distinct geographies to women's health, whether this is analyzed at local or global levels. Whatever the geographical scale, the simultaneity of local and global relations plays out in women's lives, shaping their health experiences, their access to resources for promoting a healthy life or managing disease or trauma, and their ability to use quality health care services. The inclusion of gender in analysis reveals how socially defined gender relations and discourses frame women's access to health and health care.

The chapters of this book suggest that distributions of power that shape gender as a determinant of health (cf. Doyal 1995) are nuanced and will play out in diverse, and perhaps unanticipated, ways. How and where women are marginalized in ways that are detrimental to their health show us not only the conditions and power relations producing illness, but also the capacities of women to reach out, often to other women, in developing strategies of "resistance" to systems and categories of health and disease that constrain women's potential to achieve health and live satisfying lives. Women develop social and spatial strategies in managing health problems, dealing with reproductive issues and caring for others. The authors show how this may be achieved or sought after at different scales, ranging from managing personal body boundaries for women with agoraphobia (Davidson) to crossing national borders in seeking prenatal care (Pope). Several of the chapters illustrate women's health and health care seeking strategies in situations of social and spatial dislocation, whether as university students leaving home in Britain or undocumented immigrants in the US. Consideration of movement and relationship to place – whether as a "newcomer" or established community member – provides a useful lens through which to further layer our understanding of women's health. Places themselves are in continuous process (Massey 1993), and how health is understood, experienced, and managed will similarly be embedded in the particularities and processual dynamics of place as several chapters suggest. The ability to "achieve health" is differentially distributed across time, space, and citizenship, as well as located within the intersections of gender, class positioning, "race," and other social locations that are given particular meaning in a variety of social and geographical locales.

The range of topics covered in this volume is not, and cannot be, exhaustive. There are evident omissions. Not all regions of the world are represented, and accounts are missing of the effects of unhealthy or degraded environments on health more common in developing and war-torn countries. The exacerbating conditions of poverty on women's health and their ability to access health care are only touched upon. Elderly women are mainly absent, as are those suffering from domestic violence. The self-surveillance and self-abuse reflected in eating disorders, drug addiction, and alcohol dependency are not covered. The efforts of women to define and manage their health through collective action and the increasing use of alternative medicine are not reflected in the collection, although the active and innovative strategies of women seeking to care for themselves and others are evident in many chapters. The omissions are important ones, and reflect the limitations of an edited volume as well as the state of development of the field – particularly as this relates to elaborating the distinctive geographies of women's health. Other topics that could have been included may well come to the reader's mind.

Several directions for further research can be suggested. For example, at scales from the global to the local, geography's contribution and potential is increasingly recognized for exploring the interconnections between global change, political ecology, and emerging infectious disease (Liverman 1999; Mayer 1996). Certainly gender needs to be privileged in such approaches, responding, albeit belatedly, to a call for more gender sensitive approaches to diseases of the developing world (Vlassoff and Bonilla 1994). Geographers have a long tradition of natural hazards research, although health risks as hazards and, to a lesser degree, the health implications of natural hazards have often been ignored (Lewis and Mayer 1998). Gender needs to be explicitly incorporated into these analyses as well. Geographers are also being challenged to explore vulnerability to environmental and technological risks, looking at not only gender, but age, class, and ethnicity (Cutter 1995). It is important, however, perhaps particularly with respect to gender, that we frame our questions in terms not only of vulnerability but also of resiliency. In this regard, more research is needed to understand how social and spatial processes, regionally within countries and cross-culturally, are involved in women's ability to manage local environments as they seek to achieve health or cope with illness. The health of immigrants, refugees, and Indigenous people is a further area of concern as global movements of people signal social and economic change and cultural transformations of major cities. How do resettlement issues and citizenship status affect health and health care access? Gender analyses are critical in investigating the links between what women do, where they live, and their health, but as chapters in this book show, gender intersects with class and other social locations in shaping health and illness.

In concluding this introduction we wish to emphasize that, while many of the chapters of this volume show the resourcefulness of women in managing health and illness, messages from the chapters should give those concerned with equity and the health of women pause. The current era of global neo-liberalism has political and financial implications for the health of women, structural adjustment policies imposed by the International Monetary Fund (IMF) being only one example. Increased societal conservatism in many parts of the world affects many domains of life including women's right to choose, women's access to social and economic supports, and women's role as caregivers in formal and informal health care systems. In health research, the primacy of the epidemiological paradigm persists. Coupled with the diplomatic imperatives of national and international organizations, this may hinder comparative analysis, critical for effective policy development. Furthermore, as we move to the geographical scale of the workplace, neighborhood, and home, we see that decisions made nationally and internationally filter down to affect women's everyday activities and how they manage health and illness. People are inserted differentially within the social relations and uneven distributions of power operating over space, so that some women will have greater control over their local conditions – and their health – than others (Massey 1993). Methods are needed that center women's perspectives if we are to discover what these differences mean for women's day-to-day experiences of health and how policy change can be translated into terms that make sense in the context of the particularities of place. There are many directions in research on women's health still to be pursued and, as this volume shows, different approaches that can be usefully drawn on in developing a holistic understanding of women's health and its constitution and reproduction. Feminist theories and methodology, while only recent introductions to health geography, suggest ways of bringing gender to the forefront of critical analysis. We hope this volume provides a beginning point from which to develop a vibrant scholarship on the geographies of women's health.

References

Abel, S. and Kearns, R. (1991) "Birth places: a geographical perspective on planned home birth in New Zealand," *Social Science and Medicine* 33: 825–34.

Arnold, K. and Eckstein, D. (2000) "Genetics may explain women's higher risk of smoking-related lung cancer," *Journal of the National Cancer Institute* 92: 1.

Asthana, S. (1996a) "The relevance of place in HIV transmission and prevention: geographical perspectives on the commercial sex industry in Madras," in R. Kearns and W. Gelser (eds) *Putting Health into Place: Landscape, Identity and Well-Being*, Syracuse, NY: Syracuse University Press: 1–14.

—— (1996b) "Women's health and women's empowerment: a locality perspective," *Health and Place* 2, 1: 1–14.

Bird, C. and Rieker, P. (1999) "Gender matters: an integrated model for understanding men's and women's health," *Social Science and Medicine* 48: 745–55.

Butler, R. and Parr, H. (eds) (1999) *Mind and Body Spaces: Geographies of Illness, Impairment and Disability*, London and New York: Routledge.

Caldwell, J. (1993) "Health transition: the cultural, social and behavioral determinants of health in the Third World," *Social Science and Medicine* 36: 125–35.

Caldwell, J. and Caldwell, P. (1994) "Patriarchy, gender and family discrimination, and the role of women," in L. Chen, A. Kleinman, and N. Ware (eds) *Health and Social Change in International Perspective*, Cambridge, MA: Harvard University Press: 339–71.

Caldwell, J., Findley, S., Caldwell, P., Santow, G., Cosford, B., Baird, J., and Broers-Freeman, D. (1990) *What Do We Know About Health Transition: The Cultural, Social and Behavioral Determinants of Health*, Canberra: Australian National University Press.

CEC (1997) *The State of Women's Health in the European Community*, Report from the Commission to the Council, the European Parliament, the Economic and Social Committee and the Committee of the Regions. European Commission, Directorate-General for Employment, Industrial Relations and Social Affairs, Unit V/F.1 (Public Health).

Chen, L., Kleinman, A., and Ware, N. (eds) (1993) *Advancing Health in Developing Countries: The Role for Social Research*, New York, Westport, CT and London: Auburn House.

Cornwell, J. (1984) *Hard-earned Lives: Accounts of Health and Illness from East London*, London: Tavistock.

Cutter, S. (1995) "The forgotten casualties: women, children and environmental change," *Global Environmental Change* 5, 3: 181–94.

Donovan, J. (1986) *We Don't Buy Sickness, It Just Comes: Health, Illness and Health Care in the Lives of Black People in London*, Aldershot: Gower.

Dorn, M. (1998) "Beyond nomadism: the travel narratives of a 'cripple,'" in H. Nast and S. Pile (eds) *Places Through the Body*, New York: Routledge: 183–206.

Dorn, M. and Laws, G. (1994) "Social theory, body politics, and medical geography, extending Kearns's invitation," *Professional Geographer* 46: 106–10.

Doyal, L. (1995) *What Makes Women Sick: Gender and the Political Economy of Health*, London: Macmillan.

Dyck, I. (1995a) "Putting chronic illness in place. Women immigrants' accounts of their health care," *Geoforum* 26, 3: 247–60.

—— (1995b) "Hidden geographies: the hidden lifeworlds of women with multiple sclerosis," *Social Science and Medicine* 40: 307–20.

—— (1998) "Women with disabilities and everyday geographies: home space and the contested body," in R. Kearns and W. Gelser (eds) *Putting Health into Place: Landscape, Identity and Well-Being*, Syracuse, NY: Syracuse University Press: 102–9.

—— (1999) "Body troubles: women, the workplace and negotiations of a disabled identity," in R. Butler and H. Parr (eds) *Mind and Body Spaces: Geographies of Illness, Impairment and Disability*, London and New York: Routledge: 119–37.

Dyck, I. and Kearns, R. (1995) "Transforming the relations of research: towards culturally safe geographies of health and healing," *Health and Place* 1: 137–47.

Elliot, S. (1995) "Psychosocial stress, women and heart health: a critical review," *Social Science and Medicine* 4: 105–15.

Elliott, S. and Gillie, J. (1998) "Moving experiences: a qualitative analysis of health and migration," *Health and Place* 4, 4: 293–311.

Environment and Planning D: Society and Space (1997) Guest edited issue: "Geographies of Disability," *Environment and Planning D: Society and Space* 15: 379–480.

Epp, J. (1986) *Achieving Health for All: A Framework for Health Promotion*, Ottawa: Health and Welfare Canada.

Feachem, R., Graham, W., and Timaeus, I. (1989) "Identifying the health problems and the health research priorities in developing countries," *Journal of Tropical Medicine and Health* 92: 133–91.

Flad, M. (1995) "Tracing an Irish widow's journey: immigration and medical care in the mid-nineteenth century," *Geoforum* 26, 3: 261–72.

Garvin, T. (1995) "We're strong women. Building a community–university partnership," *Geoforum* 26: 272–86.

Geoforum (1995) Special issue: "Geographies of Women's Health," *Geoforum* 26, 3: 239–323.

Gober, P. (1994) "Why abortion rates vary: a geographical examination of the supply and demand for abortion services in the United States in 1988," *Annals of the Association of American Geographers* 84: 230–50.

Harrison, M. (1995) "A doctor's place: female physicians in Mexico DF," *Health and Place* 1: 101–11.

Hayes, M. and Dunn, J. (1998) *Population Health in Canada: A Systematic Review*, Ottawa: CPRN.

Iyun, B. F. and Oke, B. A. (2000) "Ecological and cultural barriers to the treatment of childhood diarrhea in riverine areas of Ondo State, Nigeria," *Social Science and Medicine* 50, 7/8: 953–64.

Jones, K. and Moon, G. (1993) "Medical geography: taking space seriously," *Progress in Human Geography* 17: 515–24.

Kearns, R. A. (1993) "Place and health: towards a reformed medical geography," *Professional Geographer* 45: 139–47.

—— (1995) "Medical geography: making space for differences," *Progress in Human Geography* 19: 144–52.

—— (1997) "Narrative and metaphor in health geographies," *Progress in Human Geography* 21: 269–77.

Kearns, R. A. and Gesler, W. (eds) (1998) *Putting Health into Place: Landscape, Identity and Well-Being*, Syracuse, NY: Syracuse University Press.

Kreiger, N. and Fee, E. (1994) "Man-made medicine and women's health: the biopolitics of sex/gender and race/ethnicity," in E. Fee and N. Kreiger (eds) *Women's Health, Politics and Power: Essays on Sex/Gender, Medicine and Public Health*, Amityville, NY: Baywood: 11–30.

Lewis, N. (1998) "Intellectual intersections: gender and health in the Pacific," *Social Science and Medicine* 46, 6: 641–59.

Lewis, N. and Kieffer, E. (1994) "The health of women: beyond maternal and child health," in D. Phillips and Y. Verhasselt (eds) *Health and Development*, London and New York: Routledge: 122–37.

Lewis, N. and Mayer, J. (1998) "Disease as a natural hazard," *Progress in Human Geography* 12, 1: 15–33.

Lewis, N., Huyer, S., Kettel, B., and Marsden, L. (1994) *Safe Womanhood: A Discussion Paper*, Toronto: International Federation of Institutes of Advanced Study Gender Science and Development Programme.

Litva, A. and Eyles, J. (1995) "Coming out: exposing social theory in medical geography," *Health and Place* 1: 5–14.

Liverman, D. (1999) "Geography and the global environment," *Annals of the Association of American Geography* 89, 1: 107–20.

McDowell, L. (1999) *Gender, Identity and Place*, Minneapolis: University of Minnesota Press.

Macintyre, S., Hunt, K., and Sweeting, H. (1996) "Gender differences in health: are things really as simple as they seem?" *Social Science and Medicine* 42: 617–24.

McLafferty, S. and Templaski, B. (1995) "Restructuring and women's reproductive health: implications for low birthweight in New York city," *Geoforum* 26, 3: 309–23.

Massey, D. (1993) "Power-geometry and a progressive sense of place," in J. Bird, B. Curtis, T. Putnam, G. Robertson, and L. Tickner (eds) *Mapping the Futures: Local Cultures, Global Change*, London: Routledge: 59–69.

Matthews, S. (1995) "Geographies of women's health," *Geoforum* 26, 3: 239–45.

Mayer, J. (1996) "The political ecology of disease as one new focus for medical geography," *Progress in Human Geography* 20: 441–56.

Moss, P. (1997) "Negotiating spaces in home environments: older women living with arthritis," *Social Science and Medicine* 45: 23–33.

Moss, P. and Dyck, I. (1996) "Inquiry into environment and body: women, work and chronic illness," *Environment and Planning D: Society and Space* 14: 737–53.

—— (1999) "Body, corporeal space, and legitimating chronic illness: women diagnosed with ME," *Antipode* 31: 372–97.

Pearson, M. (1989) "Medical geography: genderless and colourblind?" *Contemporary Issues in Geography and Education* 3: 9–17.

Professional Geographer (1996) "Focus: should women count? The role of quantitative methodology in feminist geographic research," *Professional Geographer* 47: 426–66.

—— (1999) "Focus: qualitative approaches in health geography," *Professional Geographer* 51: 240–320.

Reinharz, S. (1992) *Feminist Methods in Social Research*, Oxford: Oxford University Press.

Rich, A. (1986) *Blood, Bread and Poetry: Selected Prose 1979–1985*, New York: Norton.

Rosenberg, M. (1988) "Linking the geographical, the medical, and the political in analysing health care systems," *Social Science and Medicine* 26: 179–86.

—— (1998) "Medical or health geography? Populations, peoples, places," *International Journal of Population Geography* 4: 211–26.

Rosenberg, M., Rootman, I., Munson, P., Taylor, S. M., Dyck, I., and Eyles, J. (1990) "Focus: achieving health for all: the geographer's role," *Canadian Geographer* 34: 331–46.

Rosenfield, P. (1992) "The potential of transdisciplinary research for sustaining and expanding linkages between the health and social sciences," *Social Science and Medicine* 35, 2: 1343–58.

Ross, N., Rosenberg, M., and Pross, D. (1994a) "Siting a women's health facility: a location-allocation study of breast cancer screening services in eastern Ontario," *Canadian Geographer* 38: 150–61.

—— (1994b) "Contradictions in women's health care provision: a case study of attendance for breast screening," *Social Science and Medicine* 39: 1015–25.

Ruzek, S. (1993) "Towards a more inclusive model of women's health," *American Journal of Public Health* 83: 6–8.

Senior, M. and Williamson, S. (1990) "An investigation into the influence of geographical factors on attendance for cervical cytology screening," *Transactions, Institute of British Geographers* NS 15: 421–34.

Social Science and Medicine (1992) Special issue: "Gender, Health and Environment," *Social Science and Medicine* 35, 6.

—— (1996) Special issue: "Women and Health Policies in Developing Countries," *Social Science and Medicine* 37, 11.

Timyan, J., Griffey Brechin, S., Measham, D., and Ogunleye, B. (1993) "Access to care: more than a problem of distance," in M. Koblinsky, J. Timyan, and J. Gay (eds) *The Health of Women: A Global Perspective*, Boulder, CO: Westview Press: 217–34.

United Nations (1991) *The World's Women 1970–1990: Trends and Statistics*, New York: United Nations.

Vlassoff, C. and Bonilla, E. (1994) "Gender related differences in the impact of tropical diseases," *Journal of Biosocial Science* 26: 37–53.

von Reichert, C., McBroom, W., Reed, F., and Wilson, P. (1995) "Access to care and travel for birthing: native American–white differences in Montana," *Geoforum* 26, 3: 297–308.

Whelehan, P. and contributors (1988) *Women and Health: Cross-cultural Perspectives*, Granby, MA: Bergin & Garvey.

World Health Organization (WHO) (1986) *Evaluation of the Global Strategy for Health for All by the Year 2000*, Geneva: WHO.

Young, R. (1999) "Prioritising family health needs: a time–space analysis of women's health-related behaviors," *Social Science and Medicine* 48: 797–813.

Part I

Globalization, structural change, and political realignment

Implications for women's health

2 Women's health in Europe

Beyond epidemiology?

Carol Thomas and Jan Rigby

Introduction

This chapter arises from our involvement in the European Women's Health Project (EWHP) in 1996. The EWHP was a European Commission (EC)[1] funded project, directed by a researcher based at the University of Limerick, Ireland.[2] A key feature of the project was the production of national reports on women's health by "Coordinators" based in each of the fifteen European Union (EU) Member States. In fact, there were two Coordinators in the United Kingdom because Northern Ireland was reported on separately. One of the authors, Carol Thomas, was the UK (England, Wales, Scotland) Member State Coordinator, with research support provided by Jan Rigby.

Our intention is to use the EWHP and its published output, *The State of Women's Health in the European Community* (CEC 1997, hereafter referred to as the *Report*), as an example of wider problems in research on women's health. The problems we want to focus on are the dominance of an epidemiological paradigm in population health research, a paradigm which privileges individual behavioral and lifestyle risk factors over socio-structural processes in disease etiology, and the failure of official and governmental organizations in most countries to take women's health needs sufficiently seriously. The EWHP makes for a particularly interesting case study in this respect because it *started out* as a policy-oriented attempt to generate a socio-political rather than a narrowly epidemiological account of women's health in Western Europe. That is, it sought to collate data on aspects of women's health which went beyond a description of patterns of mortality and morbidity, and went further than a focus on the standard behavioral risk factors as explanatory variables: smoking, diet, alcohol consumption, and exercise. As we outline below, the perspective on women's health adopted by the project Director and most of the national Coordinators involved the recognition of the need to locate women's health experiences in the social fabric of their daily lives, taking account of socio-economic factors, gender role responsibilities and inequalities (among women and between women and men); of the importance of seeking out data on issues such as domestic violence and the experiences of particular groups of women including those on low income, older women, and travelers; and of the extent to which health policies and health care systems within European Member States did or did not consider the particular health care and health promotion needs of women. In this context, we were very pleased to be involved in the EWHP, at least for the first five months.

Despite the fact that the national Coordinators worked to a project Protocol which was broad in scope, producing national reports which attempted to provide information on a wide range of health-related social, cultural, and political factors as well as on patterns of mortality, morbidity, and standard behavioral risk factors, the final *Report* (CEC 1997) released by the European Commission office was a very traditional epidemiological account of the health of women in the European Member States. Whilst, as we shall show later, the *Report* did contain some useful summary data it bore little resemblance to the type of women's health report that we were expecting. What it did contain was comparative data on mortality and morbidity patterns in EC States at the national level (including recent trend data), some interesting but limited information on "social and demographic trends" (population size, "family life," "working life," and "gender-related development indices"), and data on variations in women's smoking behavior, alcohol consumption, diet, weight, and exercise. The *Report* also included a chapter on "special issues in women's health" which provided brief numerical descriptions of the following problems and issues: eating disorders, HIV/AIDS, family planning, abortion, and the menopause. What it did not contain was any information or discussion on health policies and health care systems in Member States, or any discussion about socio-economic and socio-cultural determinants of health; in fact *explanation* for health variations was entirely limited to biological (especially age) variables and a limited range of behavioral risk factors. The larger literatures on health inequalities and on gender and health may as well not have existed.

What had happened? We can only speculate about this although we feel sure that the project initiator/Director was as disappointed in the project's outcome as we were. Perhaps the project was much too ambitious? Perhaps the quality of the data produced by the national Coordinators was of such poor or uneven quality that little use could be made of them, so that the author(s) of the *Report* had to fall back on routinely collected data on mortality, morbidity, and health-related behaviors? Certainly, as discussed below, we had great difficulty in tracking down many of the UK data demanded by the project Protocol, especially in the limited time available, and it is likely that other Coordinators faced greater data availability problems than we did. Such difficulties may well have played a role, but we suspect that two more powerful sets of forces were at work. In our view, one set of forces was associated with the political and administrative imperatives of diplomacy: the EC office could not release a *Report* which highlighted gender- or class-related health and social inequalities and which was implicitly or explicitly critical of past or present governments of EU Member

States. We would suggest that the other set of forces was bound up with the continuing general dominance, not least in EU public health circles, of the positivistic epidemiological paradigm in health research (Dean 1993; Popay *et al.* 1998). This dominance meant that only a particular kind of health status report was deemed to be acceptable, authoritative, and legitimate, the type of report which replicates traditional public health formats and interests.

We will return to a discussion of these forces in the final section of the chapter, drawing on recent literature on women's health research and policy making. In the next section we outline the original perspective of the EWHP in more detail, then move on to discuss some of the data that were presented in the *Report* (CEC 1997). The *Report* appears to have had a very limited circulation,[3] and thus it may be of interest to outline some of its findings here.

The European Women's Health Project

Project aims

The EWHP was of only five months' duration (that is in its first, and as it turned out its only, phase) and Coordinators were only modestly resourced (amounting to a small fee to Coordinators' institutions plus travel expenses to enable Coordinators to attend two international project meetings). Member State Coordinators were not required to generate new data. Rather, their task was to quickly collate available data on women's health status and relevant health policies within their own countries, working to a Protocol proposed by the project Director, but later agreed to by the Coordinators. The first stated aim of the project was to use these national reports, together with data from a range of central sources, to feed into the production of a report on the health status of women in Europe for the Commission of the European Communities, Luxembourg. These central data sources were as follows: the WHO Health for All Database 1996 (see WHO 1996); various reports and data published by the Statistical Office of the European Communities (Eurostat); data from the first (1994) wave of Eurostat's European Community Household Panel (ECHP) survey; The World's Women 1970–90 statistics published by the UN (1991); data provided by different monitoring centers, such as the International Agency on Research on Cancer (IARC) in Lyon and the European Centre for the Epidemiological Monitoring of AIDS in Paris; and an EC-wide Eurobarometer survey carried out in 1996. The latter survey "asked a representative sample of non-institutionalized persons (about 1,000) in each Member State a number of questions on health, including attitudinal questions, self-reported health status, and preventive health services received in the past year" (CEC 1997: 14). The stated aims of the EWHP were as follows:

This project entails a study of the status of women's health in the European Union both on a national and community level. Health policies and health promotion/prevention strategies and evolving trends with regard to women's health in the Member States of the European Union will be reviewed and compared including age specific health issues and those relating to particular groups. Existing information will be analyzed; key areas for concern and priorities for Community actions, which could complement national measures, will be identified. Within this context relevant health, demographic and socio-economic indicators will be utilized and compared.

(EWHP 1995: 1)

The project guidelines went on to highlight the following: there may be a stagnation in the growth of women's life expectancy (for example, in Denmark) due to a variety of interrelated paid work, unpaid work, and behavioral factors; women's longer life expectancy is bound up with high levels of morbidity with advancing age; health promotion and disease prevention initiatives for women should not focus only on their reproductive and maternity roles; and women's health interests are under-represented in almost all areas of public health including policy design and service provision (EWHP 1995).

The project "Protocol" had a particular focus on age-related women's health issues (such as breast cancer/ovarian cancer, screening/tests, menopause, coronary heart disease), the needs of vulnerable groups (such as migrants, sex workers, single mothers, women in the labor market), whether women's health is identified as a priority (or as an issue at all) for health policy by Member States, and whether women were targeted in disease prevention initiatives.

The Protocol required Member State Coordinators to find and summarize information in a number of areas. The first involved information about the health care systems operating in Member States and the place of women's health in health policy developments, together with information on health data sources within countries. The second area related to information on gender patterns of mortality, morbidity, and other health status indicators; this included a focus on socio-economic health differentials. The third area involved information on health determinants, especially smoking, alcohol consumption, illegal drug use, diet and weight, exercise, stress levels, employment and unemployment rates, poverty, and health service usage including availability and use of screening services. The final area was to provide data that would enable detailed analyses of specific women's health issues to be undertaken. These included data on sexual health, eating disorders, reproduction and maternity issues, cancer (breast, cervix, lung), coronary heart disease, menopause, elderly women's health and health care problems, domestic violence, rape and sexual harassment, mental health issues including stress and depression, and the health needs of disadvantaged women (such as disabled women, poor women, single parents, sex workers, women in rural areas).

Despite a number of shortcomings, for example the absence of any specific mention of lesbian women or minority ethnic women (although reference was made to migrant women), it can be seen from the foregoing that the EWHP did adopt a broad based socio-political perspective on women's health. If the *Report* (CEC 1997) had addressed all of the themes identified in the Protocol then it would certainly have been a valuable and politically significant document. Instead, the *Report* covers a narrow selection of politically "safe" themes, and relies overwhelmingly on statistical data from the central data sources listed earlier. Very little reference is made in the *Report* to the national Coordinators' reports, although some reports do feature in footnotes. Any reader of the *Report* who is unfamiliar with the EWHP could be forgiven for thinking that the whole exercise was simply a review of central statistical sources on women's health by staff in the EC offices in Luxembourg.

The health status report on women

We have indicated that this *Report* (CEC 1997) was not widely circulated and that despite its serious limitations it does contain some very interesting comparative summary data on variations in women's health across Western Europe. For these reasons we will refer to some of the *Report*'s data here. Unless otherwise attributed, all the statistics are from the *Report* and the tables and figures are derived from the *Report*.

Infant mortality

This is a widely used indicator of health. In the developed world, improvements in basic housing and sanitation have been reflected in dramatic falls in infant mortality (deaths under 1 year of age). In 1970, female infant mortality varied from almost 50 deaths per 1,000 live births in Portugal to 11 per 1,000 in Sweden. In 1992, the highest rate was still in Portugal, at 9.3, and the lowest in Sweden at 5.2. The continued improvement is now thought to relate to more general social and economic improvements reflecting improved maternal health, in addition to better ante- and neo-natal care. Although there is still some variation, when compared with the rates in, for example, India (79.0) or Brazil (54.0) (WHO 1996), the EU situation is not a cause for major concern.

Long-term illness

This was assessed from the Eurobarometer study, which analyzed responses to the question "Do you have any long-standing illness, health problem or handicap that limits, to some extent or severely, your work or daily activities? This includes all types of health problems as well as those due to old age. If yes, to some extent or severely?" The results can be seen in Table 2.1. These

Table 2.1 Percentage of women aged 15 and over with disability due to long-standing illness

Country	Yes, some	Yes, severe
Finland	20.1	9.5
United Kingdom	20.1	5.6
Denmark	19.2	9.1
Austria	18.8	4.4
France	18.4	8.6
Greece	18.1	6.0
W. Germany	17.7	7.2
Portugal	17.2	12.4
Sweden	17.1	8.0
E. Germany	16.9	8.5
Ireland	16.5	2.6
Spain	15.8	4.8
Belgium	15.6	3.5
Italy	14.6	2.8
Netherlands	13.6	6.9
Luxembourg	10.6	4.2

Source: CEC (1997).

are the percentages of women, and hence the difference between the highest and lowest figures represents a large number of women. It is notable that, despite the EWHP's Protocol, there was no discussion of the particular needs and interests of disabled women in the *Report* (Thomas 1999).

Ischaemic heart disease

This is the largest single cause of mortality in women in the EU. It generally occurs at a later age than in men, as pre-menopausal hormones are thought to confer a protective effect. Figure 2.1 shows, for most countries, a decline in the rates between 1970 and 1992. It is also clear that the higher rates tend to be in the more northern countries.

Breast cancer

Breast cancer is the most common cause of mortality in the 35–55 age group, and is also the most common cancer that occurs in women, accounting for 21 percent of cancer deaths overall. The mortality rates in Denmark and the United Kingdom are the highest in the world. Incidence is more difficult to ascertain, as problems of recording and data collection vary widely. Incidence rates in the United States are substantially higher than in the United Kingdom, affecting one woman in nine compared with one in twelve (Ursin *et al.* 1994), yet mortality rates are lower. The graph (Figure 2.2) shows the considerable variations in mortality across the EU countries.

   It is regrettable that the only visual forms of illustration used in the *Report* were statistical graphs. Had any of the data been mapped, some geographical

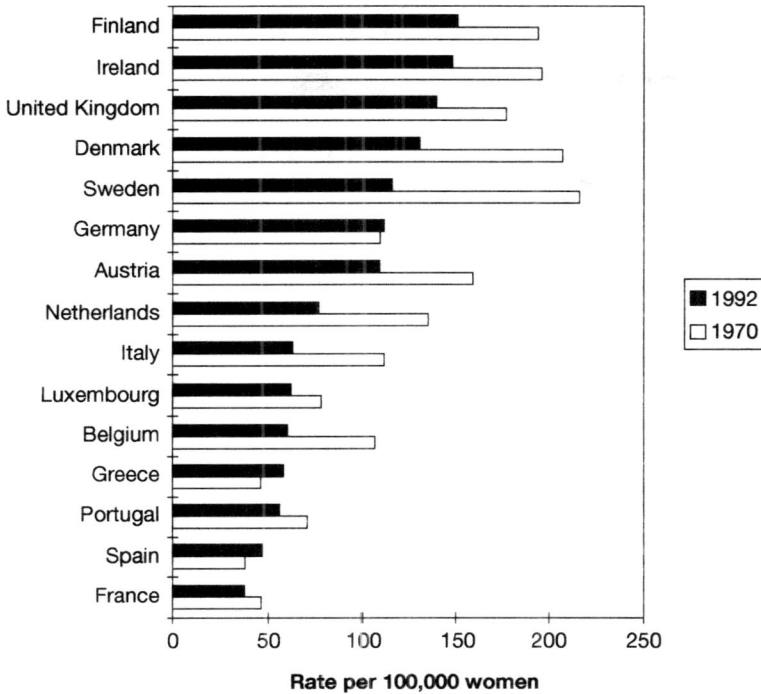

Figure 2.1 Standardized mortality rates for ischaemic heart disease, all women.
Source: CEC (1997).

patterning might have been observed. With breast cancer mortality, as with ischaemic heart disease, quite a strong north/south divide becomes apparent, with rates particularly low in the Mediterranean countries.

Suicide

The statistics for suicide and self-inflicted injury mortality show a decrease in rates between 1970 and 1992, but with considerable variations across the EU, with higher rates generally in the north. However, there is no mention of particular problems in connection with the death certification of suicide, which may be particularly relevant in countries with a high proportion of women of the Roman Catholic faith. Nor is there discussion of the wider issues relating to mental health, where women form the majority of the sufferers.

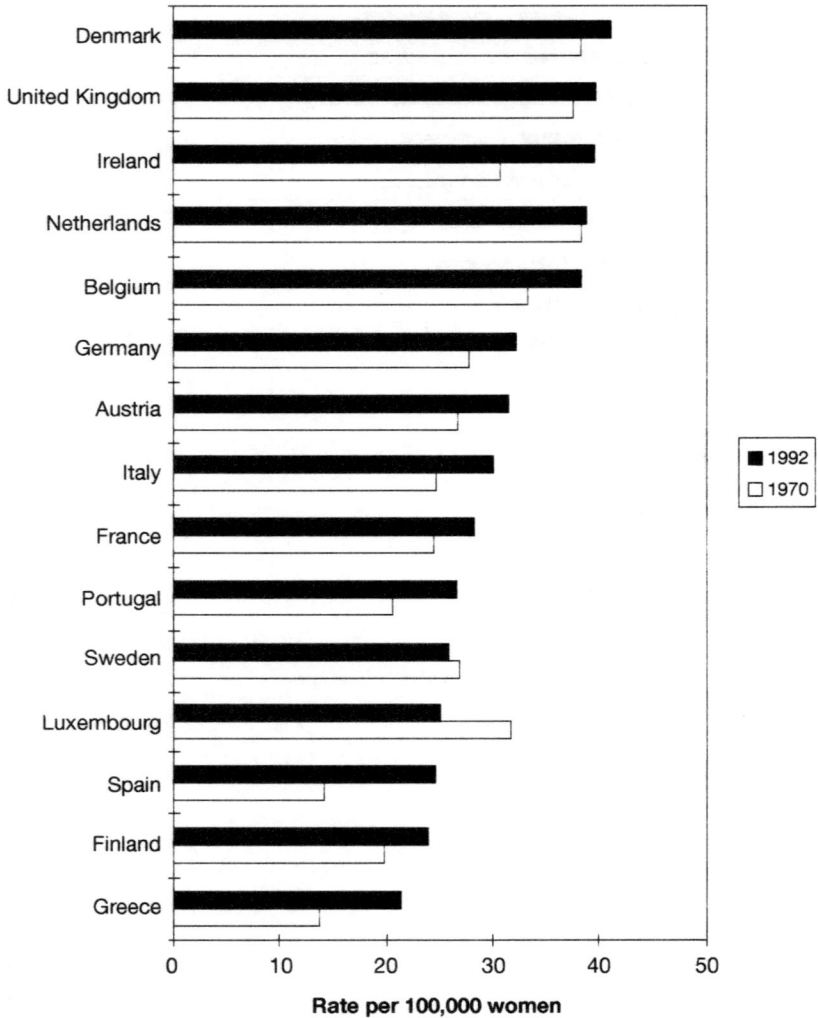

Figure 2.2 Standardized mortality rates for breast cancer, all women.

Source: CEC (1997).

Smoking

The *Report* made few attempts to compare outcomes that might be related. Figure 2.3 displays the rates of respiratory cancers along with the percentage of women in each country who smoke.

Some interesting differences are apparent, from the high rates of both smoking and mortality in Denmark to the low mortality, yet high smoking rates in Spain and France. It can also be observed that France also has

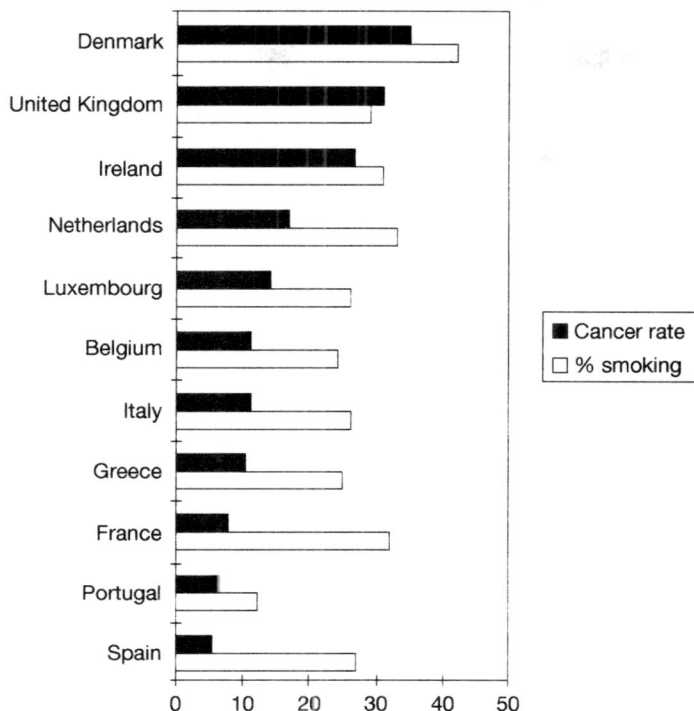

Figure 2.3 Percentage of women smoking alongside standardized mortality rates from cancers of the respiratory system, 1992.

Source: CEC (1997).

comparatively low rates of cerebrovascular disease (stroke) and ischaemic heart disease whereas Portugal has similarly low rates of heart disease, yet high rates of stroke. In the *Report*, the health effects of smoking were restricted to links with heart disease and cancer, with no consideration of the effects on reproductive health, which could have emphasized the importance of health promotion amongst younger women. This is particularly important in view of the increasing numbers of teenage girls who are smoking.

The balance of the *Report* was the implication that many aspects of women's ill-health are largely attributable to the choices they make in terms of lifestyle factors, and not the environment in which they have to live; for example, there was no consideration of housing quality or access to health care. Of even greater concern was the absence of indicators relating to poverty and welfare support. Poverty indicators are available from Eurostat, one of the data sources used extensively within the *Report*. Their omission underlines the benign approach to considerations of policy.

Special issues

It was encouraging to see the inclusion of issues such as eating disorders and violence in the *Report*. Statistics are particularly difficult to obtain, as many women prefer not to reveal information on sensitive topics. Additionally, there are more formal problems of identification and recording, with, for example, mortality from anorexia nervosa being recorded as suicide, and morbidity in terms of resultant health conditions, or as attempted suicide.

Findings in the *Report* indicated that around one-third of women in the 15–24 age group reported being dissatisfied with their body weight and about 25 percent had dieted in the previous year. Incidence rates of anorexia nervosa varied considerably, from 0.45 per 100,000 women in Sweden to 8.1 per 100,000 in the Netherlands, and estimates suggested that a further 2 percent were bulimic.

Violence against women

Again, accurate statistics are unavailable, but the *Report* acknowledges increasing concern across the EU. Where indicators were available, these suggested incidents of domestic violence affected as many as one in three women in Portugal and Germany. Reported incidence of rape is substantially less than the actual incidence, and the extent of rape within marriage cannot be established, partly because of variations in legal systems.

Reproductive issues

Statistics relating to contraception and abortion are not uniformly available, attributable in part to the considerable variability in the availability of abortion. Abortion remains illegal in Ireland and Northern Ireland. In other countries the legislation permitting abortion has only been passed recently, hence procedures for the compilation of statistics are only just emerging. The criteria for eligibility for abortion also vary. Table 2.2 indicates the use of contraception, availability of abortion, and an indication of the proportion of young mothers.

Health status

Table 2.3 uses a range of gender-related development indices (United Nations Development Programme 1995) to illustrate aspects of gender inequality. The Human Development Index ranks countries by social and economic indicators of health, income, and education. The first three countries worldwide are Canada, the United States, and Japan, with the Netherlands ranked as fourth. However, when this index is adjusted for gender, the rankings for this gender-development index show Sweden and Finland as the first two countries, with the level of gender inequality moving the Netherlands

Table 2.2 Reproductive statistics for Member States

	% women using contraception	% live births to mothers under 20	Year abortion legislation passed	Abortion rate per 1,000 women	
Austria	71	5.76 (1992)	1975	n/a	
Belgium	79	3.69 (1986)	1990	n/a	
Denmark	78	2.73 (1988)	–	14.3	(1993)
Finland	80	2.70 (1992)	1970	7.9	(1994)
France	81	2.40 (1991)	1975	13.0	(1990)
Germany	75	3.36 (1991)	1992/96	n/a	
Greece	n/a	5.82 (1992)	1986	n/a	
Ireland	n/a	4.35 (1987)	Illegal	n/a	
Italy	78	3.00 (1994)	1978	8.6	(1994)
Luxembourg	n/a	2.62 (1989)	1979	n/a	
Netherlands	76	1.87 (1992)	1984	6.0	(1994)
Portugal	66	10.35 (1985)	1984	n/a	
Spain	59	5.20 (1989)	1985	5.4	(1994)
Sweden	78	3.11 (1986)	1938	18.3	(1994)
United Kingdom	81	8.13 (1989)	1968	12.2	(1994)

Source: CEC (1997).

Table 2.3 Development indices

Member State[a]	Human Development Index (HDI)	Gender-related Development Index (GDI)		Gender Empowerment Measure (GEM)		Female share of earned income (%)[b]
Sweden	10	0.919	(1)	0.757	(1)	41.6
Finland	5	0.918	(2)	0.722	(3)	40.6
Denmark	16	0.904	(4)	0.683	(4)	39.8
France	8	0.898	(7)	0.433	(31)	35.7
Austria	14	0.882	(10)	0.610	(9)	33.6
United Kingdom	18	0.862	(13)	0.483	(19)	30.8
Italy	20	0.861	(14)	0.585	(10)	27.6
Belgium	12	0.852	(18)	0.479	(21)	27.3
Netherlands	4	0.851	(20)	0.625	(7)	25.2
Portugal	36	0.832	(25)	0.435	(30)	29.9
Greece	22	0.825	(27)	n/a		22.2
Ireland	19	0.813	(30)	0.469	(24)	22.2
Spain	9	0.795	(34)	0.452	(26)	18.6
Luxembourg	27	0.790	(35)	0.542	(13)	23.1

Source: United Nations Development Programme (1995).

Notes
a   No figures for Germany.
b   Latest available year.

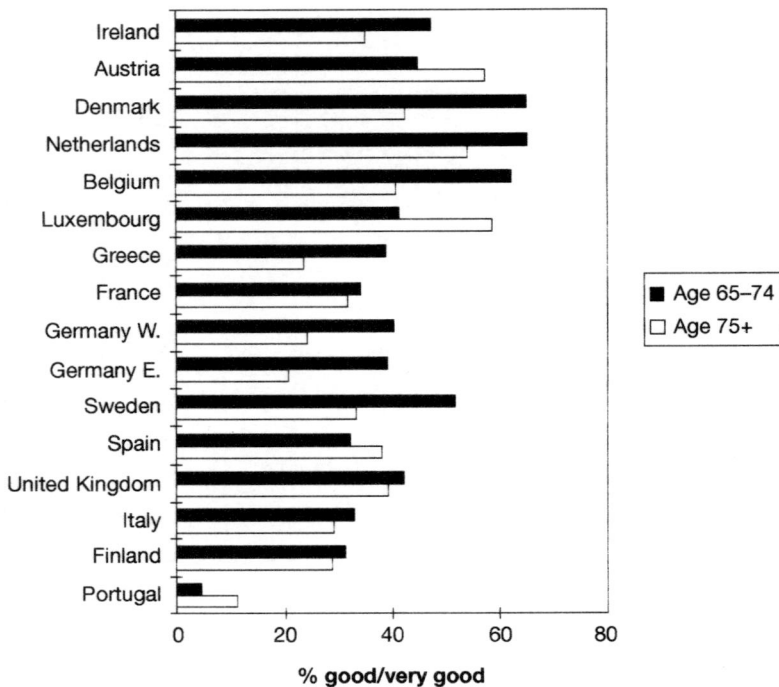

Figure 2.4 Self-perceived health status of women aged 15 and over, 1996.
Source: CEC (1997).

down to ninth. Sweden and Finland also perform well in the measure of gender empowerment (assessing economic and political decision-making).

The *Report* explored the self-perceived health status of women, as determined by the Eurobarometer study. Figure 2.4 shows the results from this for women aged 15 years or over. For some countries, a marked contrast can be seen when the results are presented for women aged 65 and over (Figure 2.5), with particular concern in Portugal.

The Conclusion of the *Report* was a particular disappointment. Statements such as "it is clear that women in the EC are quite healthy. . . . On average, more than 60 percent of women in the EC report being in good or very good health" (CEC 1997: 115) are generalizations which are hardly justifiable from the sampling used to obtain the underlying statistics. The tone is reactive, and thus the *Report* is unlikely to form the basis for support for future research into many aspects of women's health, which was one of the intended outcomes from the project. The *Report* avoids issues of culture, ethnicity, mental health, health inequalities and, most importantly, poverty, leaving us with the impression of a somewhat "sanitized" document.

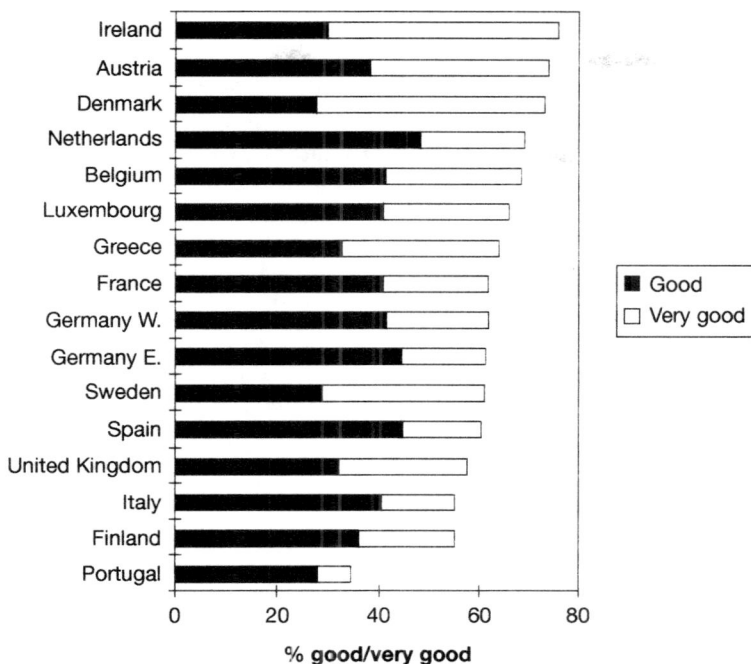

Figure 2.5 Self-perceived health status of women aged 65–74, and 75 and over, 1996.

Source: CEC (1997).

Beyond epidemiology?

There is no doubt that the EWHP was confronted with serious data-related problems. For example, as the UK (England, Wales, Scotland) researchers we quickly found that there were innumerable difficulties with the collection and collation of data from secondary sources for comparative purposes, at all scales. Such data vary across categories such as age groups, time periods, geographical area, and format (that is, raw figures or percentages). The EWHP required the rapid collection of data across a wide variety of health and social indicators and it became apparent that these data are held by a considerable number of official and voluntary bodies, with no overall coordination or collective reference. Our approaches to agencies for information on women's health and/or health policies, for example the Department of Health (England) and the corresponding bodies in the Scottish and Welsh Offices, seldom met with a confident and direct identification of an appropriate individual or department. Government agencies were unable to route either verbal or written requests, and we were taken down a number of culs-de-sac. Charitable/voluntary groups were more responsive, possibly because their focus was narrower but also because they were often supportive of an initiative which was about prioritizing women's health issues. We are certain that Coordinators in other EU Member States had similar, if not greater, difficulties accessing the information required on women's health and health policies in their own countries. The reunification of Germany, for example, placed the German Coordinator in the unenviable position of having to find trend data for both the former Federal Republic of Germany and the former German Democratic Republic. It is likely that the national reports from Coordinators were very patchy and incomplete. Whilst this may go some way towards explaining the overwhelming reliance on central statistical sources in the *Report* – especially the WHO Health for All Database, Eurostat sources, and the Eurobarometer survey – it does not excuse the narrowness of the range of health and social indicators actually selected for the *Report*, nor the complete omission of discussion on health policies in Member States.

We suggested earlier that in addition to data availability and quality difficulties there may have been two sets of forces operating to limit the *Report* to a standard epidemiological document. First, in our view, there was the pressure felt by EC staff to produce information on women's health across EU Member States in as politically neutral a fashion as possible. This meant leaving out discussion of Member States' health policies, health care systems, and socio-economic and health inequalities profiles. It was safer to describe national-level mortality and morbidity data with no examination of causal mechanisms beyond the prevalence of individual risk factor behaviors, such as smoking and lack of exercise, together with the presence or absence of preventive screening programs. Second, we believe that EC staff who worked on the *Report* were embedded in an epidemiological paradigm which privileges individual behavioral risk factors in the chain of ill-health causation, and fails to locate disease etiology in a broader socio-structural context. These two constraining "forces" will now be considered in turn, drawing on recent literatures on women's health and health determination.

The unwillingness to engage with issues associated with EU Member States' health policies and health care systems in the *Report*, presumably for reasons of diplomacy, is particularly unfortunate in the arena of women's health because there has been a long-standing policy neglect of matters relating to women's health at national and international levels in Europe and elsewhere (Doyal 1995, 1998a). Among EU Member States at the time of the EWHP, only the Irish Republic was moving in the direction of a national women's health policy (Irish Department of Health 1995). As Lesley Doyal has noted in relation to Britain, "As yet there has been little debate in the UK on possible frameworks for managing policy development and implementation in the area of women's health" (Doyal 1998b: 241). Feminist researchers have established that there is a need for greater attention to be paid to women's health issues both in research (biomedical and social scientific) and in health promotion and health care policy making and practice (Doyal 1985, 1993,

1995, 1998a; Foster 1995; Roberts 1985; *Social Science and Medicine* 1993, 1999; Stacey 1985). For example, in Britain:

> Women's health advocates and their supporters have long claimed that the NHS [National Health Service] treats women unfairly. . . . They have amassed considerable evidence to show that women are treated differently from men in ways that objectively disadvantage them and have campaigned for the removal of discriminatory practices.
>
> (Doyal 1998c: 4)

The EWHP represented an opportunity to review evidence on the degree to which health policies and health care systems in EU Member States were "gender sensitive" and took account of the health needs of women and, had the evidence been reported upon, could possibly have contributed to new EC policy frameworks on these matters. In the event the opportunity was missed, and with it the chance to compare the social and political conditions in Europe with those elsewhere that *have* given rise to national women's health policies, most notably in Australia (Broom 1991; Doyal 1998b; Gray 1998; Wainer and Peck 1995). In this respect it can be argued that the *Report* reinforced the longer-term tendency to avoid a serious policy oriented engagement with women's health needs in Europe.

The dominance of an epidemiological paradigm in population health research also has a long history (Dean 1993; Popay *et al.* 1998). The legacy of positivist philosophical foundations and empiricist methods is clearly evident in contemporary epidemiology: the isolated "risk factor" approach remains supreme. Risk factors, particularly behavioral or lifestyle risk factors such as smoking, poor diet, lack of exercise, and excessive alcohol consumption, are separated from their socio-material and environmental context such that their complex relationship with underlying social structures and relationships is lost from view. What is so disappointing about the outcome of the EWHP is that it started out with a clear commitment to a broad socio-structural and socio-cultural perspective on women's health and its determination. If this commitment had been seen through to the *Report* stage and beyond,[4] then the comparative social and health status data and discussion could perhaps have contributed to recent and future social science debates about the factors and processes which shape women's health (both in relation to gender differences and differences among women), debates which have moved well beyond a concentration on risk behaviors *per se* as the major causal factors (Doyal 1998a; *Social Science and Medicine* 1993, 1999). For example, in the early 1990s Sara Arber's (1990) research on health inequalities among women highlighted the need to adopt an integrated "role" and "structural" framework in understanding women's health determination: "it is essential to consider *both* women's roles *and* their material circumstances within which those roles are enacted" (Arber 1990: 41). A focus on domestic roles is particularly necessary in Britain where, compared with countries such as France and Sweden, a relatively high proportion of women are full-time housewives and mothers (Bartley *et al.* 1992).

In her examination of women's health globally, Doyal (1995) emphasized the need to understand women's health in the context of the structured inequality that characterizes their lives. Her approach was to identify the economic, social, and cultural determinants of women's health by focusing on "the major areas of activity that constitute women's lives" (1995: 21). These activities include domestic labor and resource distribution within households, sexual activity, reproductive and motherhood activities, paid work, and health-related behaviors: "It is the cumulative effects of these various labors that are the major determinants of women's states of health. This is true even in old age, when many of these activities have ceased but their impact on well being becomes increasingly evident" (Doyal 1995: 22). Even when the focus is on health-related behaviors such as smoking, we know from work by feminist researchers such as Hilary Graham (1993a, 1993b) that behaviors are linked in fundamental ways to socio-structural environments and cannot simply be understood as misinformed lifestyle choices. However, in its Conclusion, the *Health Status Report on Women* simply has this to say:

> a large number (and percentage) of women report unhealthy life styles (e.g. smoking, drinking, sedentary life styles and unhealthy diets). Combined, these factors contribute to (much of) the disability, morbidity and premature mortality among women in the EC.
>
> The main causes of death for women are cardiovascular disease and cancer. Both of these diseases also result in significant amounts of premature mortality, which to a considerable extent may be prevented either through primary prevention, improved life-styles, or secondary prevention (early detection of disease through, for example, screening). Unfortunately, there seems to be a considerable misconception among women about the extent to which they are at risk for heart disease and what are the main risk factors for the disease.
>
> (CEC 1997: 115)

Thus in the *Report* the problem is couched in terms of unhealthy lifestyles and women's lack of knowledge, and the solutions are to change lifestyles/ knowledge and to increase preventive medicine. The narrow epidemiological paradigm which determined the form and content of the *Report* is clearly inadequate and, as we have indicated, has been surpassed conceptually by feminist and other social science researchers. The worrying lesson from the EWHP is that this paradigm remains entrenched in centers of power, and acts as a block to the advancement of women's health interests.

Notes

1 The project was funded by the EC Directorate-General for Employment, Industrial Relations and Social Affairs: Unit V/F.1 (Public Health).
2 We have decided not to disclose the name of the project Director here. However, it is important to stress that we have the greatest respect for her and we believe that she did not carry responsibility for the project's outcome as outlined here.
3 Despite being one of the Member State Coordinators, Carol Thomas was not sent any official notification that the *Report* had been produced and, having heard of its publication by chance, she had to request a copy in writing.
4 The production of a health status *Report* was originally seen as only the first phase of the EWHP. It was envisaged that a second report containing an in-depth analysis of the data would follow.

References

Arber, S. (1990) "Opening the 'Black Box': inequalities in women's health," in P. Abbott and G. Payne (eds) *New Directions in the Sociology of Health*, London: Falmer Press: 37–56.

Bartley, M., Popay, J., and Plewis, I. (1992) "Domestic conditions, paid employment and women's experience of ill-health," *Sociology of Health and Illness* 14: 313–43.

Broom, D. (1991) *Damned If We Do: Contradictions in Women's Health Care*, Sydney: Allen & Unwin.

CEC (1997) *The State of Women's Health in the European Community*, Report from the Commission to the Council, the European Parliament, the Economic and Social Committee and the Committee of the Regions. European Commission, Directorate-General for Employment, Industrial Relations and Social Affairs, Unit V/F.1 (Public Health).

Dean, K. (1993) *Population Health Research: Linking Theory and Methods*, London: Sage.

Doyal, L. (1985) "Women and the National Health Service: the carers and the careless," in E. Lewin and V. Oleson (eds) *Women, Health and Healing: Towards a New Perspective*, London: Tavistock: 236–69.

—— (1993) "Changing medicine? Gender and the politics of health care," in J. Gabe, D. Kellahar, and G. Williams (eds) *Challenging Medicine*, London: Tavistock: 140–59.

—— (1995) *What Makes Women Sick: Gender and the Political Economy of Health*, London: Macmillan.

—— (ed.) (1998a) *Women and Health Services. An Agenda for Change*, Buckingham: Open University Press.

—— (1998b) "Conclusions: the ways forward?" in L. Doyal (ed.) *Women and Health Services. An Agenda for Change*, Buckingham: Open University Press: 238–50.

—— (1998c) "Introduction: women and health services," in L. Doyal (ed.) *Women and Health Services. An Agenda for Change*, Buckingham: Open University Press: 3–21.

EWHP (1995) "European Women's Health Project: Summary," unpublished paper: University of Limerick.

Foster, P. (1995) *Women and the Health Care Industry*, Buckingham: Open University Press.

Graham, H. (1993a) *Hardship and Health in Women's Lives*, London: Harvester.

—— (1993b) *When Life's a Drag: Women, Smoking and Disadvantage*, London: HMSO.

Gray, G. (1998) "How Australia came to have a national women's health policy," *International Journal of Health Services* 28, 1: 107–25.

Irish Department of Health (1995) *Towards a Health Policy for Women*, Dublin: Department of Health.

Popay, J., Williams, G., Thomas, C., and Gatrell, A. (1998) "Theorising inequalities in health: the place of lay knowledge," *Sociology of Health and Illness* 20, 5: 619–44.

Roberts, H. (1985) *The Patient Patients: Women and their Doctors*, London: Pandora.

Social Science and Medicine (1993) Special issue: "Women, Men and Health," *Social Science and Medicine* 36.

—— (1999) Special issue: "Gender and Health," *Social Science and Medicine* 48.

Stacey, M. (1985) "Women and health: the United States and the United Kingdom compared," in E. Lewin and V. Oleson (eds) *Women, Health and Healing: Towards a New Perspective*, London: Tavistock: 270–303.

Thomas, C. (1999) *Female Forms: Experiencing and Understanding Disability*, Buckingham: Open University Press.

United Nations (1991) *The World's Women 1970–1990, Trends and Statistics*, New York: United Nations.

United Nations Development Programme (1995) *Human Development Report 1995*, New York: Oxford University Press.

Ursin, G., Bernstein, L., and Pike, M. C. (1994) "Breast cancer," in R. Doll, J. F. Fraumeni, and C. S. Muir (eds) *Trends in Cancer Incidence and Mortality*, London: Imperial Cancer Research Fund: 241–64.

Wainer, J. and Peck, N. (1995) "By women for women: Australia's national women's health policy," *Reproductive Health Matters* 6: 114–21.

World Health Organization (1995) *Highlights on Women's Health in Europe*, Copenhagen: WHO Regional Office for Europe.

—— (1996) *Health for All Database*, Copenhagen: WHO Regional Office for Europe.

3   Scales of justice

Women, equity, and HIV in East Africa

Susan Craddock

Introduction

One of the themes of the 12th World AIDS Conference in 1998 was "Bridging the Gap" between industrialized and nonindustrialized countries in availability of drugs and other resources to combat the transmission of HIV. The idea is an admirable one in many respects. It also glosses over the complex geopolitical causes and context of the AIDS epidemic that have arguably acquired particular patterns in nonindustrialized countries. The reasons can, in part, be found in the long history of inequitable encounters with industrial economies, encounters which persist today in the form of foreign loans that are made contingent upon "structural adjustments" of receiving economies. The call to "bridge the gap" is thus an ironic one for the degree to which it belies the underlying realities of political economies on a global scale.

While bringing attention to those regions of the world increasingly stricken with the burden of AIDS, the conference theme also highlighted the primacy of biomedical research and pharmaceutical solutions in the fight against HIV. Biomedical research is accomplishing many desirable goals in better understanding of the nature of the virus and in searching for vaccines that might go a long way in preventing further transmission. But the emphasis on biomedicine in AIDS research is closing off avenues of enquiry into behaviors that put people at risk for HIV, and more importantly, into the social, political, cultural, and economic contexts of those behaviors. With or without a vaccine, an understanding of behavioral patterns and their causes is critical to prevention efforts. It is also critical to understanding the embeddedness of diseases including AIDS in social inequities and power relations that have both distal and proximate causes, and that manifest in regionally specific ways.

In this chapter I look at some of these issues as they pertain to women in East Africa. Known as the "AIDS belt," East African countries have some of the highest rates of HIV and AIDS in the world (WHO 1998), yet projections do not predict any plateauing of new cases in the foreseeable future (Bongaart 1996; WHO 1998). The reasons for focusing on women within these regions are threefold: because in many areas within East Africa women are at higher risk of HIV than are men (Helitzer-Allen 1994; Schoepf 1993); because there has been disproportionate focus so far in the African AIDS literature on high HIV rates among prostitutes without concomitant explanations of the social and economic conditions of commercial sex work; and because even in areas of equal HIV ratios, inquiry is necessary into the discrepant paths that lead men and women into vulnerability.

This chapter however is not meant as a conclusive study that presents a definitive theoretical framework backed by empirical research. It is meant, rather, as an interrogation of risk and the various scales at which risk is determined. Though the focus here is HIV/AIDS, a political and social economy framework can be useful in locating more broadly defined vulnerabilities in gendered social relations, access to resources, economic constraints, cultural codes of conduct, discursive meanings, and individual responses. Examples are given where possible, usually for Malawi, but my agenda is to raise questions and indicate areas of inquiry that have received inadequate attention by scholars investigating HIV and other risk. My intent is for this to be taken as part of a conversation that was begun by scholars inside and out of geography, is added to here, and will be continued by others in the future. My own part of the conversation is to expand upon the theoretical frameworks that have been offered so far, particularly for investigating HIV and AIDS, and especially within geography,[1] and to suggest an expanded scale of inquiry, moving from one that focuses primarily on the local to one that incorporates analysis at the international as well as regional scales.

Toward a more effective theory of risk

Biomedical research still dominates investigations into HIV and AIDS, setting the agenda for funding and consequently determining in large measure the questions asked and the types of solutions sought in AIDS research (Singer 1998). The questions are aimed primarily at determining transmission routes of the virus, focusing attention upon individuals or "risk groups" and their sexual practices.[2] Behaviors are largely atheorized in these studies, the only important point being seen as the types of sex being practiced, how often, and with whom.[3] Prevention programs derived from such approaches consequently hinge upon behavior modification strategies that treat individuals as autonomous beings in an apolitical world who just need to be apprised of the need for condom use.

An alternative to these ineffective models of prevention lies in the interrogation of those complex institutional, structural, and discursive factors that determine the possible avenues of behavior in every individual. Schoepf, for example, acknowledges that HIV transmission results in large measure from conditions of poverty and gender relations as defined by "the processes, structures, and institutions by means of which societies order sex differences and invest them with cultural meanings for the people who act them out in daily life" (1993: 53).[4] This recognition that HIV lies embedded in social economies of impoverishment and gendered inequity is a huge step towards an understanding of risk, and of why women are vulnerable to HIV for reasons different from men. Yet there are questions about the exact configurations of poverty and why it places some individuals at risk for HIV that need further elaboration.

One way to do this is by investigating empowerment and entitlement at the household, regional, and state levels, including access to resources such as education, health care, and job opportunities, and encompassing historical political economies that have mobilized particular social patterns such as gendered migration and structures of employment (Jochelson *et al.* 1991; Schoepf *et al.* 1991; Watts and Bohle 1993). "Empowerment" is a word used often enough to diffuse its meaning, but a useful definition is that of Watts and Bohle who see it as being located in "politics and a theory of power" (1993: 49) and as speaking of "who gets what benefits and how [that is] decided" (Kent 1991: 194 quoted in ibid.). Power is not manifested solely through legal or juridical channels, in other words, but through a more variegated network of "customary" practice, cultural codes of behavior, social location, or political expediency. Gender, generation, and physical location all inform degree of individual empowerment because these factors often determine, *inter alia*, availability of community and government resources, degree of control over income, decisions concerning family mobility, social practice, and even sexual exchange. Particularly within the context of HIV/AIDS, empowerment suggests having sufficient command over educational, institutional, and financial resources (i.e. entitlement, cf. Sen 1981, 1990) and over personal behavior and social practices to avoid situations of risk. A recent report with implications for gendered risk, for example, finds that girls in Malawi are not expected to obtain education beyond the primary level because of pressures to marry. As one informant in the study stated, "girls leave school as soon as they start menstruating, which is at 12–14, to get married . . . so we find it useless to educate girls" (Helitzer-Allen 1994: 28). The valuation of girls as wives rather than as citizens contributing to local or national economies then plays out in household relations allocating primacy to male decision making and privileging male control over income (Carney 1993; Stichter and Parpart 1988).

Government channels may also legitimize cultural parameters of behavior and power inequity. Malawi's late president, Kamuzu Banda, derived a carefully constructed state taxonomy of gendered social hierarchy based on a vaguely pre-colonialist mythology of village life. Men were construed as agricultural producers as well as political figures, while women "could expect to remain under the guardianship of all the nkhoswe – male members of a Chewa family . . . with Banda even declaring himself to be the 'Nkhoswe No. 1'" (Forster 1994: 491). The reciprocal nature of multi-level analysis and the impossibility of separating cultural constructions of power at the household, local, or state levels are evident here. So, too, is the inseparability of material and discursive performances of power. Yet the emphasis of Kent (1991) and Watts and Bohle (1993) on how decisions are made in questions of power speaks to the dynamic nature of power relations and the fact that they are constantly being negotiated and renegotiated. One of the benefits of an empowerment optic, then, is to determine those faultlines of power that are more resistant to change, and those that are more responsive to external stimuli and internal contestation.

The primary benefit of breaking poverty into investigations of empowerment and entitlement is to show that not all impoverished individuals are equally at risk for HIV. Poverty is too vague a category to be entirely useful, because gearing prevention programs at the poor does not necessarily take into account the highly differential nature of poverty, and the varied capacity of impoverished individuals to access resources, negotiate choices of employment, be mobile, or mobilize a range of social and economic assistance in times of scarce income (Watts and Bohle 1993). Women tend to have a more constrained capacity in all of those examples, but within this generalization it must be recognized that some women have much greater entitlements than others. A focus on access to resources and empowerment rather than on poverty *per se* produces a more accurate assessment of risk by recognizing that middle- and upper-class women may also be disempowered in ways that render them vulnerable to HIV. Access to money does not necessarily equal entitlement. The picture is a much more complex one involving women's control over income, their leverage in marital decision making, the degree to which wives of wealthy men have access to political power, and the sexual economies open to, and even expected of, wealthy men (Schoepf 1998). Several studies in fact have found that women of higher socioeconomic and educational status are more likely to be HIV positive (Slutsker *et al.* 1994; cf. Akeroyd 1997). Poverty in this framework thus becomes a variable in the analysis of vulnerability, but no longer a critical determinant of risk.

Apart from empowerment and entitlement, the examination of historical political economies aids assessments of risk by illuminating the broader trajectories of state relations with other states and with particular groups, and determining how present economic patterns came into being. Outlining a colonial history of Africa is beyond the scope of this chapter, but it is none the less important to note that present social economic patterns in many regions of Sub-Saharan Africa have their roots in colonial policies that restructured regional economies and the location of different communities within them. More will be said about this with respect to Malawi. The point here is that attention to historical precedent aids in the process of demystifying risky behavioral patterns, introduces the notion of changes over time, and elucidates the rootedness of regional social economies in transnational administration, state politics, and local need. It assists in bringing to light the point that individuals do not act autonomously but rather *vis-à-vis* their shifting relationship to a number of institutional and social contingencies from the household to the global level.

A potential problem inherent in analyses based upon power relations is that individual responses are lost in the examination of institutional authority and, especially for gendered analyses of power, that women are presented as passive victims rather than individuals with the capacity for negotiation and action (Mohanty 1991). Poststructuralism has been instructive in this regard by recognizing the location of power in dispersed practices of everyday life, in the control and contestation of knowledge (Foucault 1979), and in representational practices that shape understandings of sex, gender, and disease and consequently inform public awareness of, and institutional responses to, issues such as HIV/AIDS (Wilton 1997). It has also arguably been instrumental in bringing attention to voices of the "other" not commonly recognized in political economic analyses intent upon illuminating the larger brushstrokes of class and institutional relations.[5] Equally germane to an analysis of institutional parameters of social practice is the acknowlegment of latitude within some but not all of these parameters for individuals to make decisions, negotiate responses, or construct resistant practices and productions of knowledge.

The examples given in the analysis thus far have not always related directly to HIV transmission. The sections that follow relate the above discussion to several areas of inquiry that are critical to a better understanding of risk and which may point toward more fruitful arenas of research and prevention.

Structural adjustment and the burden of AIDS

Even within literature focusing on the social contexts of HIV risk there has been less attention paid to the impact of structural adjustment programs, or SAPs. Structural adjustment was instituted in the 1980s by the International Monetary Fund and the World Bank to stimulate the export sectors of nonindustrialized countries and to strengthen their economies enough to provide export markets for Western commodities. More specifically, SAPs came in response to the debt crisis of the mid-1980s, a crisis generated in part by an increase in bank lending to so-called developing countries in the 1970s and early 1980s, and by the emerging inability of these countries to repay loans due to a series of external shocks such as the OPEC-led rises in oil prices in the early and late 1970s, and international recessions in the mid-1970s and again in 1980-1 (Corbridge 1993; Lurie *et al.* 1995). In some countries such as Malawi, these external shocks were accompanied by drought-driven agricultural failure (Lele 1990). The result was that debtor countries could not repay their loans, nor could they contract for further loans from private banks. They were forced to turn to the IMF for loan agreements, but these agreements incorporated severe austerity measures as contingencies for further borrowing.

It is the nature of these contingencies that warrants further examination in an analysis of HIV risk. Though differing somewhat according to country, the basic requirements for approval of IMF and World Bank loans include relaxing import restrictions, focusing resource allocation toward export rather than local markets, curtailing government subsidization of commodities, increasing personal income and consumption taxes, and reducing government spending on service sectors including education and health (Lurie *et al.* 1995). The rationale of austerity measures lies in the undying faith of agencies such as the IMF in the power of the market to generate financial returns, and equal faith in the ability of these cash flows to trickle down to all sectors of a population. In reality the results of SAPs have been largely deleterious. A brief glance at the list of austerity measures would allow one to accurately predict that the poor if not the middle classes of debtor countries would suffer as a result of their implementation.

Lele's analysis of Malawi's structural adjustment programs, for example, found that the requirement of donors to withdraw fertilizer subsidies negatively impacted smallholder farmers who did not have sufficient cash to purchase nonsubsidized fertilizer for growing corn, and also did not have adequate resiliency to risk acquiring fertilizer on credit (Lele 1990: 1214). Twice the Malawian government withdrew from the subsidy agreement. The first time was in 1984–5, when a devalued currency and increased transport costs drove up the price of fertilizer imports. The second was in 1987, when reduced government food stocks and a large influx of Mozambican refugees forced the government to shift back to incentives for fertilizer adoption. To further provide incentive for maize production, the government in the next year raised the maize producer price by 44 percent; while good for producers, this increase made it difficult for those households dependent on buying their maize in local markets to purchase adequate food supplies (ibid.).

The points to be made here are several. Lele's agenda was to analyze neither the impact of all areas of structural adjustment in Malawi nor the impact of structural adjustment on HIV risk, yet her findings can be extended in those directions. If smallholders were suffering from the withdrawal of fertilizer subsidies, then this suffering was undoubtedly compounded by the simultaneous elimination of consumer price subsidies, a rise in public utility and service fees, and cuts in public expenditures (ibid.: 1211). Though not stated explicitly by Lele, her claim that government maize stocks were low in 1987 suggests that smallholders were unable to grow enough corn to sell, even if they had enough for their own needs. Lack of access to fertilizer places in jeopardy the capacity of poorer farmers to grow a crop on which they are dependent for subsistence and for income. Inability to grow and consume maize means dependency on the market for food, but the elimination of consumer price subsidies means higher prices for maize at a time when cash in poorer rural households is in short supply.

Reduced income as a result of structural adjustment thus indicates the possibility of nutritional deficit, a condition that makes individuals more susceptible to seroconversion in the case of HIV exposure (Lurie *et al.* 1995). It also makes more likely the inability to keep children in schools, both because (increased) school fees can no longer be met, and because older children may now be depended upon for wage labor. Inability to pay school fees is the most frequently cited reason for leaving school early in Malawi (Kishindo 1995), in addition to cultural impediments to educating girls. But lack of schooling reduces the kinds of employment open to men and women, and especially women. Lower educational levels increase the likelihood that girls will turn to commercial sex work of some type if other means of employment are unavailable or inadequate (Schoepf 1993).[6] The subject of commercial sex work will be returned to, but suffice it to say here that most forms of commercial sex practice in Malawi and other regions of East Africa vastly increase risk of HIV.

Second, further investigation is needed into which households are impacted more significantly by structural adjustment. Lele mentions that the small-holder sector in Malawi is divided between those farmers with large enough holdings to produce crops for the market as well as for consumption, and those households dependent on the market for food and employment. Of these poorer smallholder households, approximately half are headed by women (Lele 1990: 1209). Yet Lele does not go on to analyze whether these female-headed households are more severely impacted by SAPs, and if so, in what ways. Since many women are already less entitled through restricted access to agricultural extension programs or to employment opportunities (Chirwa 1996; Hirschmann 1984), it is possible that structural adjustment affects them more drastically by increasing the price of food while reducing wages and constricting still further the opportunities for generating income. Structural adjustment's further impoverishment of smallholder households means that the main avenues of income generation for women, namely selling beer, crafts, or small household items, diminish because few households have the disposable income to purchase these items.

At issue here is what Watts and Bohle discuss as resilience in the face of deepening crisis (1993). Structural adjustment programs impact the poor in general by making them poorer, but it is those households with fewer resources to begin with and fewer resources to call upon in the face of increased poverty that will suffer the most. The decisions these households are forced to make need further investigation, such as whether women in female-headed households decide to migrate, and if so where and for what purposes; whether they enter into commercial sex work, and if so what type; or whether they enter into arrangements with one or two men who might pay rent for them or bring them gifts in return for sex (Schoepf 1993, 1998). Any of these decisions potentially places women at greater risk of HIV exposure.

A third point is that the compound nature of structural adjustment not only increases vulnerability to HIV, it also reduces the ability to confront this problem (Lurie *et al.* 1995). The irony of international calls at AIDS conferences to address the health care problems of AIDS patients becomes more obvious in the context of SAP mandates to reduce spending on health care in countries facing multiple health burdens including rising numbers of AIDS cases. Spending on health, education, and welfare as a whole in Sub-Saharan Africa declined 26 percent between 1980 and 1985 (ibid.: 543). Thus the negative impact of structural adjustment is not limited to increasing risky behavior by making more likely a choice of migration or commercial sex work in the face of increasing impoverishment. It also reduces the possibility of monitoring HIV status or of getting care in the event of HIV seroconversion. Facilities for testing HIV are extremely limited in East Africa and are unlikely to increase in the near future with no allocation of funding. This makes knowledge of HIV status virtually impossible, with an unfortunate consequence of more extensive HIV transmission.

With funding for health care reduced, attempting to care for the rising burden of AIDS patients in East Africa is proving to be a losing battle. In Malawi, a third of beds are occupied by AIDS patients, and the occupancy rate in hospitals overall is 200 percent; in the southern city of Zomba, the bed occupancy is 350 percent in the TB ward, and the vast majority of these patients have AIDS (Wilbrink 1995: 311). Space to care for AIDS patients is thus an increasingly trenchant problem. Average per capita health care expenditure for African governments in general was $2.00 at the beginning of the 1990s, and spending on AIDS patients was $400 (Lurie *et al.* 1995: 543–4).[7] Not only are AIDS patients thus taking a disproportionate allotment of a diminishing health care budget, but even this relatively large portion is inadequate to buy drug treatments or other therapies that could prevent opportunistic infections and prolong lives. Drug shortages in many East African countries can be attributed not only to declining health care expenditures, but to other SAP conditionalities such as currency devaluation and foreign exchange shortages (ibid.: 544).

Pharmaceuticals are another area needing closer examination, however, because it is not just SAPs that are making AIDS drugs unavailable in East Africa and other regions. Pricing policies of pharmaceutical companies making AIDS drugs offer an example of economic politics at the corporate scale impacting populations at local levels. The prohibitive cost of chemotherapies for AIDS in part reflects the enormous expenses of AIDS research, but also exemplifies the greed of drug companies, aware of the huge profits to be made because those with terminal AIDS have no other alternatives for prolonging their lives but the protease inhibitors or "drug cocktails" offered on the market. Even for most persons with AIDS in the US, the cost of drug cocktails is out of reach without the help of insurance; for those many without insurance, drug therapies are simply too costly to be accessible. For those in East Africa, the problem is worse since incomes are on average a fraction of those in the US and insurance is virtually unknown. In the afterglow of the Geneva AIDS conference, some pharmaceutical companies moved to offer drugs free or highly discounted to countries such as Uganda as part of a UN AIDS program. While seemingly beneficent, this gesture accomplishes much more in the way of international public relations than it does in the way of AIDS treatment: the call to "bridge the gap" is magnanimously answered, while at the same time international criticism of price gouging is offset. One account of the conference described the anger of some AIDS activists at seeing pharmaceutical companies use these philanthropic activities "to obtain a hold on what is [*sic*] seen as enormous emerging markets with significant profit potential" (Schoofs 1998: 34). The limited time for which drugs will be made available, however, is the best indication of the purely public relations nature of this offer; short-term drug therapy accomplishes nothing in terms of saving lives, but threatens instead to create drug-resistant strains of HIV.

Discussion of pharmaceuticals raises the final point about SAPs, which is that they constitute only one component among many in the analysis of risk. Not only do SAPs differentially impact every country, but the differences lie in the specificity of national and local economies, social arrangements, political structures, and cultural norms. As the next section suggests, these more localized specificities in turn need closer scrutiny in the analysis of women and HIV.

Sex, power, and survival

No analysis of HIV risk can overlook sexual practices of men and women, but there is increasing recognition that such analyses must recognize not only the myriad conditions under which sexual practices take place, but the power relations within which they are structured (Miles 1993; Schoepf 1993; Ulin 1992). The highly varied cultural embeddedness of sexual practice, together with the place-specific configurations of economic and social opportunity, makes local studies of sexual practice paramount in risk analyses. Yet there are a few themes that are common to most of East Africa and can be discussed as to their implications for future research.

Colonial legacies: poverty, migration, and commercial sex work

The East African prostitute is probably the single most studied category in international AIDS research. It is by now well known that prostitutes in urban areas such as Nairobi are up to 80 percent HIV seropositive (Mann *et al.* 1992), though prostitutes even in less urban areas such as Blantyre or Lilongwe in Malawi show rates of 60–80 percent (Kishindo 1995; Mann *et al.* 1992). Yet the visibility of these statistics is problematic for the ways in which they conflate category with serostatus, and gloss over the complex power relations within which commercial sex operates. Indeed, the different conditions under which commercial sex work is practiced, and the routes by which women enter prostitution, have received considerably less attention than has the fact that prostitution seems to be a highly risky endeavor. In the work that has been done so far in these areas either in or outside East Africa, however, it is precisely these specificities of commercial sex work that determine not only the degree of risk of acquiring HIV, but the approaches needed for prevention (Asthana and Oostvogels 1996; Murray and Robinson 1996).

Within East Africa, one theme emerging in the investigation of prostitution is the role of migration (Jochelson *et al.* 1991). The impact of SAPs has been mentioned, but for much of East Africa the patterns of gendered migration were set into motion during colonialism. The hows and whys of male migration during the late nineteenth and early twentieth centuries are the subject of some debate (Jochelson 1995), but these generally entailed a gradual tightening of colonial control over agricultural production, household taxation, and alienation of lands for estate cash crop production (Chirwa 1996; Jochelson 1995). The result was increased male migration into areas of labor demand such as the gold mines of South Africa, while women generally remained at home to continue agricultural production.

To varying degrees these patterns of migration still exist in many parts of East Africa. South African mine companies have largely stopped employing Malawian workers (Chirwa 1998),[8] but failure to find employment or to sustain agricultural production within Malawi results in a reinitiation of migration within or outside the country (ibid.). Constrained ability to continue agricultural production alone and restricted opportunities of employment outside agriculture plague many rural women in East Africa now, just as they did in the colonial period. The result is that some women have few choices but to turn to commercial sex work. The biggest difference from the colonial period, of course, is the risk of HIV exposure that this choice now entails. But to what degree this risk varies and why needs closer investigation. Some studies have begun to tease out the different forms of prostitution in East Africa with their varied potentials for risk (Kishindo 1995; Pickering *et al.* 1997), but more of these localized studies are needed if effective prevention strategies are to be negotiated.

The common assumption about prostitutes anywhere, including East Africa, is that they are relatively helpless victims of circumstance, caught in a life-and-death struggle between short-term financial survival and longer-term risk of death from AIDS. There is much truth to this scenario in its recognition that commercial sex work is not the choice many women would make given viable options. It may often be the most viable option precisely because of severe gender inequities in labor markets, and because the inequitable power relations within which much commercial sex takes place leave women with little leverage to insist upon the use of condoms. The contextualization of commercial sex work within relations of power and inequitable social economies is an important break from the standard biomedical portrayal of the prostitute-as-HIV-vector, and an important step toward understanding why sex workers do not always adopt the use of condoms even when they are made readily available. Yet there are two basic areas of investigation here: the first is why women choose commercial sex work in the first place, and the second focuses on the possibility of HIV prevention strategies once women become prostitutes.

For the latter, more of the kind of detailed work done by Asthana and Oostvogels (1996) and Murray and Robinson (1996) on commercial sex workers in Madras and Australia, respectively, is needed for East Africa. These authors situate their analyses of prevention strategies in the specific organization of prostitution and the differential relations of production that characterize it. Commercial sex workers in Sydney, for example, have lower HIV rates than the general population because they are well organized and able to control the conditions under which sexual exchange occurs (Murray and Robinson 1996). Commercial sex workers in Madras, on the other hand, are substantially more disempowered on a number of levels including inequitable relations with pimps, greater dispersion throughout the city, increased surveillance by police, the role of middlemen in procuring contacts, and the greater social condemnation and thus secrecy surrounding their work. The result is a much higher level of HIV transmission, a low level of condom use, and greater difficulty in deploying effective prevention strategies (Asthana 1997; Asthana and Oostvogels 1996).

What this work shows is the necessity of knowing not just the power relations between prostitutes and their clients, but the many other contingencies and power relations within the larger spectrum of commercial sex work that determine the parameters within which women can negotiate the conditions of sexual exchange. But these studies also show the high degree of geographic variability of the social and economic relations of production in commercial sex work. As Asthana points out in her study of Madras prostitutes (1997), the characteristics of commercial sexual exchange in Madras differ greatly from those of Bombay or Calcutta, two cities with distinct red light districts, less police surveillance of commercial sex workers, and less social conservatism than characterizes southern India. The result is a differential risk of HIV among the sex workers of these cities.[9]

More investigation is needed, too, into the reasons why women end up in commercial sex work. Migration is not the only driving force behind this choice, although some degree of disentitlement and/or disempowerment usually is involved, including reduced income, divorce, lack of education, shrinkage of the job sector, and restricted access to what jobs are available. Yet some authors have pointed out that desperation is not necessarily the determining factor in going into commercial sex work, and that sex workers are not necessarily hapless victims of inequitable economies, bad relationships, or state neglect. In her review of four historical accounts of women in colonial East Africa, Jochelson commends one of them, White (1990), for its more nuanced treatment of female migration and prostitution.[10] "For White, the conventional historical view of prostitutes as victims is a leftover of nineteenth century moralism" (Jochelson 1995: 326). The prostitutes she focuses on in her study were resourceful entrepreneurs "attuned to the needs of [their] natal family or [their] own progeny, and to the resources and possibilities of the city" (ibid.). Many of these women migrants moved from prostitution to property ownership in Nairobi, choosing to establish successful, independent lives for themselves in the city rather than return home to constrained lives as daughters or wives in rural villages.

This latter view of resourceful women using prostitution as a means for accumulating wealth, supporting their families, or disengaging from more constrained village lives is reflected in Akeroyd's overview of studies on prostitution in Africa (1997). Some commercial sex workers, as evidenced by these studies, come from relatively well-off families, or enable their families to live more comfortably than the average urban or rural resident because of the wages they remit home from commercial sex work. Schoepf (1993: 57) also notes that prostitution can be a means toward a large income, glamor, and the ability to buy a home or a small business. Reflecting White's comment on the inappropriateness of nineteenth-century moralism, studies are also finding that some prostitutes go home to warm welcomes in their natal families. As summarized by the authors of a study on prostitution in The Gambia, "Most [prostitutes] enjoyed a higher than average standard of living. . . . The rural families were not impoverished. Their well-being and warm welcome for the visiting daughter proved that she had not faced a dramatic choice of prostitution or poverty" (Pickering *et al.* 1997: 79, cited in Akeroyd 1997: 19).[11]

For the purposes of risk analysis, what these studies tell us is that commercial sex work is highly varied in its practices and causes, and that more work needs to be done in teasing out the difference these variations make for vulnerability to HIV. Strategies aimed at preventing women from entering commercial sex work may not always be appropriate, at least when the decision to engage in prostitution was not made from a lack of other options. A more nuanced analysis of condom use is appropriate, however, since too little is known about correlations between condom use, socioeconomic status of prostitutes, and the conditions under which sex work is practiced. Reasons for low condom use in fact are as varied as the structures and conditions of sex work itself, encompassing but also extending beyond issues of power. In Kishindo's study of 540 bar girls in Malawi (1995), the reasons given for low condom use (23 percent) included clients' negative attitudes, but also the prostitutes' own dislike of condoms based in part on a fear that they dislodge during sex and eventually cause sterility in women (1995: 158). Waldorf's study of one township in Malawi showed a variety of negative attitudes toward the condom from both men and women. These included beliefs that condoms promoted promiscuity, their negative association with past family planning programs, the difficulty of use and disposal in circumstances of little privacy, reductions in pleasure during sex, and their association with recreational sex (Waldorf 1997: 140). The inability of many women to demand condom use among their clients is a very real issue, but so too is the regionally specific cultural iconography of the condom.

Adolescence and HIV

A discussion of sex and HIV risk that concentrates only on commercial sex work would be incomplete, if not stereotypical, in its assumptions that only commercial sex workers are at risk of infection. Another cohort worthy of mention is adolescents. National AIDS prevention programs do not exclude adolescents in their pro-condom radio broadcasts, billboards, and newspaper ads, but to what extent adolescents are actually targeted in prevention campaigns is less clear. Based on several studies of adolescent sexual practices and attitudes undertaken in Malawi, it seems clear that better risk-prevention strategies are needed.

Five studies have recently been conducted in Malawi that examine the knowledge of AIDS and the sexual practices of youths of various age groups and geographic locations (urban, peri-urban, or rural) (Bandawe n.d.; Centre for Social Research 1994; Helitzer-Allen 1994; Msapato *et al.* 1990; UNICEF-Malawi 1994). The general finding of these studies is that while awareness of AIDS is high among teenagers (around 96 percent), awareness of risk is low even though a significant proportion of those interviewed were sexually active. Part of this lack of awareness of personal risk stemmed from somewhat faulty understandings of HIV transmission, but it stemmed as well from more complex attitudes regarding the visibility of disease, the perceived nature of sexual encounters, and the (non-)respectability of individuals. In one study, for example, over 90 percent of those interviewed stated that AIDS could be avoided by not having sex with an "easy" partner (Helitzer-Allen 1994: xii), and that AIDS only afflicted bar girls or truck drivers (ibid.: 96). As for individuals everywhere, AIDS for these youths is stigmatized enough to necessitate various "othering" processes that involve ascribing risk only to those who are considered promiscuous or otherwise morally questionable. Blaming thus becomes an almost inevitable component of this equation. As one youth stated it, "I would not care for an AIDS victim because it was his fault to acquire the disease" (Msapato *et al.* 1990: 14).

Yet the studies which inquired about the reasons for having sex revealed the gendered realities behind the nature of sexual encounters and the patterns of blame that have evolved out of the uncertain terrain of AIDS knowledge and avoidance. Both boys and girls in the studies expressed ideas about the desirability of sex and their readiness to explore it (Centre for Social Research 1994; Helitzer-Allen 1994; UNICEF-Malawi 1994), yet the reasons did not stop there. For girls in particular, other less voluntary factors informed decisions to have sex. Pressure from families to obtain money from boyfriends or to get married spurs some girls into sexual exchanges (Centre for Social Research 1994: 7), while for others the need to obtain money for school fees or books dictates transactions with older men who in local parlance are called "sugar daddies," that is older men who have sex with young school girls in exchange for money or gifts (UNICEF-Malawi 1994: 8; WHO 1994). Over half of the girls interviewed in one study mentioned money as the main reason girls engage in pre-marital sex (Centre for Social Research 1994: 7), while 66 percent of girls in another study stated they had been offered money or gifts in exchange for sex (Helitzer-Allen 1994: 78).

One result of this gendered sexual economy is that girls are placed at higher risk for HIV than are boys because the conditions under which they engage in sex are less often of their own choosing. Young girls are picked by sugar daddies because they are more likely to be HIV negative, yet the status of the sugar daddy himself is less often questioned. Negotiating condom use is invariably more difficult in sexual situations involving some degree of pressure rather than mutual desire, whether that pressure is towards marriage or money. That a full 55 percent of girls interviewed in one study said they had been forced to have sex at some point in their lives (Helitzer-Allen 1994: 78) evidences unequal sexual economies in these regions as anywhere in the world, but unfortunately AIDS prevention programs are not responding effectively to this. Making condoms available or educating about their efficacy in preventing HIV is not going to help as long as young girls are engaging in sex characterized by inequitable power relations and external contingencies. That reported cases of AIDS among 10–19 year-olds are almost four times higher among girls than boys in Malawi, however, suggests the urgent need for prevention strategies that recognize the role of power relations and socioeconomic contingencies in the sexual practices of young boys and girls.[12]

Another result of girls being pressured into various sexual situations such as sugar daddy relationships is that they consequently get blamed for higher HIV rates. Part of this blame centers on the sexual availability of girls in general, with a majority of respondents in one study agreeing with the statement that "if girls would just say no there would not be a problem of HIV/AIDS among youth" (UNICEF-Malawi 1994: 8). But part of the blame centers as well on the sugar daddy relationship itself, a relationship that is seen as risky but in which girls, and not the men, are blamed, for "making themselves easily available to older men" (ibid.: 12). The iconography of female promiscuity and its relationship to sexually transmitted diseases is clearly deeply entrenched and geographically pervasive.

Conclusion

International calls for bridging the gap in resources for preventing HIV, and in transmission of HIV itself, have little relevance when not informed by the sociopolitical complexities involved in that undertaking. Too much rhetoric has been generated and too many studies conducted that rely upon simplistic thinking about the AIDS situation in regions such as East Africa. At best, public relations are given prominence in highly visible arenas such as international AIDS conferences at the expense of true prevention efforts in countries needing assistance with AIDS programs. At worst, stereotypes of the promiscuous African and the prostitute-as-vector are perpetuated with the end result being education programs that achieve little in the way of prevention (Packard and Epstein 1992). Fortunately an increasing number of AIDS studies depart from these characteristics. However, more studies are needed that dispense with simplistic thinking and analyze the highly contingent, variable, and dynamic conditions under which sexual exchanges take place for men and women of all classes, socioeconomic status, and ages in East Africa and elsewhere.

Gender sensitivity in these studies is paramount given the different routes by which men and women become vulnerable to HIV in East Africa, but sensitivity in itself is not enough. Neither is situating women's vulnerability in poverty without further disaggregation of this characteristic. A framework of empowerment, political economy, and cultural dynamics is useful in recognizing that it is access to resources, location in decision making processes, and the interconnected relationships among institutions, the state, households, individuals, and representational practices that largely determine vulnerability to HIV. Impoverishment may increase the chances of being disempowered but, particularly among women, it is not a necessary qualification. A social and political economy of risk framework also helps to highlight those areas in which power relations are more effectively negotiated in prevention efforts, versus those areas in which changes in social practices or institutional policies are less likely to occur (Kesby 1999).

There is also inadequate attention being paid to the effects of international practices such as structural adjustment programs and pharmaceutical pricing policies on the patterns of HIV and AIDS in affected countries. While such studies might be more difficult to navigate because of their political sensitivity, initial reports make it clear that longstanding and therefore largely accepted practices undertaken by powerful institutions cannot escape the scrutiny of AIDS researchers if they are serious about deriving more effective formulas for prevention. AIDS is nothing if not a political phenomenon embedded in many sensitive political dynamics from sex to statesmanship, and none of these issues can be avoided if the subject is to be taken seriously. The most effective way to examine the effects of international institutional practices, however, is to increase attention toward localized studies. The location of HIV risk in such highly contingent relations of power, social economy, and individual identity make local studies a necessity, especially when dealing with the personal-yet-political and economic dynamics of sexual practice.

There are of course many areas needing study that I have not focused on, but what I have tried to do is to point out larger arenas within which there are numerous possibilities for investigation. One example that comes to mind under the auspice of international institutional practices is the recent move the United Nations has taken to encourage mothers in Africa to feed their babies formula rather than breast milk (Specter 1998). The recommendation, made in an attempt to stem the tide of mother-to-baby transmission of HIV, represented an "either-or" choice between AIDS and diarrheal diseases, rather than the more complicated geopolitical picture which included the possibility of placing pressure on pharmaceutical companies to make AZT available and affordable to more pregnant women, on international lending agencies to subsidize AZT in affected regions, or on the IMF to curtail its demands for structural adjustment in order to make health care funding more readily available in debtor countries. Few organizations have such visibility and leverage as the United Nations, but the will for a more politically charged act of pressuring powerful corporate entities is clearly lacking. The call to stop breast feeding is arguably another judgment lapse on the part of public health advisors who place one deadly and internationally highly visible disease ahead of one much more deadly but less visible. Mothers who follow the recommendation of the United Nations face a three times greater risk of their babies dying from diarrheal diseases than they did of dying of AIDS (Specter 1998).

The lives of these babies, their mothers, and other women in East Africa recall the words of the late Jonathan Mann when he stated that "Never before has the importance of articulating a clear image of health problems, and the dire consequences of fuzzy or simplistic thinking, been so clearly demonstrated" (Mann *et al.* 1992: 12). If it takes the United Nations and the World Bank to point clearly towards the imperative for clear thinking on the AIDS issue, then maybe they have served a useful function after all.

Notes

1 With a few notable exceptions (Asthana 1997; Asthana and Oostvogels 1996; Brown 1997; Murray and Robinson 1996) geographers have been slow to venture out of diffusion models of AIDS and into analyses of risk that attempt to account for its social complexities. This is especially mystifying given geography's focus on place-specificity of vulnerability.

2 I mention sexual practices only here because it is heterosexual sex that causes the vast majority of HIV cases in Sub-Saharan Africa. Most attention has been paid to heterosexual and vertical transmission and very little to male–male or female–female sex, intravenous drug use, or other routes of transmission of HIV in Africa.

3 The epidemiological studies of HIV/AIDS in Sub-Saharan Africa that fit this description are too many to cite, but a few examples would include J. Bwayo *et al.* 1994; J. O. Ndinya-Achola *et al.* 1997; H. Pickering *et al.* 1997; and L. Slutsker *et al.* 1994.

4 See also Akeroyd 1997 for gendered political ecologies of HIV in Africa.

5 See Parpart and Marchand 1995 for an overview of postmodernism's influence on feminist development theory, including the claim that postmodernism has not added anything new to feminist analyses of social practice, and the counterclaim that postmodernism has opened avenues of research into marginality and focused attention on the voices of the traditionally disenfranchised.

6 This point needs to be qualified, however, because like so many associations it is more complicated than a simple association of low educational levels with prostitution. In his study of 540 bar girls in Malawi, Kishindo found that none of the girls had gone beyond eight years of primary school (1995: 155). As Kishindo observes, this suggests on the one hand that these "girls" found commercial sex

work the most profitable means of employment given their levels of education, and indeed the author claims that few options outside menial labor for below minimum wage would have been open to them. On the other hand, eight years of education is relatively high in a country which does not value education for women, and which still had a 36 percent literacy rate for women as of 1991 (Malawi Government 1991:10, cited in Kishindo 1995: 155). Relative to most women in Malawi then these bar girls were quite educated, but not educated enough to earn them higher paying jobs outside commercial sex work.

7 This is compared with the $32,000 per year that the US spends on each AIDS patient (Lurie *et al.* 1995: 543–4).

8 The reason given by the South African government for not employing Malawians is their high rates of HIV, but as Chirwa (1998) argues, a more likely reason is the mining industry's retrenchment and its need to employ more South Africans.

9 Largely as a result of a public health project in Calcutta to organize commercial sex workers around condom implementation, condom use among sex workers has risen from 2.7 percent in 1992 to 90.5 percent in 1998. As far as statistics can ascertain, only 5.5 percent of sex workers in Calcutta are HIV positive. The different political economy of sex workers in Bombay does not lend itself so readily to sex worker organization, and sex workers there have HIV rates of around 50 percent (Dugger 1999: A8).

10 Jochelson also commends a second book, Belinda Bozzoli's *Women of the Phokeng* (1991), for its portrayal of women migrants as something other than hapless victims of unfortunate circumstance as well. Bozzoli focuses on women from relatively prosperous peasant households who migrated to cities in pursuit of adventure and their own ambitions. Migration was a way to attain adult status, earn some money, and perhaps find a husband within whom to begin a household. As Jochelson puts it, Bozzoli's study "reveals that migrancy takes on a different meaning in different social contexts," and that "the category of 'women migrants' is not homogenous, but must be historically and regionally contextualised" (Jochelson 1995: 326).

11 Contrast this, however, with Kishindo's study of Malawian bar girls, in which only 24 percent of the prostitutes interviewed stated that their parents were aware of how they were earning a living and were able to send money home (1995: 158).

12 For more analysis of these studies, their uses and limitations, see Craddock 1996.

References

Akeroyd, A. V. (1997) "Sociocultural aspects of AIDS in Africa: occupational and gender issues," in G. Bond, J. Kreniske, I. Susser, and J. Vincent (eds) *AIDS in Africa and the Caribbean*, Boulder, CO: Westview Press: 11–30.

Asthana, S. (1997) "The relevance of place in HIV transmission and prevention: the Commercial Sex Industry in Madras," in R. Kearns and W. Gesler (eds) *Putting Health into Place: Landscape, Identity, and Well-being*, Syracuse, NY: Syracuse University Press: 168–87.

Asthana, S. and Oostvogels, R. (1996) "Community participation in HIV prevention: problems and prospects for community-based strategies among female sex workers in Madras," *Social Science and Medicine* 43, 2: 133–48.

Bandawe, C. R. (n.d.) "Preliminary recommendation to the Malawi Government Ministries of Health and Education and Culture, following a study of AIDS-related behaviours among secondary school students in Malawi," Zomba: Department of Community Health, University of Malawi College of Medicine.

Bongaart, J. (1996) "Global trends in AIDS mortality," *Population and Development Review* 22, 1: 21–45.

Bozzoli, B. with the assistance of M. Nkotsoe (1991) *Women of the Phokeng: Consciousness, Life Strategy, and Migrancy in South Africa 1900–1983*, London: James Currey; Portsmouth: Heinemann Educational Books.

Brown, M. (1997) *RePlacing Citizenship: AIDS and Activism in Vancouver*, New York: Guilford.

Bwayo, J., Plummer, F., Omari, M., Mutere, A., Moses, S., Ndinya-Achola, J., Velentgas, P., and Kreiss, J. (1994) "Human immunodeficiency virus infection in long-distance truck drivers in East Africa," *Archives of Internal Medicine* 154: 1391–6.

Carney, J. (1993) "Converting the wetlands, engendering the environment," *Economic Geography* 69, 4: 329–49.

Centre for Social Research (1994) *Baseline Survey: Youth and AIDS*, Zomba: University of Malawi.

Chirwa, W. (1996) "The Malawi government and South African labour recruiters, 1974–92," *The Journal of Modern African Studies* 34, 4: 623–42.

—— (1998) "Aliens and AIDS in southern Africa: the Malawi–South Africa debate," *African Affairs* 97: 53–79.

Corbridge, S. (1993) *Debt and Development IBG Studies in Geography*, Oxford: Blackwell.

Craddock, S. (1996) "AIDS in Malawi: a critical analysis of transmission and prevention," *African Rural and Urban Studies* 4, 3: 35–60.

Dugger, C. (1999) "Calcutta's prostitutes preach about condoms," *New York Times* 4 January: A1, A8.

Forster, P. (1994) "Culture, nationalism, and the invention of tradition in Malawi," *Journal of Modern African Studies* 32, 3: 477–98.

Foucault, M. (1979) *Discipline and Punish*, trans. S. Sheridan, New York: Vintage.

Gilman, S. (1988) *Disease and Representation: Picturing Disease from Madness to AIDS*, Ithaca, NY: Cornell University Press.

Helitzer-Allen, D. (1994) *An Investigation of Community-Based Communication Networks of Adolescent Girls in Rural Malawi for HIV/STD Prevention Messages*, Washington, DC: International Center for Research on Women.

Hirschmann, D. (1984) *Women, Planning, and Policy in Malawi*, Addis Ababa: UN Economic Commission for Africa.

Jochelson, K. (1995) "Women, migrancy and morality: a problem of perspective," *Journal of Southern African Studies* 21, 2: 323–32.

Jochelson, K., Mothibeli, M., and Leger, J. P. (1991) "Human immunodeficiency virus and migrant labor in South Africa," *International Journal of Health Services* 21, 1: 157–73.

Kent, G. (1991) "Children's rights to adequate nutrition," unpublished manuscript, University of Hawaii.

Kesby, M. (1999) "Participatory diagramming as a means to improve communication about sex in rural Zimbabwe: a pilot study," unpublished manuscript, University of St Andrews.

Kishindo, P. (1995) "Sexual behaviour in the face of risk: the case of bar girls in Malawi's major cities," *Health Transition Review*, Supplement to Volume 5: 153–60.

Lele, U. (1990) "Structural adjustment, agricultural development and the poor:

some lessons from the Malawian experience," *World Development* 18, 9: 1207–19.

Lurie, P., Hintzen, P., and Lowe, R. (1995) "Socioeconomic obstacles to HIV prevention and treatment in developing countries: the roles of the International Monetary Fund and the World Bank," *AIDS* 9: 539–46.

Mann, J. (1992) "Introduction," in J. Mann, D. Tarantola, and T. Netter (eds) *AIDS in the World*, Cambridge, MA: Harvard University Press: 1–12.

Mann, J., Tarantola, D., and Netter, T. (eds) (1992) *AIDS in the World*, Cambridge, MA: Harvard University Press.

Miles, L. (1993) "Women, AIDS, and power in heterosexual sex: a discourse analysis," *Women's Studies International Forum* 16, 5: 497–511.

Mohanty, C. (1988) "Under Western eyes: feminist scholarship and colonial discourses," *Feminist Review* 30: 61–88.

—— (1991) "Cartographies of struggle: Third World women and the politics of feminism," in C. Mohanty, A. Russo, and L. Torres (eds) *Third World Women and the Politics of Feminism*, Bloomington: Indiana University Press: 1–47.

Msapato, K. M., Kumwenda, K. M., Chirwa, B. Z., Chalira, A. M., and Mzembe, C. P. (1990) *Study of Knowledge and Aspects of Attitudes of School Teenagers in Mzimba District about HIV Infection/AIDS*, Lilongwe: Health Research Unit, Ministry of Health.

Murray, A. and Robinson, T. (1996) "Minding your peers and queers: female sex workers in the AIDS discourse in Australia and Southeast Asia," *Gender, Place, and Culture* 3, 1: 43–59.

Ndinya-Achola, J. O., Ghee, A. E., Kihara, A. N., Krone, M. R., Plummer, F. A., Fisher, L. D., and Holmes, K. K. (1997) "High HIV prevalence, low condom use and gender differences in sexual behaviour among patients with STD-related complaints at a Nairobi primary health care clinic," *International Journal of STD and AIDS* 8: 506–14.

Packard, R. and Epstein, P. (1992) "Medical research on AIDS in Africa: a historical perspective," in E. Fee and D. Fox (eds) *AIDS: The Making of a Chronic Disease*, Berkeley: University of California Press: 346–76.

Parpart, J. and Marchand, M. (1995) "Exploding the canon: an introduction/conclusion," in M. Marchand and J. Parpart (eds) *Feminism/Postmodernism/Development*, New York: Routledge: 1–22.

Pickering, H., Okongo, M., Ojwiya, A., Yirrell, D., and Whitworth, J. (1997) "Sexual networks in Uganda: mixing patterns between a trading town, its rural hinterland and a nearby fishing village," *International Journal of STD and AIDS*, 8: 495–500.

Schoepf, B. G. (1993) "Gender, development, and AIDS: a political economy and culture framework," *Women and International Development Annual* 3: 53–85.

—— (1998) "Inscribing the body politic: women and AIDS in Africa," in M. Lock and P. Kaufert (eds) *Pragmatic Women and Body Politics*, Cambridge Studies in Medical Anthropology, Cambridge: Cambridge University Press.

Schoepf, B. G., Walu, E., Rukarangira, S. N., Payanzo, N., and Schoepf, C. (1991) "Gender, power, and risk of AIDS in Zaire," in M. Turshen (ed.) *Women and Health in Africa*, Trenton, NJ: Africa World Press: 187–203.

Schoofs, M. (1998) "Bazaar science," *POZ* 39: 34.

Sen, A. (1981) *Poverty and Famines*, Oxford: Clarendon Press.

—— (1990) "Food, economics, and entitlements," in J. Dreze and A. Sen (eds) *The Political Economy of Hunger*, Vol. 1, Oxford: Clarendon Press: 34–52.

Singer, M. (1998) "Forging a political economy of AIDS," in M. Singer (ed.) *The Political Economy of AIDS*, Amityville, NY: Baywood Publishing.

Slutsker, L., Cabeza, J., Wirima, J., and Steketee, R. (1994) "HIV-1 infection among women of reproductive age in a rural district in Malawi," *AIDS* 8: 1337–40.

Specter, M. (1998) "Breast-feeding and HIV: weighing health risks," *New York Times* 19 August: A1.d.

Stichter, S. B. and Parpart, J. L. (eds) (1988) *Patriarchy and Class: African Women in the Home and the Workforce*, Boulder, CO: Westview Press.

Ulin, P. (1992) "African women and AIDS: negotiating behavioral change," *Social Science and Medicine* 34, 1: 63–73.

UNICEF-Malawi (1994) *HIV/AIDS Prevention Through Information and Education for Youth*, Lilongwe: Government Printing Office.

Waldorf, S. (1997) "Mchape: a wake-up call for AIDS control programs in Africa (a case history from Malawi)," *AIDS and Public Policy Journal* 12, 3: 136–43.

Watts, M. and Bohle, H. (1993) "The space of vulnerability: the causal structure of hunger and famine," *Progress in Human Geography* 17, 1: 43–67.

White, L. (1990) *The Comforts of Home. Prostitution in Colonial Nairobi*, Chicago: University of Chicago Press.

Wilbrink, J. (1995) "Letter to the editors," *Tropical and Geographical Medicine* 47, 6: 310–11.

Wilton, T. (1997) *EnGendering AIDS: Deconstructing Sex, Text and Epidemic*, London: Sage.

World Health Organization (WHO) (1994) *AIDS: Images of the Epidemic*, Geneva: WHO.

—— (1998) *Update on the AIDS Epidemic*, Joint Publication of UN AIDS/WHO, Geneva.

4 Women workers and the regulation of health and safety on the industrial periphery

The case of Northern Thailand

Jim Glassman

Introduction: worker health and safety in the era of "globalization"

In *Justice, Nature, and the Geography of Difference*, David Harvey discusses the September 1991 fire at the Imperial Foods chicken processing plant in Hamlet, North Carolina, which claimed the lives of twenty-five workers and injured fifty-six more (Harvey 1996: 334–6). Harvey notes that the recent growth of rural industries in the United States has swollen the numbers of factories attempting to take advantage of a "relatively isolated industrial reserve army" left behind by the decline of agricultural employment (ibid.: 336–7). He suggests that this expansion of industrial capital into rural areas is part of a broader historical tendency of capital to seek out lower wage locations and non-union workforces, thus undermining the ability of larger groups of workers in core industrial areas to place regulatory constraints on the accumulation process. The result of this geographically based attack by capital on labor regulation is the re-emergence within the United States of "a totally unsubtle form of coercive exploitation which is pre- rather than post-Fordist in form" (ibid.: 337). Like earlier pre-Fordist forms of exploitation, the new pre-Fordism makes ample use of the vulnerabilities and disempowerment of groups such as women and people of color: eighteen of the twenty-five workers who died at Hamlet were women, and twelve were Black. Thus, the Hamlet victims are descended from the 146 workers, most of them women and all of them recent immigrants, who died in the Triangle Shirtwaist Company fire of 1911 on the Lower East Side of Manhattan (Harvey 1996: 336; Greider 1997: 337–8).

Events in Thailand – the site of a recent pre-Fordist industrial growth boom – bear comparison with those in Hamlet and reinforce the claim that industrial expansion has in part been a tool for evading regulation. On 10 May 1993, a fire in the Kader toy factory – located in Nakhon Pathom province, just outside Bangkok – took at least 188 lives and injured at least 469 others. All but fourteen of the dead and injured were women workers, some as young as thirteen years old (Greider 1997: 337). Most were recent migrants to Bangkok from rural areas that could not provide jobs paying as much as those in the factories around Thailand's capital city – again the "industrial reserve army." The factory was in violation of numerous (poorly enforced) Thai safety codes – as, reportedly, were 60 percent of the large factories in the Bangkok area investigated after the fire (ibid.: 340). Many of the women died in the rapid collapse of the cheaply built four-story structure, while others died pounding at locked exit doors or jumping to the pavement below (ibid.: 338–40). The fire was the worst of its kind ever recorded, surpassing the record previously held by the Triangle Shirtwaist fire.

As with the textile mills of Manchester and Lowell a century earlier, the textile manufacturers of the global periphery today continue to employ primarily women workers – favoring them because of their ostensibly "nimble fingers" and greater docility. Thus, in rapidly industrializing places such as the Bangkok Metropolitan Area (BMA), women bear an increasing burden of occupational illness and mortality, rooted in their selective recruitment to sweatshops which offer wages otherwise unavailable to the rural poor.

But it is not only in Thailand's major metropolitan region that such problems are evident. This chapter discusses occupational health problems which have surfaced in the northern region of Thailand (Figure 4.1) as the Thai state and international capital have collaborated to spur the growth of manufacturing industries "up-country." The case of worker health problems in Thailand generally, and in Northern Thailand in particular, demonstrates the scope of the pre-Fordist industrialization pattern Harvey describes and the health concerns which it brings to workers in various types of global peripheries. As this chapter will suggest, events like those in Hamlet, Bangkok, and Northern Thailand are all linked together by the "logic" of a gendered, capitalist industrialization project which brings labor processes in disparate places under the same broad array of constraints and pressures, creating similar patterns of work and workplace injury around the world.

In his discussion of this industrialization dynamic, Harvey notes the salience of a class-based analysis, arguing that in Hamlet a strong workers' movement would have done more to protect the interests of women and people of color than has the "militant particularism" of women's and civil rights struggles based around a politics of identity (Harvey 1996: 338–41). One could interpret Harvey's claim in one of two ways.[1] One way would be to read it as an orthodox Marxist argument that class is a more fundamental category of analysis than gender or race and thus is the most powerful tool for understanding most social realities. A different, and in my view more compelling way – one consonant with "dual systems theory" approaches (Hartmann 1981; Walby 1990) – would be to suggest that while working-class men and women of all races and ethnicities may indeed experience shared forms of exploitation and oppression through "raw class politics" (Harvey 1996: 338), none the less the historical process of class formation is gendered and racialized in specific ways. Particular kinds of subordinate class positions and occupations tend to be filled disproportionately by women

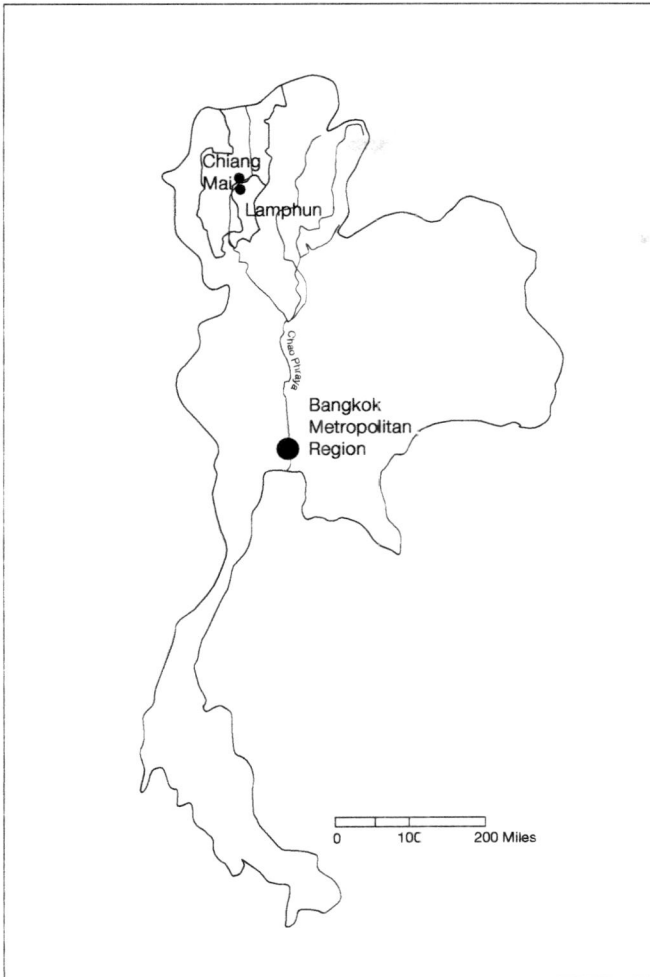

Figure 4.1 Map of Thailand.

and people of color, so that a full-fledged class analysis should at the same time be an analysis of gender relations and issues of race/ethnicity.

Moreover, as Harvey's analysis suggests, class formation and the structuring of occupations are not only gendered and racialized but simultaneously "spatialized" in particular ways. Thus, the return to pre-Fordist industrial forms throughout much of the global periphery (including the periphery developing within the United States) compounds labor force fragmentation by extending production processes territorially. This may weaken the bargaining power of labor organizations in core areas and deprive new industrial laborers of contact with larger and more experienced groups of workers.

A geographically informed dual systems perspective of the sort I am suggesting here has significant implications for discussions of women's health. I explore these implications by examining issues surrounding women's workplace health and safety conditions in Thailand.[2] I show that a class- and gender-based analysis – and particularly one attentive to the territorial accumulation strategies of the capitalist state in developing countries – both enhances our understanding of the kinds of health risks which confront many women in the developing world and indicates what kinds of responses are necessary to contain these risks.

This chapter is divided into four parts. In the first section, I outline the general pattern of industrial manufacturing growth in Thailand since World War II and note the gender dimensions of this growth, comparing these with what has been observed about the gender dimensions of industrial development elsewhere in the developing world. In the second section, I discuss the explosion of occupational health problems in Thailand which has occurred as a result of rapid industrialization. I place this explosion in the context of Thailand's epidemiological transition and note how political economic factors affect the transition and the attendant risks incurred by various groups of women. In the third section, I discuss the specific case of manufacturing industrialization in Northern Thailand and I examine the health problems that have developed in connection with such industrialization, placing this in the general context of Thailand's economic growth and development policies. In the conclusion, I note the theoretical and practical implications of this sort of analysis for strategies to improve women workers' health in the era of globalization.

Industrialization and the feminization of labor in Thailand

Until the economic crisis which began in 1996, Thailand was seen by most orthodox economists as one of the great economic success stories of the post-World War II era, sporting very rapid rates of industrial manufacturing growth and the highest increases in Gross Domestic Product in the world during 1988–90 (Pasuk and Baker 1998). The reasons for Thailand's rapid burst of industrial growth cannot be analyzed here, but certain basic features of the industrialization pattern need to be identified. First, low wages in the manufacturing sector, supported for many years by agricultural policies which kept rice prices low, have provided the "comparative advantage" which attracted manufacturing investment throughout most of the postwar period (Pasuk *et al.* 1996; Jomo 1997). Second, economic activity – and particularly manufacturing – has long been centered heavily around Bangkok (Dixon and Parnwell 1991; Pasuk and Baker 1995). Post-World War II growth has accentuated rather than diluted this historical legacy of Bangkok's political domination and economic primacy. For most inhabitants of relatively poor rural areas (and particularly many young women), the primary method of enhancing income has been to migrate to Bangkok or other urban centers in search of employment (Parnwell and Arghiros 1996; Mills 1999b). Third, all of the above factors have contributed to a pattern of industrial growth that is highly uneven and inegalitarian in geographical, sectoral, and social terms. This is registered, among other ways, in extreme (and growing) inequality in income distribution (Medhi 1996; Voravidh 1996).

Significantly, one general exception to the pattern of growing economic disparities is the relationship between men's and women's manufacturing earnings. Between 1983 and 1997, earnings of women working in manufacturing in urban areas increased from 70.8 to 78.6 percent of men's earnings (NSO, *LFS*, various years). This closing of the gender gap did not occur to the same extent in rural areas as it did in metropolitan areas, however. Furthermore, much of the reduction in earnings differentials which has occurred is the result of more women entering intermediate-level manufacturing industries (such as electronics) and working longer hours, a phenomenon which has had important occupational health consequences.

The entry of these women into the manufacturing labor force is part of the general movement from "private" to "public" forms of patriarchy (Brown 1981; Walby 1990) as well as the much-discussed phenomenon of women workers on the "global assembly line" (Elson and Pearson 1981a, 1981b; Nash and Fernandez-Kelley 1983). It has been common to assert that as manufacturing growth spreads globally more women are recruited into the manufacturing sector, leading to a "feminization" of the manufacturing labor process. More specifically, it has been argued that the patterns of growth which characterize the post-1973 era of global neo-liberalism are built around forms of labor market "flexibility" that hinge on this feminization of labor (Standing 1989; Lim 1993; Cravey 1998).

One notable feature regarding labor force participation by women in Thailand is that Thai women have long had a fairly large presence in manufacturing and have increased this presence gradually over the past twenty to twenty-five years. Moreover, participation by Thai women in the manufacturing labor force has increased much more rapidly than has their overall labor force participation. For example, between 1983 and 1997, the number of women working in the private manufacturing sector increased from 626,500 to 1,687,500, rising from 39.5 percent of all manufacturing employees to 47.4 percent. This meant that of all women officially in the labor force the percentage working in manufacturing increased from approximately 13 to approximately 20 percent over this period (NSO, *LFS*, various years). This high level of participation in manufacturing labor reflects the relatively minimal constraints which Thai households and specific Thai forms of patriarchy have typically placed on women's labor outside the home.

Of even more importance than their generally high levels of labor force participation is the fact that women have been the overwhelming majority of production-level employees in the manufacturing sectors which have led export growth during the Thai economic boom. In seven of the top ten export industries, women comprise over 80 percent of all employees (Sungsidh and

Kanchada 1994: 246; Bell 1996: 59). For example, the 1994 *Industrial Survey* found that over 65 percent of all non-managerial employees ("operatives") in industry were female, with women constituting over 83 percent of operatives in the food canning industry and over 93 percent in the clothing industry. Thus, many commentators argue that Thailand's rapid economic growth has taken place on the backs of women (Bell 1992: 61).

The recruitment of women to leading export sectors is a ubiquitous feature of the global assembly line, reflecting a certain homogeneity in the practices and perspectives shared by many ruling-class men around the world, who insist on women's superiority in performing tedious, repetitive, and "low skill" tasks. While these men typically insist that women are more docile, their employees sometimes confound this assumption by rebelling – in ways both big and small (Ong 1987; Porpora *et al.* 1989). Yet, as Susan Tiano notes, women frequently do in fact behave in ways that are outwardly submissive to employers' demands – despite being alienated by their work and critical of their treatment as women and as workers (Tiano 1994). The need to maintain employment in a context of limited options may for many women preclude militant forms of resistance (Theobald 1995). Working-class men face similar limitations, but women's greater household responsibilities and internalization of norms stressing duty to the family add to their constraints. For example, as has been observed in the case of Thailand, women frequently send more money home to support families than do men, and this makes the cost of job loss and the dangers of labor militance even greater for them (Porpora *et al.* 1989; Mingsarn *et al.* 1995). Thus, whatever the local resources for resistance by women in different sites along the global assembly line, it has generally been the case that states and corporations continue to deploy patriarchal recruitment and employment practices.

In Thailand, employers' assumptions about female dexterity and docility have led them to overwhelmingly recruit women for jobs in sectors such as those mentioned above (Mills 1999b). Yet Thai women have significant resources for resistance and those working in these sectors have not always confirmed the expectation that they will be docile and well-behaved employees (Porpora *et al.* 1989; Ji 1998; Mills 1999a). Thai society (like many other Southeast Asian societies) arguably has a less harsh or rigid gender hierarchy than societies such as Japan or Taiwan. This is in part because women often exercise substantial control over household economic resources, something which is frequently aided by matrilocality (Potter 1977; Reid 1988; Darunee and Shashi 1989).

One consequence of this is that as Thai women have become integrated into and acclimated to the manufacturing labor force – often after a period of adaptation that includes adjustment to geographical relocation – they have shown capacity for forms of labor militance that are disconcerting to employers. While women have fought less for unions than for specific forms of material betterment in their working conditions, their collective efforts to procure the latter have raised the possibility that more militant working-class organizations will develop – an eventuality which naturally is not favored by capitalists or the capitalist state.

Among both women and men, there was evidence of increasing labor militance in the 1990s, including a significant increase in the number of strikes (Pasuk and Baker 1998). None the less, the Thai union movement remains quite weak overall, compared with those in most other newly industrializing countries (Frenkel 1993; Hewison and Brown 1994), and thus many women workers are subject (as are many male laborers) to extremely dangerous working conditions. Despite women's local resources for resistance, then, their lack of recourse to forms of collective empowerment such as strong unions or NGO movements has so far made it difficult to change the occupational safety and health hazards they face.

Both employers and the state have used a variety of tactics to deter unionization of the labor force (Bundit 1998; Ji 1998). In general the state has repressed militant or leftist unions and, since 1972, encouraged the growth of conservative, pro-business unionism in which state enterprise union leaders – sifted for their ideological orientation – played a central role (Sungsidh 1989; Glassman 1999). This latter tactic has more or less endured to the present (though the state enterprise unions experienced a significant set-back in 1991 when they were downgraded to "associations" by the military regime and prohibited from striking). State enterprise-centered unionization has historically had a negative impact on the ability of the labor movement as a whole to represent the interests of women workers. This is because manufacturing labor in the state enterprises is primarily male while the majority of women manufacturing laborers work in the more weakly organized private sector (NSO, *LFS*, various years). Thus – in addition to the standard problems of women being underrepresented within union leadership (Pasuk *et al.* 1996) and male union leaders neglecting issues of special interest to women workers (e.g. maternity leave and sexual harassment) – the structure of organized labor insures that when state enterprise union leaders are bought out by offers which benefit their immediate constituents their gains do not automatically benefit most female manufacturing employees to the same degree.

The cooptive labor management approach centered around state enterprise unions has a geographical component, since most state enterprises are based in Bangkok.[3] Though somewhat schematic, one could identify three broad geographic manufacturing zones in relation to the state's labor relations strategy. Within Bangkok, while underregulated and often small-scale factory labor is still prevalent, there is a higher degree of semi-regulated state enterprise activity. On the periphery of Bangkok, there has been a burgeoning of poorly regulated and lower wage manufacturing industries, including much of the production for export which employs the lion's share of women workers. In up-country regions, there is comparatively little manufacturing activity, but what exists is usually very small-scale and even more poorly regulated than on the Bangkok periphery. It is important to recognize zonal structure since, as will be noted below, the increased wages and labor militance seen in the BMA during the 1990s have sent certain manufacturers in search of a more docile labor force outside the BMA. For some of the firms which settled in Northern Thailand, the desire for women workers and for cheaper, less militant labor came together in the decision to expand production up-country.

Thailand's epidemiological transition and the health of workers

Studies of developing countries have noted that epidemiological transition in such countries today seems far less straightforward than was the case for many of the early industrializing countries, with both "traditional" and "modern" diseases coexisting at relatively high levels among many of today's industrializing nations (Phillips and Verhasselt 1994). Thailand's epidemiological transition, like those of a number of other newly industrializing countries (NICs), illustrates another dimension of this story. As Figures 4.2 and 4.3 illustrate, "traditional" sources of mortality in Thailand have indeed been replaced by "modern" killers, but these killers now include a very large number of deaths due to accidents. This broad category – which includes transport accidents, workplace accidents, and all other accidents which take place at home or in public places – accounted for 61.5 deaths per 100,000 persons during both 1994 and 1995 and is now the second leading cause of death in Thailand (Ministry of Public Health, various years). The significance of this for the notion of epidemiological transition is that, unlike other "modern" killers, accidents tend to kill people at relatively young ages. For example, the average age of death from traffic accidents – which account for the majority of deaths due to accidents – is 30 years (calculated from Ministry of Public Health, various years).

Work-induced mortality and morbidity need to be discussed in the context of decreased infectious disease and increased accident mortality because this epidemiological pattern reflects directly on the nature of the Thai development process and the power relations in which it is embedded. Specifically, the reduction in "traditional" sources of mortality and morbidity such as infectious diseases owes much to the concerted effort of the US and Thai states during the Cold War era to expand health services in rural areas (Muscat 1990: 86–92, 216–20). This was part of a broader project by which the Thai state extended its presence more fully into remote regions which were seen as susceptible to Communist infiltration. Campaigns against malaria both provided an opportunity to test the World Health Organization (WHO) strategy of DDT-based mosquito control and limited the potential of epidemics in militarily sensitive areas (ibid.: 86–92). In addition, the provision of such services as modern sanitation and childhood nutrition programs improved rural living standards in relatively poor communities which might otherwise support radical social change (Muscat 1990: 216–20; 1994: 238).

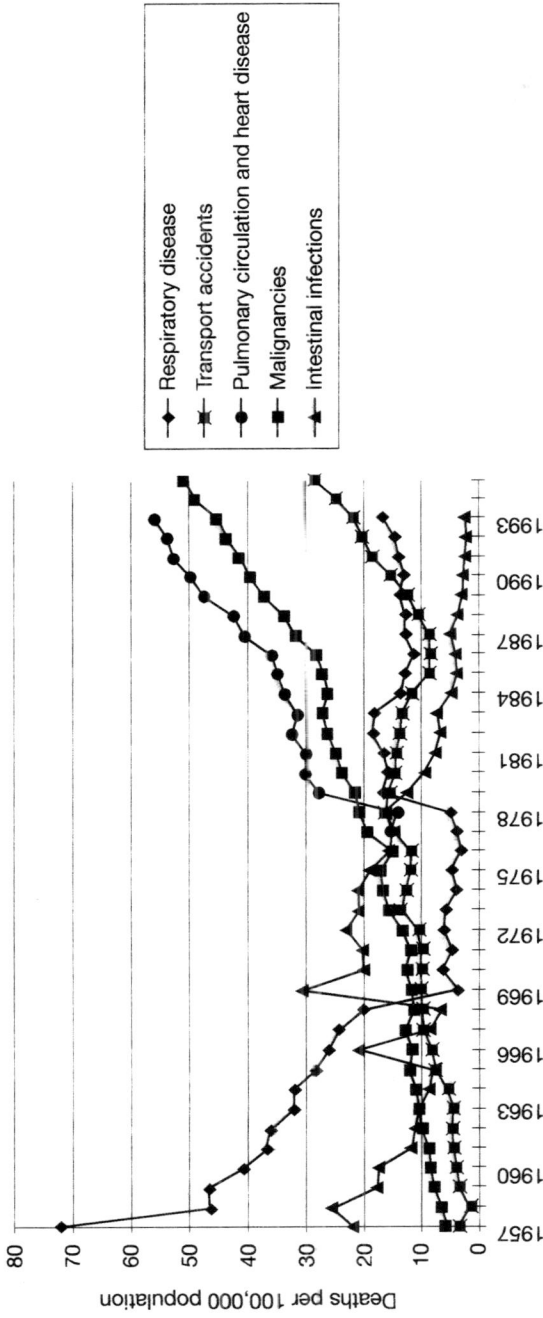

Figure 4.2 Death rates for major cause groups, whole kingdom, 1957–95.

Source: Ministry of Public Health, various years.

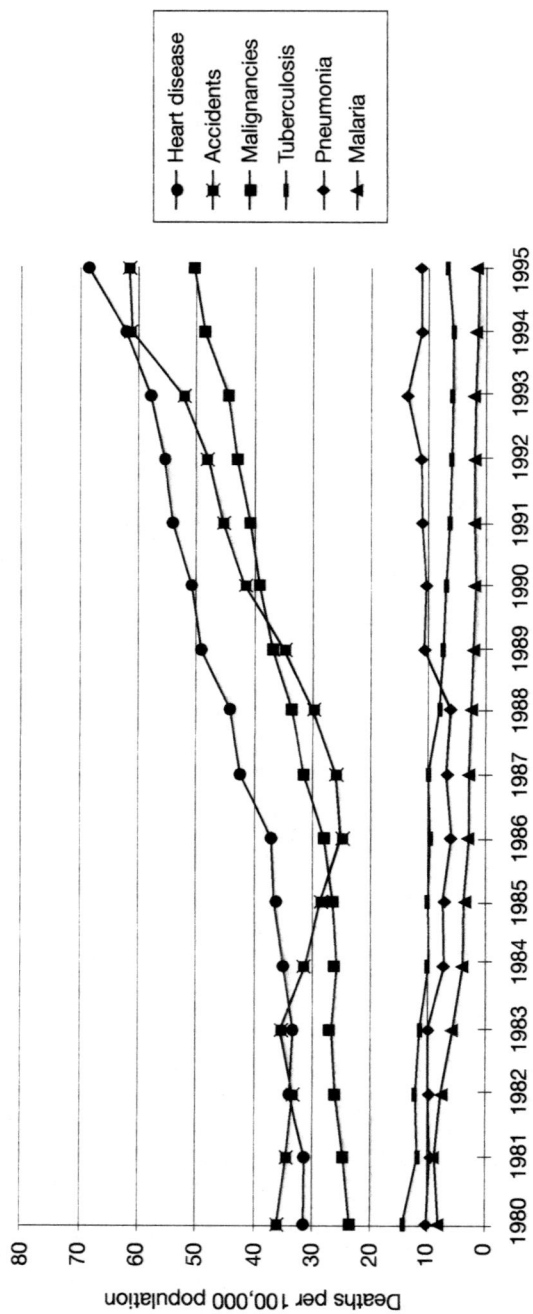

Figure 4.3 Death rates for major causes of mortality, whole kingdom, 1980–95.

Source: Ministry of Public Health, various years.

State efforts in reducing infectious diseases contrast substantially with state efforts to reduce either accidents generally or occupational accidents more specifically. While reduction of infectious diseases was both politically acceptable and relatively low-cost (especially where subsidized by the US Agency for International Development or the WHO), prevention of accidents requires both greater expenditures by the state (e.g. for upgrading of the transportation system) and more interference with what are taken to be the prerogatives of capital (i.e. more factory regulation). Neither high levels of state spending nor strong regulations are generally viewed favorably by most capitalists or international aid organizations, and in the era of global neo-liberalism they are particularly disdained.

This political economic context provides the backdrop for the development of occupational health and safety problems connected with manufacturing growth in Thailand. The annual number of occupational fatalities in Thailand rose steadily from 640 in 1990 to 980 in 1993 with a slight decline to 820 in 1994. Figures 4.4 and 4.5, which show morbidity and mortality *rates*, illustrate that while Thailand's official workplace mortality rate is not substantially different from those of other NICs its injury rate is exceptionally high and has been increasing dramatically in recent years. Given that injuries are less likely to be reported than deaths, the actual injury rate in Thailand may be much higher than indicated here. Moreover, it is widely understood that neither official injury rate nor official death rate figures are adequate, since they only include the injuries and deaths occurring in registered factories with ten or more workers – smaller factories are not required to participate in worker compensation schemes. The actual levels of morbidity and mortality may be as much as five times higher, according to the head of the Labor Department's Center for the Improvement of Workplace and the Environment.

Workplace accidents are thus one of the leading causes of death and injury among the young in Thailand – comparable in impact to the much more widely publicized AIDS epidemic. It should be noted that the official Thai data on workplace accidents are not broken down by gender so that it is not possible to say precisely how many workplace deaths there have been among females. None the less, we can construct a reasonable proxy for this figure by assuming that 34 percent of all workplace fatalities occur among women. This is the average for the years 1980–95 in the three International Classification of Disease (ICD) categories subsuming most workplace deaths – "falls," "exposure to smoke, fire, and flames," and "accidental poisoning by and exposure to noxious substance." On the basis of this extrapolation, it appears that workplace mortality is responsible for as many or – if the estimate of actual fatalities being five times the recorded number is accurate – even far more deaths among women during recent years than is AIDS (Table 4.1).

It should also be noted that figures on work-related accidents do not include most illnesses that may be caused by workplace hazards such as

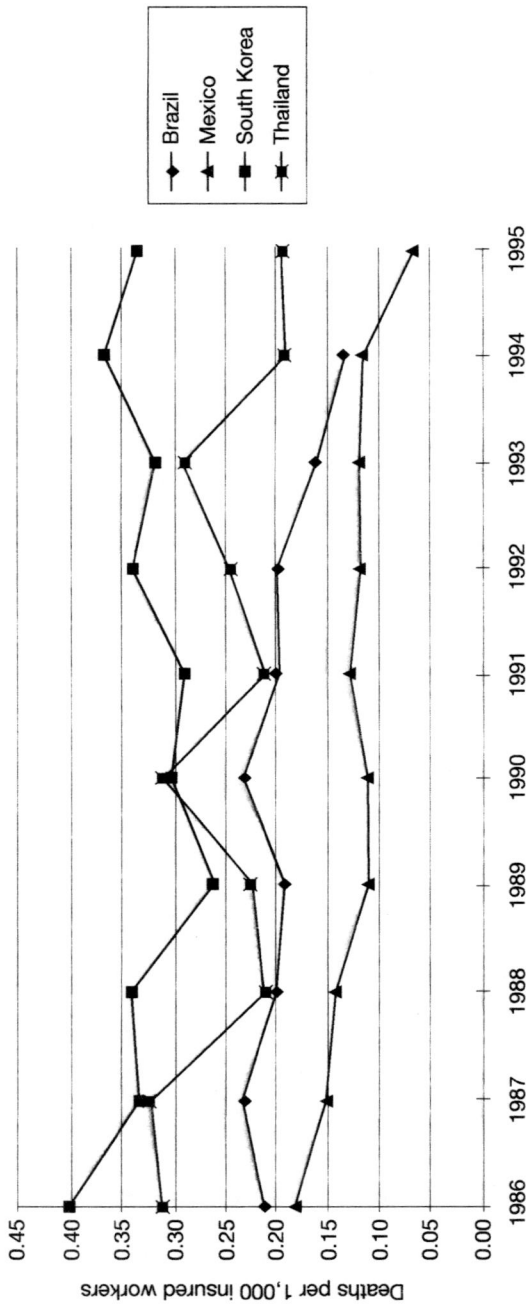

Figure 4.4 Rate of fatal occupational injuries, by country, 1986–95.

Source: ILO, various years.

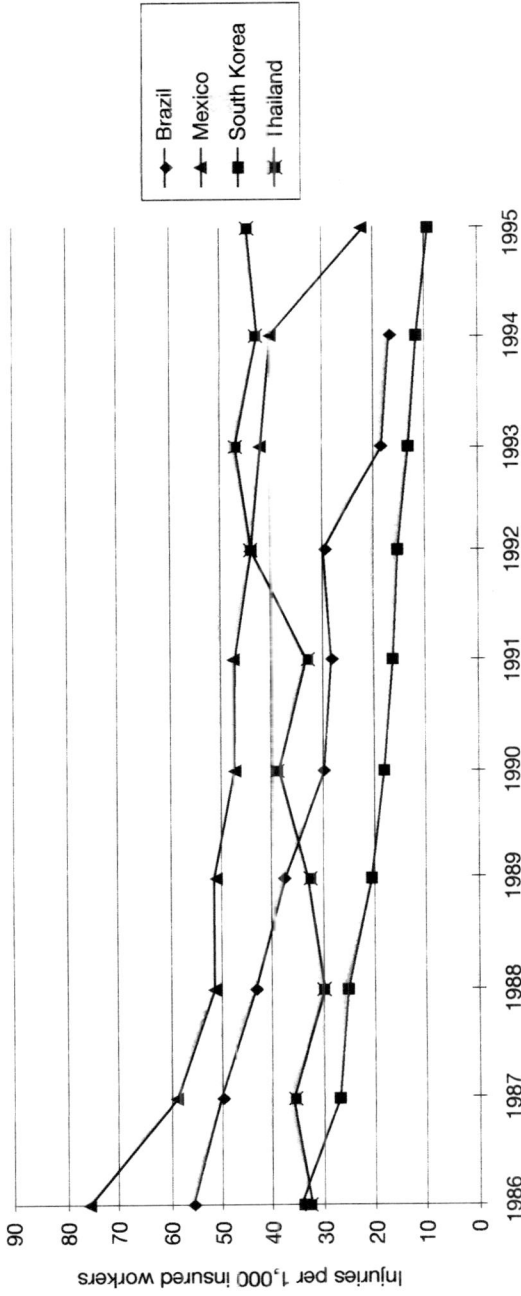

Figure 4.5 Occupational injury rate, by country, 1986–95.

Source: ILO, various years.

Table 4.1 AIDS and workplace accident mortality, Thailand and Chiang
          Mai-Lamphun, 1984–96

	AIDS deaths	Workplace accident deaths
All persons	15,420	8,159
Women	2,512	2,774

Sources: Ministry of Public Health, various years; Alpha Research (1997); Center for the
Improvement of Working Conditions and the Environment, various years; DLSW (1996).

chemical exposures. These are extremely hard to document, given inadequate
scientific research on workplace hazards and employer refusal to acknowledge chemical-caused illness or to release information on chemicals being
used in production. One estimate of the number of industrial workers
suffering from environmental illness placed this figure at 150,000 during
1996 (Pasuk and Baker 1998: 292). However, many such work-induced
health problems may not be diagnosed and/or may not appear for years.
The official figures on workplace morbidity and mortality are thus best
considered an extremely conservative minimum estimate. For example,
women in the textile industry are susceptible to a severe respiratory condition
called byssinosis, which results from inhalation of cotton dust particles and
leads to breathing problems, weariness, chest pains, and disability or death
in extreme cases. A 1995 survey showed that as many as 307,725 workers
in 3,080 factories are at risk from the disease, and as many as 30 percent of
all Workers' Compensation Fund claims may be by people suffering from
byssinosis. Yet standard diagnostic procedures such as chest X-rays do not
identify the condition (*Bangkok Post*, 9 August 1998).

Diagnostic inadequacies of the state's medical system aside, it is clear that
neither women nor men are well-served by the state regulatory apparatus
ostensibly designed to prevent accidents or exposures in the first place.
Statistics on factory inspection produced by the Department of Labor and
Social Welfare indicate that between 1984 and 1996 only around 14 percent
of all officially registered factories in the country were inspected annually.
The inspection rate was somewhat higher in Bangkok (17 percent) but lower
in up-country regions such as the North (11 percent). Nation-wide, over 50
percent of those factories inspected were found to be in violation of one
or another provision of the labor law, and the North had an even higher
rate of violations – over 60 percent. Despite the prevalence of labor law
violations, few factory owners are ever punished: over the time period in
question, only 0.2 percent of those factories found in violation of labor laws
were prosecuted, most factories merely being given advice on how to improve
the situation (DLSW, *YLS*, various years).

According to the Department of Labor and Social Welfare's own published
statistics, violation of health and safety regulations is extremely common.
For example, in 1995 over 61 percent of all establishments inspected had

safety violations, with the figure among those which were inspected because of accident reports being over 88 percent (DLSW, *YLS*, 1996). Again such statistics only tell a minimalist version of the story. Most factories are not registered and are never inspected, a problem which is particularly acute in up-country regions. For example, the head of the Chiang Mai Provincial Department of Labor and Social Welfare estimates that there are more than twice as many factories in the province as officially registered, and his inspection staff is far from sufficient even to cover the number of factories officially registered. Lack of adequate regulatory staff arguably indicates a lack of commitment to effectively regulating industry. Moreover, when workers are injured, the state has shown limited interest in providing compensation or in forcing companies to do so. For example, in 1995 there were over 200,000 injuries resulting in compensation claims but only some 100 claims for which compensation was awarded (Voravidh 1998).

Problems of inadequate workplace health and safety measures are due to more than state neglect or lack of interest, however, as can be illustrated by a conflict over worker health and safety concerns which centers directly on the experiences of women in manufacturing industries. Dr Oraphan Methadilokun is one of the few physicians working in Thailand who has training in occupational health and illness.[4] In the 1990s, she began diagnosing and treating patients with workplace-related illnesses from exposure to materials such as asbestos and lead, and she also testified in a number of legal cases involving such illness (*Bangkok Post*, 22 December 1991; 9 October 1993; *The Nation* [Bangkok], 19 April 1992). One case involved women workers from the Seagate company, a US-based firm which assembled disk drives in a Samut Prakan plant (near Bangkok) and at that time was one of the largest single employers in Thailand. In 1991, four Seagate workers died after incurring what Dr Oraphan determined to be higher-than-permissible levels of lead exposure, and possibly exposures to other unidentified chemicals as well. While carrying out the investigation at Seagate, however, she reportedly received a threatening phone call from the head of the powerful Thai Board of Investment (BoI) – a body connected with the Prime Minister's office which promotes both foreign and domestic investment in Thai industry – and subsequently the agency she headed, the National Institute of Occupational and Environmental Medicine, was shut down by the Ministry of Health (Forsyth 1994: 30–4).

Dr Oraphan's marginalization can be taken as an indicator of the even more extreme marginalization of her patients, women workers with no professional training (and thus potential political clout) and with little in the way of either strong labor organizations or an effective state regulatory apparatus to rely upon. Significantly, however, these industrial accident victims have not been acquiescent and have fought with at least limited success to improve workplace regulation. In 1994, a woman named Somboon Srikhamdokkhae, who suffers from byssinosis, formed an organization called the Network of Sick Persons from Work and Environment of Thailand, comprising largely women workers. During 1996 and 1997, the Network mobilized within a nation-wide umbrella organization called the Assembly of the Poor, successfully pressing the Thai state and private employers on several occasions to compensate injured workers who had received no payments. In addition, members of the Network worked with a Thai labor NGO to demand restructuring of the Labor Department's Institute for Occupational Health and Safety so that it would provide more compensation to injured workers (Voravidh 1998).

Beyond the workers in the Network, women elsewhere in the Bangkok area have shown significant ability and willingness to lead labor struggles for improved working conditions (Pasuk *et al.* 1996: 98–9). Thus, for example, women have effectively extended locally based labor unions throughout the Omnoi-Omyai area of Nakhon Pathom and Samut Sakorn provinces, one of the central textile and garment manufacturing regions within the BMA (Bundit 1998; Ji 1998). However, precisely because workers have made some organizational inroads in the BMA, there is currently a threat that manufacturers are going to use the economic crisis as an excuse to restructure and relocate older factories to areas outside the BMA, or even outside Thailand. Indeed, establishment of facilities in regions where labor is less organized is not new for BMA textile, garment, and electronics firms, in spite of the general tendency of investment to cluster around Bangkok.[5]

Occupational morbidity and mortality in Northern Thailand

As part of its response to the over-concentration of manufacturing and economic activity in Bangkok, the Thai state has promoted the development of industrial estates in various up-country locations. To facilitate growth of manufacturing in the upper North, the Thai state's Industrial Estate Authority (IEAT) built the Northern Region Industrial Estate (NRIE) in Lamphun province, which was completed in March 1985. The estate is located 23 kilometers south of Chiang Mai province's municipal district along the Chiang Mai–Lampang superhighway and just 2 kilometers east of Lamphun's municipal district by rail. This enables it to tap Chiang Mai city's substantial labor market and international airport while paying Lamphun's lower minimum wage (Glassman 1999).

When Thailand's economy boomed in 1988–90 and production costs began to rise in Bangkok, a number of investors began to look to the North for a lower cost production site, leading to rapid growth in investment at the NRIE by 1992. As of February 1997, over 90 percent of the NRIE's 100 available units of land had been sold, and sixty-two of the factories slated for these plots were in operation while another nineteen were under construction. Of the sixty-two factories in operation, sixteen were producing or assembling electronics components, and twelve of these were Japanese-owned or were joint ventures involving Japanese owners. Overall, as of 1995, the NRIE was estimated to be employing 22,000 persons, with electronics and machinery firms responsible for over 60 percent of this employment.

Though the IEAT does not release figures on the percentage of industrial estate workers who are female, electronics firms which I visited during 1996–7 had the standard profile of such firms throughout Thailand, employing almost exclusively women in the assembly jobs. Confirmation of this impression comes from a French research team's survey of sixty-three Northern Region manufacturers, fourteen of these from the NRIE, carried out during 1995–7. The survey found that women constituted 75 percent of all employees in the sampled firms. Women made up 82 percent of electronics employees and 91 percent of textile employees, most of the latter working outside the NRIE (ORSTOM 1997). The rationale given by electronics firms for hiring women assemblers was stereotypical and straightforward: women were regarded as having better manual dexterity of the sort needed in the assembly operations and, as one Japanese plant manager put it, they "are easier to control." Similar sentiments have been expressed by other managers of electronics, textile, and garment firms in the region (Gray 1990: 193; Theobald 1995: 27–8).

While Thai state policies promoting manufacturing decentralization have thus helped capitalists find the kind of labor force they seek in the North, state policies have hindered union attempts to organize this labor. The state's endorsement of conservative, Bangkok-centered state enterprise unions, and its simultaneous repression of other labor organizations, has done much to limit the growth of unions in regions such as the North, since development of up-country unions in the face of local business opposition is dauntingly difficult without national solidarity. In part because of this, Chiang Mai and Lamphun provinces have had no unions whatsoever throughout most of their history. Given this complete lack of unions, it is not surprising that these provinces have also had very few strikes or work stoppages. Workers do, as will be seen, utilize the "weapons of the weak," through slowing down the work pace or even simply leaving their jobs. However, they are so disinclined to act confrontationally that throughout the economic boom of the late 1980s there was not a single strike in all of Northern Thailand (DLSW, *YLS*, various years).

One labor organization in Bangkok did attempt briefly to address this problem of low labor militance in the North by sending a representative to the Chiang Mai-Lamphun area to organize at the NRIE. He found, among other problems, that laws requiring union promoters to be at least 20 years old posed a huge hurdle, since most of the large factories which would be the obvious target of unionization campaigns were employing many women under that age. He thus left after only three months, a period which some local activists considered insufficient and a reflection of minimal interest on the part of the national unions. Beyond this fledgling effort, it appears that the unions in Bangkok have not shown signs of being concerned about the prospects of companies moving to such places as the North and so have not committed resources to the organizing effort there.

Union-hostile capital, a capital-friendly state, and weak labor organizations all conspired in laying the foundations for the NRIE tragedies of 1993–4. Beginning in 1993, a number of workers at NRIE electronics firms, almost all of them women, began to die from unexplained causes which involved headaches, inflamed stomachs, and vomiting. The exact number of workers who died is uncertain but by 1994 the total may have reached as high as twenty-three (Forsyth 1994: 35; Theobald 1995: 18).[6] The causes of the deaths have not been definitively determined but both local NGOs and health officials believe that they were probably the result of exposure to heavy metals such as lead. This was a particularly salient problem for the young women working long hours in the electronics factories, who were suffering sustained exposures to chemicals by working overtime in order to earn bonus pay (Forsyth 1994: 36).

Local NGOs reacted to the deaths with concern, and related them to environmental problems which had developed in Lamphun since the opening of the NRIE. For example, Lamphun activists had been complaining that waste and untreated water from the NRIE were being dumped into local fields and streams, causing deaths of fish and other problems (*Bangkok Post* 1 May 1994). When the worker deaths occurred, the two sets of concerns synergized and led to an outpouring of public anger over the effects of the NRIE on Lamphun.

The reaction of leading institutions of the Thai state was defensive. The head of the IEAT, Somchet Thinaphong, claimed that the deaths were caused by AIDS, a claim that could not be sustained by medical records (Forsyth 1994: 36). Local regulators with the Department of Labor and its Center for the Improvement of Working Conditions and Environment felt besieged by the NGOs and contended that the outpouring of concern actually damaged their ability to conduct inspections of the factories. For its part, the local medical system was in over its head, since it was reported that no hospital in the North even had the medical equipment necessary to test for heavy-metal poisoning (Forsyth 1994: 35–6; 1997: 195).

Workers responded in their own way. None were unionized, and between this and the limitations of state regulation, there were few potential avenues of direct protest. Nor were any involved at this time with NGOs, and most both wanted and needed to keep some sort of employment, so they could not directly confront management and risk being blacklisted. Instead, when they felt that work conditions were getting too bad, they simply began to quit and seek work elsewhere. A Chiang Mai doctor who had investigated some of the cases of worker illness estimated that after the deaths as many as 50 percent of the workers at the NRIE may have quit because of the fear that they would be next to die.[7] This was in any event a strategy more consistent with the strategies workers at the estate had already learned to utilize; indeed, despite their reputation for passivity, there had been a number of cases where workers who were not granted wage increases or holiday leaves they requested quit and went to other firms in the estate, sometimes moving in groups.[8] While the workers' strategy was non-confrontational, it was not carried out without at least nascent awareness of the conflictual relationship between workers and management. For example, in a series of interviews and focus group studies with workers from the NRIE, Sally Theobald found that workers consistently complained of long hours, health problems, boredom, and strict rules and regulations, although they regarded these as annoyances which "we have to put up with to get the money" (Theobald 1995: 30). The women also worried about chemical poisoning at work but found it difficult to get information about the materials they had to work with. They noted that "we're afraid to ask our boss as we'd be seen as trouble makers and he'd say there's nothing wrong anyway" (ibid.: 48; cf. Varunee and Benja 1994: 48–50). Thus, the relatively meek response of labor should not be interpreted as reflecting a complete lack of political consciousness or resistance but, rather, as reflecting the awareness which members of the "industrial reserve army" have of their extremely weak bargaining position.

A prominent court case involving a woman who worked at the NRIE reinforces the view that northern workers have good reason to doubt the merits of fighting the system on its own terms. Mayuree Tewiya was employed at the Japanese joint-venture firm, Electro Ceramics.[9] She began working in 1988, at the age of 24, preparing ceramic-alumina plates for soldering before their installation in television sets. In early 1993 she took sick leave from the company after suffering from head and body aches, but she refused to resign unless she received compensation from both Electro Ceramics and the Social Security Office. After a doctor at Chiang Mai's McCormick Hospital diagnosed her as suffering from alumina poisoning, she returned to the company with the diagnosis in hand to demand compensation, but the company refused to accept the diagnosis as valid and eventually terminated her employment in April 1994 (Forsyth 1994: 35–6; Theobald 1995: 51). Mayuree had written to Dr Oraphan for advice before going to McCormick, and after the company released her Dr Oraphan began helping her prepare a legal case against the company. The case went before the Central Labor Court and was decided in late 1996, with the court ruling that the evidence on the cause of Mayuree's illness was inconclusive (*Bangkok Post* 29 October 1996).

The case had been billed as a crucial one for both employers and employees since success for Mayuree might open the door for legal claims by other workers. Workers at the NRIE thus could not have missed the significance of the court's ruling for legal fights over health and safety. Yet if Mayuree's case suggests that northern workers are justified in feeling disempowered, a contemporaneous event suggests they could learn from Bangkok workers that powerlessness is in part the result of failure to organize and act with militance. The day after the Central Labor Court decided against Mayuree, 200 members of the Assembly of the Poor waged a protest outside the Ministry of Labor in Bangkok. They received a 4 million *baht* compensation payment for twenty-five members of the Network of Sick Persons from Work and Environment of Thailand who were suffering from byssinosis (*The Nation* [Bangkok] 30 October 1996).

It is noteworthy, too, that even given the serious structural limitations to effective resistance by northern workers, the outpouring of concern by the NGOs over the NRIE deaths may not have gone entirely unrewarded. Both some of the factories and the Labor Department regulatory bodies claim to have taken more aggressive measures to ensure that workers wear protective gear and that tighter safety precautions are maintained. They lament that popular attention has focused on the NRIE firms when, they point out, conditions are worse and more difficult to regulate outside the estate – a perception that is simultaneously self-serving and accurate. Nevertheless, the fear of having a bad public image – and perhaps of having greater difficulty maintaining workforce stability – seems to have had a few salutary, if limited or potentially transient, effects.[10] Moreover, the struggle over health at the NRIE continues. Local NGOs and their supporters are attempting to create a health center for workers at the estate that would disseminate information and train workers in identifying health hazards.

Conclusion: implications of gendered industrial growth on the periphery

Viewing Thai women workers' health and safety problems through the lens of a gendered and geographical class analysis brings into focus issues of social power which are always at work in the production of health and disease but which sometimes remain buried when discussion turns to what is to be done. These issues include the places and the ways in which women enter the industrial labor force; the kinds of health problems they face there; the resources which they have available for resistance to imposition of dangerous work; the constraints placed on their actions by both the structure of gender relations within society (including within labor unions) and the power of the capitalist state; and the constraints and enablements created by their connections (or lack of connections) with broader social groups and other workers across national and international spaces. The complexities of women's positions in such a multi-faceted process as industrialization does not suggest simple answers to the questions of how specific groups of women in these contexts use, confront, or are repressed by power. A gendered and geographical class analysis none the less provides a framework for understanding certain broad tendencies in both the experiences and actions of various groups of women workers. Thus, rather than being at odds with an analysis of the complexities of gender identity and the political ramifications of this complexity, I suggest that a dual systems approach can be used to help identify a crucial general context for the particularities of worker health and illness – and the struggles of specific groups of women workers around these.

Occupational injuries and diseases are somewhat unique as a health phenomenon in that they are highly discriminating in whom they target, affecting very few privileged workers or employers and preying openly on the least powerful segments of the working class. While diseases such as malaria and AIDS also prey disproportionately on the poor and marginal, privileged people such as military officers stationed up-country or business-men who visit brothels have reason to fear them as well. Thus, the state has backing from certain elites for dedication of resources to the containment or eradication of such diseases. By contrast, few if any Bangkok professionals or factory owners are likely to die of the workplace hazards which threaten most shopfloor workers. It would seem to be as a consequence of this that a health problem comparable to AIDS in its severity in Thailand has by comparison received so little attention or publicity (especially outside national borders).

Unlike many other health threats, therefore, occupational health hazards are unlikely to be addressed seriously in the absence of a strong working-class social movement. Since women are disproportionately represented among the most marginalized workers – and are also experiencing particularly rapid increases in injuries and fatalities, due to their rapid proletarianization – they are likely to play a pivotal role in any such movement. The case of worker mobilization around health issues in Thailand points in this direction, for while both men and women are active in labor issues more generally, it has been women who have played the leading role in health struggles. Moreover, it is women such as those in the Network of Sick Persons from Work and Environment of Thailand who have – through participation in the Assembly of the Poor – helped carry workers' issues beyond the narrow boundaries of the unions' annual wage negotiations and into a broader arena of social concerns which link workers, farmers, environmentalists, and other groups. Thus, even though class-based activism is often declared to be in retreat globally, the experiences of Thai (and other) women who are being subjected to new industrial health risks continue to provide a stimulus to working-class politics – albeit of a different sort than has often issued forth from male-dominated union movements (Rowbotham and Mitter 1994).

Yet the situation of Northern Thai workers shows that the territorial dimension of workers' social struggles is crucial and cannot be neglected. Gains for Bangkok workers do not automatically result in comparable gains for workers elsewhere; and a geographically limited labor movement may possibly prove a liability not only to women working in places such as the NRIE but also to Bangkok workers themselves, insofar as many capitalists are willing to keep seeking out the less-regulated peripheries in order to reduce costs. Thus, an effective, gendered working-class movement for occupational health would ultimately seem to require that workers in the BMA and places such as Lamphun build cohesive national organizations and strategies. Indeed, given the international mobility of capital, the day may well have arrived when these workers will need to find ways of organizing and strategizing collaboratively with workers in places such as Tokyo, Taipei, Jakarta, Vientiane, and perhaps even Hamlet, North Carolina.

This latter challenge brings to the fore a central issue which has always confronted left and labor politics – and which will not disappear in an increasingly feminized and social movement-oriented post-communist labor politics. Capitalist development is inherently uneven and has bestowed certain limited privileges on groups of workers in particular locations. These privileges, which are often enabled and reinforced by imperialism, have historically given rise to various implicitly or explicitly racist practices on the part of privileged workers, including collaboration with US state repression of labor organizations in developing countries. Such practices make the formation of a unified and militant global workers' movement impossible. The era of "globalization" has brought the collapse of the "labor accord" which linked the interests of privileged (and primarily male) workers within the global core to those of capital, and has thus created new possibilities for bringing together groups of workers who might have formerly seen their interests as antagonistic (Moody 1997). Yet such coalitions are as yet more potential than actual, and a global movement for workers' health will have much work to do confronting the historical legacies of imperialism within the labor movements of core countries if it is to succeed in actualizing these potentialities.[11] Thus, while the health problems faced by women workers on the global assembly line may well reinvigorate and feminize class politics, such a politics will need spatial strategies which can overcome the divisions between various communities of workers which have been created or exacerbated by uneven capitalist development.

Acknowledgments

I would like to thank Richa Nagar, Thitiya Phaobtong, and the editors of this volume for comments on earlier drafts of this chapter, and I would like to extend special thanks to Voravidh Charoenloet and the many other labor activists and scholars who helped me with research carried out in Thailand. I would also like to thank the Geography Department and the MacArthur Program at the University of Minnesota for research support.

Notes

1 For debates about this issue of interpretation, see Braun 1998; Corbridge 1998; Hartsock 1998; Harvey 1998; Young 1998.
2 I note that there are many aspects of dual systems analysis, including a focus on how the household division of labor affects gender relations and processes of exploitation in the workplace (Walby 1990). While the perspective employed here is indebted to this sort of household-level analysis, I do not directly discuss issues of "private" patriarchy or the gender division of labor within the household. Instead, I focus on the points at which realities created by these "domestic" processes intersect with processes in such "public" spheres as factories and state agencies.
3 When labor unions were first legalized in 1972, they were originally prohibited from organizing across provincial boundaries. This prohibition was eventually

lifted, and the more left-leaning unions indeed tried to organize not only across boundaries but in solidarity with activist students and rural groups such as peasant organizations. This activity was suppressed by state violence in the mid-1970s, however, and the unions which survived tended to recede into the role of "bread and butter" unions, limiting their activities to supporting the wage demands of local workers. For analysis of these issues, see Mabry 1979; Wehmhörner 1983; Sungsidh 1989; Brown and Frenkel 1993; Hewison and Brown 1994; Glassman 1999.

4 Information in the following paragraphs is based in part on interviews by the author.

5 For example, the executive director of a BMA factory which opened a Chiang Mai branch in the 1990s indicated to me in an interview that the company had done so in response to rising wages and production costs in Bangkok. Furthermore, it avoided locating in the Northern Region Industrial Estate (NRIE) because of reports of labor conflict there – conflicts which will be discussed below. The director also made it clear to me that the company is strongly opposed to anything but in-house unions and is proud of the fact that its workers are not unionized.

6 The deaths were reported in a number of stories in the Thai English-language press throughout 1994. See, e.g. *Bangkok Post* 24 and 27 February, 28 April, and 1 May, and *The Nation* (Bangkok) 27 February and 1 May.

7 Author interview.

8 Author interviews, NRIE factory managers. This strategy was not available to all workers and only succeeded in cases such as those involving electronics employees, since there are a large number of electronics factories in the estate, each hiring large numbers of workers.

9 Mayuree's case is discussed in a number of articles from the Thai English-language press. See, e.g. *The Nation* (Bangkok) 27 February 1994.

10 One observer has noted that the apparent decline in deaths at the estate after 1994 could be because workers have started using protective gear more regularly, because the companies became more conscientious, or merely because the heavy metals which may have caused the deaths need a number of years to accumulate in the body before they are deadly, and the workers who died in 1993 had put in the requisite amount of time whereas, with the subsequent departure of many workers, most of the current workforce had not (at the time of our interview) been employed for more than two years. (Author interview.) Moreover, many workers appear to be leaving jobs at the NRIE more quickly since the 1993–4 deaths. Local NGOs working on NRIE health issues are concerned that many workers will only become ill after leaving their jobs at the estate and will not be diagnosed as suffering from the effects of workplace chemical exposures. (Author interview, NGO worker.)

11 It is particularly noteworthy that the challenges of building international solidarity include, in some cases, abandonment of precisely the kinds of tools which might facilitate effective localized resistance – e.g. the use of a local language or dialect by workers to forge solidarity against employers who are foreign or who do not speak the same dialect.

References

Alpha Research (1997) *Pocket Thailand Public Health 1997*, Bangkok: Alpha Research.

Bell, P. F. (1992) "Gender and economic development in Thailand," in P. and J. Van Esterik (eds) *Gender and Development in Southeast Asia (Proceedings* of the Twentieth Meetings of the Canadian Council for Southeast Asian Studies, York University, October 18–20, 1991)*, Montreal: Canadian Council for Southeast Asian Studies: 61–81.

—— (1996) "Development or maldevelopment? The contradictions of Thailand's economic growth," in M. J. G. Parnwell (ed.) *Uneven Development in Thailand*, Aldershot: Avebury: 49–62.

Braun, B. (1998) "A politics of possibility without the possibility of politics? Thoughts on Harvey's troubles with difference," *Annals of the Association of American Geographers* 88, 4: 712–19.

Brown, A. and Frenkel, S. (1993) "Union unevenness and insecurity in Thailand," in S. Frenkel (ed.) *Organized Labor in the Asia-Pacific Region: A Comparative Study of Trade Unionism in Nine Countries*, Ithaca, NY: ILR Press: 82–106.

Brown, C. (1981) "Mothers, fathers, and children: from private to public patriarchy," in L. Sargent (ed.) *Women and Revolution: A Discussion of the Unhappy Marriage of Marxism and Feminism*, Boston: South End Press: 239–67.

Bundit, T. (1998) *Trade Union Structure and Tripartite Systems in Thailand*, Bangkok: Arom Pongpangan Foundation and Friederich Ebert Stiftung.

Center for the Improvement of Working Conditions and the Environment, Thailand (various years) *Statistics on Workplace Injuries and Fatalities*, Bangkok: Department of Labor and Social Welfare.

Corbridge, S. (1998) "Reading David Harvey: entries, voices, loyalties," *Antipode* 30, 1: 43–55.

Cravey, A. J. (1998) *Women and Work in Mexico's Maquiladoras*, Lanham, MD, Boulder, CO, New York, and Oxford: Rowman & Littlefield.

Darunee, T. and Shashi, R. (1989) "Dutiful but overburdened: women in Thai society," *Asian Review* 3: 41–53.

Department of Labor and Social Welfare of Thailand (DLSW) (1996) *Statistics on Workplace Hazards, 1988–1995*, Bangkok: Department of Labor and Social Welfare.

—— (various years) *Yearbook of Labor Statistics (YLS)*, Bangkok: Department of Labor and Social Welfare.

Dixon, C. J. and Parnwell, M. J. G. (1991) "Thailand: the legacy of non-colonial development in South-East Asia," in C. J. Dixon and M. J. Heffernan (eds) *Colonialism and Development in the Contemporary World*, London: Mansell: 204–25.

Elson, D. and Pearson, R. (1981a) "Nimble fingers make cheap workers: an analysis of women's employment in Third World export manufacturing," *Feminist Review* 8: 87–107.

—— (1981b) "The subordination of women and the internationalisation of factory production," in K. Young, C. Wolkowitz, and R. McCullagh (eds) *Of Marriage and the Market: Women's Subordination in International Perspective*, London: CSE: 144–66.

Forsyth, T. (1994) "Shut up or shut down: how a Thai medical agency was closed after it questioned worker safety at a factory owned by Thailand's largest employer," *Asia Inc.* April: 30–7.

—— (1997) "Industrial pollution and government policy in Thailand: rhetoric versus reality," in P. Hirsch (ed.) *Seeing Forests for the Trees: Environment and Environmentalism in Thailand*, Chiang Mai: Silkworm Books: 30–7.

Frenkel, S. (1993) "Variations in patterns of trade unionism: a synthesis," in

S. Frenkel (ed.) *Organized Labor in the Asia-Pacific Region: A Comparative Study of Trade Unionism in Nine Countries*, Ithaca, NY: ILR Press: 309–46.

Glassman, J. (1999) "Thailand at the margins: state power, uneven development, and industrial transformation," unpublished PhD thesis, University of Minnesota.

Gray, J. (1990) "The road to the city: young women and transition in Northern Thailand," unpublished PhD thesis, Macquarie University.

Greider, W. (1997) *One World, Ready or Not: The Manic Logic of Global Capitalism*, New York: Simon & Schuster.

Hartmann, H. (1981) "The unhappy marriage of Marxism and feminism: towards a more progressive union," in L. Sargent (ed.) *Women and Revolution: A Discussion of the Unhappy Marriage of Marxism and Feminism*, Boston: South End Press: 1–41.

Hartsock, N. C. M. (1998) "Moments, margins, and agency," *Annals of the Association of American Geographers* 88, 4: 707–12.

Harvey, D. (1996) *Justice, Nature, and the Geography of Difference*, Cambridge, MA, and Oxford: Blackwell.

—— (1998) "The Humboldt connection," *Annals of the Association of American Geographers* 88, 4: 723–30.

Hewison, K. and Brown, A. (1994) "Labour and unions in an industrialising Thailand," *Journal of Contemporary Asia* 24, 4: 483–514.

International Labor Organization of the United Nations (ILO) (various years) *Yearbook of Labor Statistics*, Geneva: United Nations.

Ji, G. U. (1998) *Thailand: Class Struggle in an Era of Economic Crisis*, Hong Kong and Bangkok: Asia Monitor Resources Center and Workers' Democracy Book Club.

Jomo, K. S. (1997) *Southeast Asia's Misunderstood Miracle: Industrial Policy and Economic Development in Thailand, Malaysia, and Indonesia*, Boulder, CO: Westview Press.

Lim, L. L. (1993) "The feminization of labor in the Asia-Pacific rim countries: from contributions to economic dynamism to bearing the brunt of structural adjustments," in N. Ogawa, G. W. Jones, and J. G. Williamson (eds) *Human Resources in Development Along the Asia-Pacific Rim*, Singapore: Oxford University Press: 175–209.

Mabry, B. D. (1979) *The Development of Labor Institutions in Thailand*, Ithaca, NY: Cornell University Press.

Medhi K. (1996) "Thailand: poverty assessment update," Bangkok: Economic Research and Training Center, Faculty of Economics, Thammasat University.

Mills, M. B. (1999a) "Enacting solidarity: unions and migrant youth in Thailand," *Critique of Anthropology* 19, 2: 175–92.

—— (1999b) *Thai Women in the Global Labor Force: Consuming Desires, Contested Selves*, New Brunswick and London: Rutgers University Press.

Mingsarn, S. K., Felt, E. O., Azumi, E. Y., Pednekar, S. S., Wijukprasert, P., and Kaewmesri, T. (1995) "Women in development: enhancing the status of rural women in Northern Thailand," Bangkok: Thailand Development Research Institute.

Ministry of Public Health of Thailand (various years) *Public Health Statistics*, Bangkok: Ministry of Public Health.

Moody, K. (1997) *Workers in a Lean World: Unions in the International Economy*, London and New York: Verso.

Muscat, R. J. (1990) *Thailand and the United States: Development, Security, and Foreign Aid*, New York: Columbia University Press.

—— (1994) *The Fifth Tiger: A Study of Thai Development Policy*, Helsinki: United Nations University Press, M. E. Sharpe.

Nash, J. and Fernandez-Kelly, M. P. (eds) (1983) *Men, Women, and the International Division of Labor*, Albany, NY: SUNY Press.

National Statistics Office of Thailand (NSO) (various years) *Industrial Survey*, Bangkok: National Statistics Office.

—— (various years) *Labor Force Survey (LFS)*, Bangkok: National Statistics Office.

Ong, A. (1987) *Spirits of Resistance and Capitalist Discipline: Factory Women in Malaysia*, Albany, NY: SUNY Press.

ORSTOM (French Scientific Research Institute for Development by Cooperation) (1997) Unpublished data from Northern industry survey.

Parnwell, M. J. G. and Arghiros, D. A. (1996) "Introduction: uneven development in Thailand," in M. J. G. Parnwell (ed.) *Uneven Development in Thailand*, Aldershot: Avebury: 1–27.

Pasuk, P. and Baker, C. (1995) *Thailand: Economy and Politics*, Oxford: Oxford University Press.

—— (1998) *Thailand's Boom and Bust*, Chiang Mai: Silkworm Books.

Pasuk, P., Piriyarangsan, S., and Treerat, N. (1996) *Challenging Social Exclusion: Rights and Livelihood in Thailand*, Geneva: International Labour Studies, United Nations Development Programme, Research Series 107.

Phillips, D. R. and Verhasselt, Y. (eds) (1994) *Health and Development*, London and New York: Routledge.

Porpora, D., Lim, M. H., and Prommas, U. (1989) "The role of women in the international division of labor: the case of Thailand," *Development and Change* 20: 269–94.

Potter, S. H. (1977) *Family Life in a Northern Thai Village: A Study in the Structural Significance of Women*, Berkeley: University of California Press.

Reid, A. (1988) "Female roles in pre-colonial Southeast Asia," *Modern Asian Studies* 22, 3: 629–45.

Rowbotham, S. and Mitter, S. (eds) (1994) *Dignity and Daily Bread: New Forms of Economic Organizing Among Poor Women in the Third World and the First*, London and New York: Routledge.

Standing, G. (1989) "Global feminization through flexible labor," *World Development* 17, 7: 1077–95.

Sungsidh, P. (1989) "The foundation of a workers strategic group," unpublished PhD thesis, Beilefeld University.

Sungsidh, P. and Kanchada, P. (1994) "Labour institutions in an export-oriented country," in G. Rodgers (ed.) *Workers, Institutions and Economic Growth in Asia*, Geneva: International Labor Organization: 211–53.

Theobald, S. (1995) "Pressure points in industrial development: a gender analysis framework of the various stakeholders in the Northern Regional Industrial Estate, Thailand," unpublished MA thesis, University of East Anglia.

Tiano, S. (1994) *Patriarchy on the Line: Labor, Gender, and Ideology in the Mexican Maquila Industry*, Philadelphia, PA: Temple University Press.

Varunee, P. and Benja, J. (1994) "Women's industrial work conditions and the changing of family relations," report submitted to the Hitachi Scholarship Foundation (March).

Voravidh, C. (1996) "A study of contract labour in the textile and garment sector in Thailand," unpublished manuscript, Faculty of Economics, Chulalongkorn University.

—— (1998) "The situation of health and safety in Thailand," unpublished manuscript, Faculty of Economics, Chulalongkorn University.

Walby, S. (1990) *Theorizing Patriarchy*, Oxford and Cambridge, MA: Blackwell.

Wehmhörner, A. (1983) "Trade unionism in Thailand – a new dimension in a modernising society," *Journal of Contemporary Asia* 13, 4: 481–97.

Young, I. M. (1998) "Harvey's complaint with race and gender struggles," *Antipode* 30, 1: 36–42.

5   Looking back, looking around, looking forward

A woman's right to choose

Patricia Gober and Mark W. Rosenberg

Introduction

The right of North American women to choose abortion as a reproductive option was dealt a grave blow on October 23, 1998 when Dr Barnett Slepian, an obstetrician/gynecologist from Buffalo, New York became the seventh casualty of anti-abortion violence since 1993. Slepian, long a target of anti-abortion protestors, was shot by a sniper through the kitchen window of his home. The shooting followed a warning by a Canadian-American task force investigating four earlier attacks in the border region on three Canadian doctors and one American doctor from Rochester, New York (Berger 1998).

We begin our discussion of abortion rights and abortion access in North America with an account of Dr Slepian's murder because it illustrates three points about the current situation in the United States and Canada. First, the right to choose abortion as a reproductive option has evoked an especially strident form of dissent which, in turn, has spawned extreme violence of the sort that claimed Slepian's life. This militant anti-abortion violence now transcends international borders. Second, Slepian's death symbolizes an expansion of the venues in the battle over abortion rights – from the courts, to the streets, and now to the homes of doctors, nurses, and other abortion clinic personnel. And third, Slepian's death underscores the growing inaccessibility of abortion services as the number of providers steadily declines. Slepian, unlike the vast majority of his colleagues in obstetrics and gynecology who choose not to perform abortions, provided the full range of obstetric and gynecological services in his private practice in suburban Buffalo and in his other work serving poor women in downtown Buffalo. In environments already short of abortion services, the loss of even one doctor can seriously jeopardize the viability of local abortion services.

Amidst this highly charged, and sometimes violent, political environment, abortion remains an important means of controlling unwanted pregnancies in the US and Canada, as in the rest of the world (Bankole *et al.* 1998; Rahman *et al.* 1998). In the US more than 50 percent of pregnancies are unintended (either unwanted or mistimed), and one-half of these are terminated by abortion (Harlap *et al.* 1991). Each year, 3 percent of women aged

15 to 44 have an abortion, and at current rates, an estimated 43 percent of women will have at least one abortion by the time they are 45 years old (Alan Guttmacher Institute 1998). In Canada, there are more than 28 abortions for every 100 live births (Statistics Canada 1997). In both countries, abortion transcends age, race and ethnicity, social class, and region.

In the remainder of this chapter, we will revisit the research of Gober (1994, 1997) and Rosenberg (1988) and others who have written about the historic struggle of North American women to gain access to abortion services and how the geography of access has changed over time (i.e. *looking back*). *Looking around*, we will examine the current geography of access to abortion services, emphasizing the roles that state and provincial governments play either by supporting women's rights to choose (e.g. paying for abortions under provincial health insurance plans and state medical programs) or by restricting access through various new legal strategies (e.g. parental consent laws, waiting periods, and notification and counseling requirements). Also in this part of the chapter, we will explore the role of violence and intimidation in restricting access to abortion services and the unwillingness of many in the medical profession to perform abortion despite its legality and widespread popular acceptance. Only 12 percent of the population in both Canada and the US hold the hardcore position that abortion should be outlawed under all circumstances (Muldoon 1991). In the final part of the chapter, *looking forward*, we will argue that North American women's ability to exercise their legal rights to have an abortion increasingly will depend upon where they live and that the only acceptable alternative to the current geography of inequality and fear is a geography of access and choice.

Looking back

The current struggles over abortion rights and access in Canada and the United States grow out of similar, but not identical, histories of abortion reform (Meyer and Staggenborg 1998). In 1973 the US Supreme Court outlawed state restrictions on abortion through the second trimester. Fifteen years later in 1988, the Canadian Supreme Court struck down a 1969 federal law making abortions a criminal offense unless they were carried out in a hospital after approval by a therapeutic abortion committee consisting of three doctors. In both countries, pro-choice groups used the language of women's rights and individual rights to support greater access to abortion services, but different political systems, cultural values, and legal systems nuanced the debate about abortion rights and the history of access to abortion services.

United States

Abortion was a legal and commonplace method to regulate the number and spacing of children in both rural and urban America until around 1860 when state legislatures, coaxed by the fledgling medical establishment, began to outlaw abortion (Gober 1994). The newly formed American Medical Association and its member physicians sought to eliminate competition from so-called "irregulars" such as midwives, herbal healers, apothecaries, and homeopaths for patients and patients' fees by seeking to outlaw the procedure that kept them in business (Mohr 1978). The prohibition of abortion came under the same anti-obscenity or Comstock laws that prohibited the dissemination of birth control information and services. Mohr (1978) and Petchesky (1990) argue that the medical debate was driven, in part, by concerns that the heavy use of abortion by native-born Protestant women was depressing their fertility relative to immigrant Catholic women. In this view, abortion threatened the prevailing religious and ethnic make-up of the United States population.

Stringent anti-abortion laws remained in effect until the early 1970s when changing social attitudes about sexuality and a growing feminist movement led to the liberalization of some state abortion codes. In 1970, state legislatures in Alaska, Hawaii, Washington State, and New York lifted all restrictions on abortion. A second group of fourteen states liberalized their codes to allow abortion in cases of rape or incest and to protect the physical and mental health of the mother. Similar legislation was introduced in almost every state in the nation. State-to-state differences in abortion regulations gave rise to a thriving interstate business in abortions centered on New York State. In 1972, 44 percent of all abortions reported to the US Public Health Service were performed on out-of-state women (US Public Health Service 1972).

On January 22, 1973, the state-dominated landscape of abortion rights theoretically was eradicated with the US Supreme Court's landmark *Roe v. Wade* decision. The Court outlawed most state restrictions on abortion and ruled that a woman has a constitutional right, in consultation with her physician, to terminate a pregnancy free of state interference during the first trimester. During the second trimester (or before viability of the fetus), states could impose only those restrictions that were reasonably related to protecting women's health such as the quality of service and the qualifications of practitioners. States were banned from imposing arbitrary restrictions such as spousal or parental consent, waiting periods, or residency requirements. During the third trimester (after fetal viability), the Court acknowledged the state's "compelling" interest in "potential life" and allowed states to prohibit abortion altogether "except when it is necessary to preserve the life or health of the mother." Immediately after *Roe*, state abortion rates converged, the traffic in interstate abortions all but ceased, and public monies were widely used to pay for abortions for poor women.

Since 1980, an increasingly conservative Supreme Court has allowed states to restrict abortion so long as they do not place an "undue burden" on the fundamental right to have an abortion. States have responded by passing a plethora of anti-abortion legislation including parental consent and notification laws, mandatory waiting periods, state-directed counseling requirements, laws to outlaw insurance coverage of abortion, laws that ban so-called "partial-birth" abortion, and laws to prohibit abortion after viability. All but sixteen states have exercised their Supreme Court-mandated option of not using state funds to pay for abortions for Medicaid recipients. The Hyde Amendment, upheld by the Supreme Court in 1980, prohibits use of federal funds for reimbursing the cost of abortions for Medicaid recipients, except in cases of life endangerment, rape, or incest.

After *Roe*, the abortion ratio (the number of abortions per 100 births) rose dramatically, peaked during the 1980s, and declined somewhat during the 1990s (Figure 5.1). The absolute number of abortions followed a similar track, increasing from 745,000 in 1973 to 1.6 million in 1990, and then falling to 1.5 million in 1992 and 1.4 million in 1994 (US Department of Health and Human Services 1998). Explanations for the decline include a decreasing number of women of 18 through 29 years of age who are at the highest risk of abortion, less acceptance of abortion as a reproductive option, greater tolerance for unwed childbearing, and the growing inaccessibility of abortion services (Henshaw and Van Vort 1994). Matthews *et al.* (1997) estimated that decreased accessibility accounted for about one-quarter of the 5 percent decline in abortion rates between 1988 and 1992.

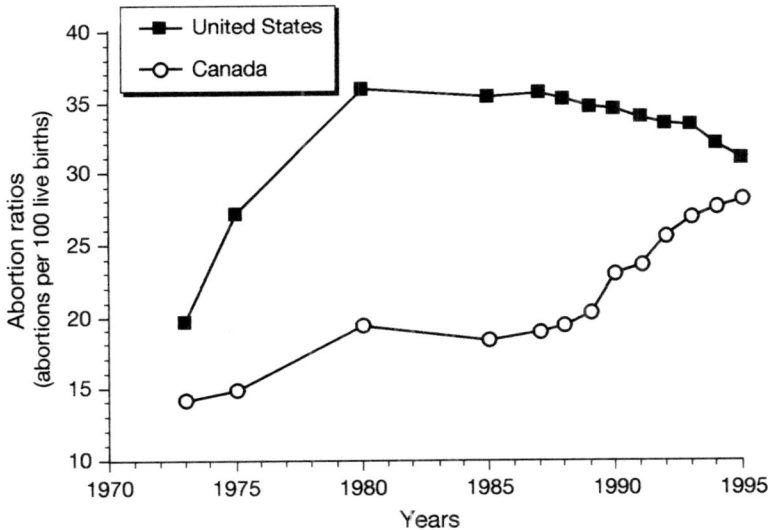

Figure 5.1 Abortion ratios (abortions per 100 live births) in the United States and Canada.

Sources: US Department of Health and Human Services (1998); Statistics Canada (1997).

Canada

Canada, as a colony of the British Empire until 1867, followed British law under which abortions carried out by a third party were made illegal in 1803. After 1861, under the Offenses Against the Person Act, it was also illegal for a woman to abort herself (McLaren 1981). By the beginning of the twentieth century many of the debates and attitudes which informed the discussion of abortion as a legal issue in the US had been imported to Canada. McLaren argues that "race suicide" and the belief that abortion was exacerbating the relative decline in birth rates of "English Canadians" in particular drove legal, moral, and medical authorities to condemn abortion as a health practice. "The concern for the 'slaughter of the innocents' at the turn of the century was sparked not so much by the fall of English Canadians' birth rate per se, but by its decline relative to that of the French Canadians and the immigrant population" (ibid.: 305).

In 1969 the federal Criminal Code of Canada was revised to allow abortions when performed in a hospital after approval by a therapeutic abortion committee consisting of three doctors. In their seminal study of abortion in Canada, the *Report of the Committee on the Operation of the Abortion Law* (1977), Badgley and his fellow committee members paint a picture of "sharp regional disparities" in accessibility because only about 20 percent of general hospitals had therapeutic abortion committees and an even smaller percentage actually carried out therapeutic abortions. Many of the physicians trained to do abortions refused to carry them out, and provincial governments and therapeutic abortion committees used varying criteria which acted as direct and indirect barriers to service (e.g. residency and patient quotas, parental and spousal consent). Badgley *et al.* (1977) also noted that a significant number of Canadian women sought abortion services in the US after the Criminal Code was revised in 1969. Using 1975 data, the committee estimated that between 15.9 percent and 17.3 percent of abortions performed on Canadian women were done in the United States and that between 45,930 and 50,106 Canadian women had abortions in the United States between 1970 and 1974 (ibid.: 80).

The same social forces, feminism and individual rights, that drove the liberalization of abortion laws in the US were also at work in Canada through the 1960s and 1970s, but reform took longer. In 1970 Dr Henry Morgentaler was charged with performing illegal abortions because he carried them out in his clinic, as an act of civil disobedience, instead of in a certified hospital with a therapeutic abortion committee (Weir 1994: 253). After three trials, where juries refused to convict Morgentaler, the Quebec government gave up its prosecution. While this established the principle of freestanding abortion clinics in Quebec, it did not invalidate the federal Criminal Code law. After a series of trials in Ontario beginning in 1982, the Supreme Court of Canada ruled in *Morgentaler, Smoling and Scott v. The Queen* that the abortion provision of the Criminal Code was unconstitutional, but "did not impose an alternative abortion regime as its American counterpart had done in *Roe v. Wade*" (Herman 1994: 272). The Canadian Parliament was unable to draft new abortion legislation, and thus the decision to seek an abortion became a decision between a woman and her physician. Significantly, in striking down Section 251, the Supreme Court of Canada also acknowledged that it was no longer necessary for women to seek abortions within a hospital setting.

After *Morgantaler*, the abortion ratio per 100 live births in Canada climbed steadily from 18.9 per 100 live births in 1986 to 28.2 per 100 live births in 1995 – very similar to prevailing levels in the United States (Figure 5.1). In absolute numbers, this represented an increase to 106,658 abortions in 1995 compared with 70,023 in 1987. Between 1978 and 1989, abortions carried out in freestanding clinics only took place in Quebec. The rate during this period was relatively constant, growing from 0.7 abortions per 100 live births in 1978 to 1.8 abortions per 100 live births in 1989. After 1989, in response to the *Morgentaler* Supreme Court decision, an increasing number of provinces began to allow freestanding abortion clinics, and the rate of abortions performed in these clinics increased to 9.4 per 100 live births. In the eighteen years from 1977 to 1995, this meant a shift from no abortions being carried out outside hospitals to about one-third being performed in clinics (Figure 5.2).

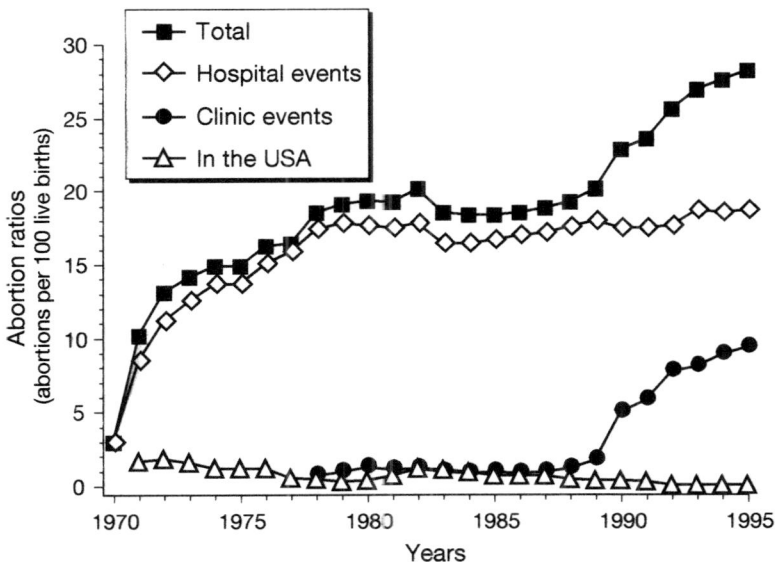

Figure 5.2 Annual therapeutic abortions to Canadian residents by location.
Source: Statistics Canada (1997).

This brief look back shows remarkable similarities and subtle differences in the struggle for abortion rights in the United States and Canada. In both countries, early abortion debates were framed by nativist concerns over fertility differentials between immigrants and English-speaking Protestant women and by efforts of formally trained physicians to restrict competition from midwives and other non-licensed healers. *Roe* in 1973 and *Morgentaler* in 1988 marked the end of highly restrictive periods, and these rulings established the universal right to abortion. This right proved to be illusory and short-lived, however, as well-defined geographies of abortion rights and abortion access evolved, due in the United States to a patchwork of state restrictions on abortion rights, and in both countries, to the lack of clinics and hospitals in some states and provinces, to the reluctance of states and provinces to pay for abortions under certain circumstances, to the medical community's reluctance to perform abortions, to its willingness to isolate abortion from other aspects of reproductive health services, and to an emerging geography of fear and violence.

Looking around

In *looking around*, we see growing tension in abortion rights – tension between national and state or provincial interests in abortion rights, tension between the rights of doctors and other health care professionals to refuse to perform abortions and the rights of women to have them, and tension between the free-speech rights of abortion activists and the rights of women and their doctors to be free from harassment and intimidation at abortion clinics and at their homes. Although these tensions have not altered the fundamental right to an abortion as established by *Roe* and *Morgantaler*, they seriously compromise the access to abortion rights for millions of North American women. Differential access to abortion services creates a highly variegated landscape in which women in some places can exercise their legal right to abortion while women in other places cannot.

United States

In the case of *Planned Parenthood of Southeastern Pennsylvania v. Casey* in 1992, the Supreme Court, while upholding a woman's constitutional right to abortion before fetal viability, allowed state restrictions on abortion so long as they do not impose an "undue burden" on women seeking abortions. "Undue burden" is defined as one that has "the purpose or effect of placing a substantial obstacle in the path of a woman seeking an abortion of a nonviable fetus." *Casey* allows states to impose a 24-hour waiting period and parental consent so long as it is accompanied by a judicial bypass which enables a young woman to demonstrate to a judge that she is mature enough to make the decision on her own. In years subsequent to *Casey*, states have designed ever-more imaginative ways to make abortions more difficult to obtain while adhering to the letter, if not the spirit, of the "undue burden" standard. During the 1998 legislative session, 305 anti-choice bills were introduced in forty states, and 46 of them were enacted in twenty-two states (NARAL 1998). Thirty states currently enforce parental consent or notification laws for minors seeking an abortion, fourteen states require waiting periods of between 8 and 72 hours, and only sixteen states continue to pay for abortions for poor women. A poor woman living in New York State can obtain an immediate, publicly funded abortion without parental consent while her counterpart in North Dakota must pay $200 to $400 for an abortion, obtain her parent's consent, make an initial appointment, and then return three days later for the procedure itself.

There is increasing concern about the interaction effects of state restrictions and the Supreme Court's interpretation of the "undue burden" standard one statute at a time. In states where restrictions on public funding coexist with waiting periods, for example, a poor woman may experience two delays, one in waiting until she can accumulate the necessary funds to make an appointment, and another in adhering to the state's waiting period. A state-mandated delay of one day can translate into an actual delay of one week or more if, as in many non-metropolitan parts of the nation, abortions are performed only once a week or an appointment is not available on the next possible date. The addition of a parental consent requirement imposes yet a third potential delay – that of obtaining parental consent or getting permission from a judge through a bypass procedure. Matthews *et al.* (1997: 59) argue that the "undue burden" standard should be broadened to include the "constellation of restrictions and factors affecting abortion access within states."

Superimposed on the whole issue of legal access is the growing vulnerability of abortion as a medical service. One aspect of this vulnerability problem is the shift in abortion services away from hospitals into specialized abortion clinics – a trend very similar to what has occurred in Canada. In 1972, 81 percent of all US abortion providers were hospital-based; just twenty years later in 1992, this figure was only 36 percent (Henshaw and Van Vort 1990, 1994). In 1992, 93 percent of abortions took place in non-hospital settings (Henshaw 1995). What has emerged is a national network in which a few specialized providers handle the vast majority of abortions in large metropolitan areas. Largely withdrawn from the scene are community-based hospitals that potentially could provide abortion services nearer to home. Especially compromised by the present system are poor women who rely on hospital emergency rooms for routine medical care and women in non-metropolitan areas where providers are scarce.

Women's access to abortion services is also threatened by a severe shortage of doctors who are willing to perform abortions. Carole Joffe (1995) argues that the medical establishment has a longstanding antipathy toward abortion. In *looking back*, we noted that physicians were in the forefront of the nineteenth-century effort to criminalize abortion. While a small number of physicians, such as Barnett Slepian, emerged from the pre-*Roe* era of botched, back-street abortions fiercely committed to performing safe and legal abortions – Joffe calls them "doctors of conscience" – the vast majority feared reprisals from unsympathetic colleagues and prosecution from hostile district attorneys. They came to view abortion as something to be avoided to the extent possible. More recently, abortion has come to be perceived as a dull and repetitive procedure in a profession enthralled by advances in molecular biology and endocrinology. This fact, in conjunction with threats to physician safety from anti-abortion violence, has led many young doctors to shy away from the practice of abortion. In addition, medical residency programs are withdrawing from training young doctors in the practice of abortion. The proportion of programs providing routine training in first-trimester abortion decreased from 23 percent in 1985 to 12 percent in 1991, and the proportion providing routine training in second-trimester abortion fell from 21 to 7 percent (MacKay and MacKay 1995).

Added to and interacting with the aforementioned environment of increased state restrictions on abortion access and drastically declining medical access is an evolving climate of fear, intimidation, and violence associated with abortion in the US. Violence against abortion providers (bombings, arson, vandalism, and death threats) and disruption at clinics (hate mail, harassing phone calls, bomb threats, and picketing) escalated rapidly during the early 1990s (Figure 5.3). Frustrated by the Supreme Court's refusal to overturn *Roe* in its 1992 *Casey* decision, the anti-abortion movement moved its battle over abortion from the courts to the streets. Intensified rhetoric emboldened more militant elements operating at the margins of the anti-abortion movement. On March 10, 1993, Dr David Gunn, a physician who performed abortions at the Pensacola Women's Health Clinic was shot and killed at an anti-abortion protest at his office. In August of that year, Dr George Tiller was shot in both arms during a similar protest in Wichita, Kansas. Shocked by these incidents, Congress passed the Freedom of Access to Clinic Entrance Act (FACE) in May, 1994, making it a federal offense to physically obstruct the entrance of an abortion clinic or to use force, threats, or tactics intended to intimidate women seeking an abortion. FACE carries stiff penalties – up to a $100,000 fine and one year in prison – for a first offense. With the passage of FACE, violence and disruption at clinics abated somewhat in 1994 and 1995 but picked up again in recent years, especially in the form of picketing (Figure 5.3). In 1995 there were 1,652 incidents of picketing at abortion clinics; in 1997 there were 7,827 such events.

To enforce the provisions of FACE, local authorities established so-called "buffer zones" to keep protestors at least 15 feet from the clinic and "bubble zones" to separate protestors from women seeking abortions and other individuals entering and leaving clinics. Protestors appealed the legality of these restrictions to the Supreme Court on the grounds that their freedom of speech was violated. In February, 1997, the Supreme Court upheld "buffer

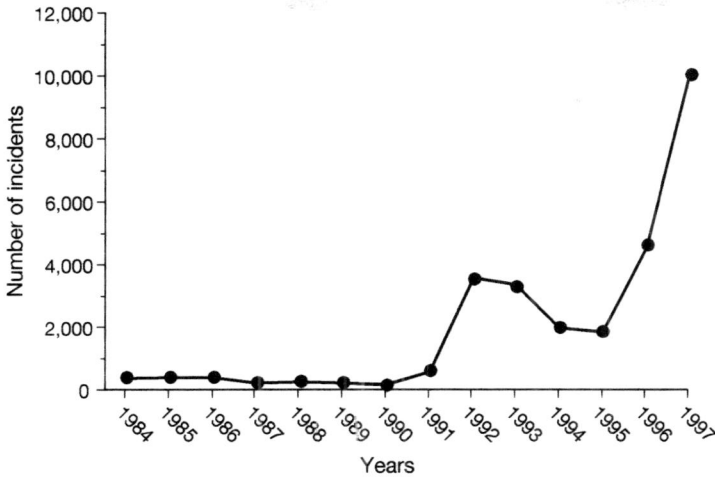

Figure 5.3 Incidents of violence and disruption at US abortion clinics.

Source: National Abortion Federation (1998).

zones" keeping protestors at least 15 feet from the clinic, ruling them necessary to protect access to services, but struck down "bubble zones" as not fixed in space and therefore difficult to maintain and enforce. With its fuzzy, middle-of-the-road position on access to clinics, the Supreme Court has allowed communities considerable latitude in how FACE provisions are enforced, thus reinforcing local differentials in abortion access.

Canada

There are many parallels between Canada and the US in the battle over abortion rights. The legal right to abortion remains intact, albeit in an environment of diminished access and a climate of escalating violence. But there are also important differences. These differences involve three societal characteristics that many would argue distinguish Canada from the US. First, support for the public, universal health insurance system under which all Canadians are guaranteed access to basic medical and hospital care is so widely supported by Canadians of all political stripes, it makes the debate over abortion, at least in part, a debate over access to the publicly funded health care system. Most Canadians are, therefore, reluctant to see any group denied access to health care services and most Canadian politicians are reluctant to be seen to be attacking the public health care system. Second, the governments of Canada, past and present, and Canadians in general have followed the British tradition in their attitudes towards violent crime and punishment, placing emphasis on strict gun control laws, the banning of capital punishment, and a general lack of sympathy towards those who

participate in violent protest activities. Third, most Canadians believe the
federal and provincial governments should play an important role in the their
lives. In the fifteenth annual *MacLean's Magazine* year end poll, when asked
the hypothetical question "if the economy were to stop growing and we
found ourselves in a recession, which of the following points of view best
reflects your idea of how the federal and provincial governments should
respond?", 37 percent of respondents said "governments should increase
spending to stimulate the economy in an effort to increase jobs"; 35 percent
said "governments should not try to create jobs, but instead spend more on
social programs and retraining programs"; and only 22 percent responded
"government can't make any difference anyway and should just let market
forces run their course." The remaining respondents either did not know or
refused to answer (*MacLean's Magazine* 1998). This is not to suggest there
are no Canadians who believe in private medicine and refusing public funds
for abortion services, who are against gun control laws, want capital punishment restored, and violently protest against abortions being carried out under
any circumstances, but to make clear that the social context in Canada is
different from that found in the US.

Anti-abortion forces have sought to block women's rights to abortions
through court cases based on fetal rights. In the first of two highly publicized
cases, *Borowski v. Attorney General of Canada*, Joe Borowski, a former
provincial politician and an anti-abortion activist, attempted to argue the
illegality of abortions based on the argument that a fetus is a human being
and therefore should be protected under Section 7 of the Canadian Charter
of Rights and Freedom. Having previously in 1988 ruled that Section 251
was unconstitutional, in 1989 the Supreme Court of Canada ruled that
Borowski had no case since there was no law (Dorczak 1991; McConnell
1989). In the second case, *Tremblay v. Daigle*, Jean-Guy Tremblay, the man
who had impregnated Chantal Daigle, applied and received lower court
injunctions prohibiting Ms Daigle from having an abortion. Tremblay's
lawyers argued that an abortion violated the rights of the fetus based on
common law, Quebec civil law, and the Charter of Rights and Freedom.
Again, the Supreme Court of Canada rejected outright the argument that
the fetus had status in common law or Quebec civil law and left the issue of
Charter Rights moot following their earlier logic in the *Borowski* case
(Shaffer 1994).

As in the United States, medical access in Canada is, for the most part,
restricted to large cities and provincial capitals. *Morgantaler* did not lead
to freestanding clinics opening their doors throughout Canada (Table 5.1).
Not all provincial governments welcomed the introduction of freestanding
clinics and used the administrative convenience of refusing to fund abortions carried out in clinics as a way of deterring women from choosing this
option. Moreover, what Table 5.1 does not show is that most hospitals carry
out very few abortions and only the largest hospitals in the major urban
centers of each province carry out the vast majority of abortions. The highly

Table 5.1 Hospital and freestanding abortion clinics in Canada, 1998

Province/ territory	Number of hospitals[a]	Number of freestanding clinics	Funding conditions of freestanding clinics	Locations of freestanding clinics
Newfoundland	1	1	Fully funded	St John's
Prince Edward I.	0	0		
Nova Scotia	5	1	$300 to $500 fees	Halifax
New Brunswick	2	1	$450 fee	Fredericton
Quebec[b]	30	5	Partially funded, some fees	Hull, Montreal, Sherbrooke
Ontario	76	6	Fully funded	Ottawa, Toronto
Manitoba	1	1	Fees up to $550	Winnipeg
Saskatchewan	2	0		
Alberta	3	2	Fully funded	Calgary, Edmonton
British Columbia	36	2	Fully funded	Vancouver
Northwest Terr.	3	0		
Yukon Terr.	1	0		

Sources: Canadian Abortion Rights Action League (1999); Sarick (1998).

Notes
a Abortions in hospitals are fully funded under provincial/territorial public health plans.
b In Quebec, there are also fourteen community health centres which are part of the provincial health care system and provide abortion services.

concentrated geographic pattern of abortion services is much the same as reported by Badgley *et al.* (1977) and Rosenberg (1988). Moreover, it contributes to wide provincial differences in the incidence of abortion. The therapeutic abortion rate as measured by the number of hospital-based therapeutic abortions per 1,000 females aged 15 to 44 years is 10.3 for Canada as a whole, but ranges from a low of 0.3 in Prince Edward Island to a high of 16.7 in the Northwest Territories. When measured as a rate per 100 live births, the therapeutic abortion rate for the country is 18.7 with Prince Edward Island again with the lowest rate of 0.5 and the Yukon having the highest rate at 27.2 (Statistics Canada 1997).

The failure of anti-abortion groups to block abortion services through either the courts or the legislatures of Canada has led them to both splinter and adopt more extremist tactics (Herman 1994). In the early 1980s, the abortion groups focused their tactics mainly on the freestanding abortion clinics in Toronto and Vancouver. The Morgentaler Clinic in Toronto, in particular, became a site of confrontation between anti-abortionists and pro-choice groups on a daily basis. In the initial stages of the confrontation, the anti-abortion groups "picketed en masse, organised marches and rallies, accosted women entering for appointments," and established an anti-abortion counseling agency next door to the abortion clinic (ibid.: 271–2). The anti-abortion groups then added to their harassment tactics following women in and out of the clinic and picketing homes of doctors, nurses, and counselors employed at the clinic. While the picketing and rallies in front of the Morgentaler Clinic frustrated others living in the neighborhood, the harassment of women, doctors, nurses, and counselors offended the wider public's "standards of decency and compassion" (ibid.: 272).

In 1985, the Toronto Women's Bookstore located underneath the Morgentaler Clinic was firebombed. This was followed in 1992 by the bombing of the clinic itself. Since then, two doctors in British Columbia, one doctor in Winnipeg, and one doctor in Hamilton have been shot and wounded by an unknown sniper(s) because they provide abortion services, the latest victim in this pattern of violence being Dr Slepian in Buffalo (*Globe and Mail*, 1998: A4).

The anti-abortionists have created a geography of fear and violence in their efforts to stop women's right to choose. What began as a highly localized geography of harassment and intimidation focused on the clinics, became a wider geography of fear linked to the homes of women, doctors, nurses, and counselors. Then it became a nationwide geography of fear and violence as the Morgentaler Clinic was burned and bombed and doctors were wounded in various parts of Canada. Now it has become a trans-border geography of fear and violence as police in Canada and the US believe that the same person(s) may be responsible for the shootings in Canada and the death of Dr Slepian in Buffalo.

Far more difficult to assess are the effects of violence on the incidence of abortion and public attitudes toward abortion. At the very least, however, violence has transformed the physical layout of abortion clinics and the public's perception of them. North American abortion clinics today are akin to fortresses. Security cameras and armed guards cover the entrances screened by metal detectors. To enter a typical abortion clinic, one must ring a bell and speak into an intercom to verify name, appointment time, and reasons for visit. The receptionist inside electronically unlocks the door so that the person may enter. The receptionists themselves are encased in bulletproof glass, as is the remainder of the waiting room (Crane 1998). These measures, although necessary to protect clinic personnel from violence, recast the public's image of abortion clinics from private and supportive places where routine medical procedures are performed into public places where privacy and confidentiality cannot be maintained, and more importantly, where personal safety cannot be guaranteed.

Looking forward

Despite the differences in their legal environments and social contexts, Canada and the United States have profound similarities in why and where women will seek abortion services and who will obtain those services. The why relates to deeper issues of women's role in society and their aspirations for fuller, deeper, richer, and more meaningful lives. When asked why they have an abortion, women give three main reasons. Three-quarters say that having a baby would interfere with work, school, or other responsibilities; two-thirds indicate that they cannot afford a child; and one-half state that they do not want to be a single parent or are having problems with their spouse or partner (Torres and Forrest 1988). These reasons go to the heart of women's changing societal role away from dependent wife, mother, and homemaker to one with greater sexual freedom and economic and personal independence (Gelb and Palley 1987; Holcomb *et al.* 1990). The economic and social advances of North American women have not been accompanied by drastic reductions in contraceptive failure rates, however, and thus the need for eliminating unwanted pregnancies remains stubbornly high. The number of abortions per 100 births hovers at around 30 in both the United States and Canada (Figure 5.1).

Women's ability to exercise their legal rights to have an abortion increasingly will depend on where they live. In the US, states will continue to place additional legal restrictions on abortion, and in Canada, provinces will continue to fund abortions selectively at freestanding clinics. In both countries, the harassment of abortion patients and medical staff will continue, marginal areas will lose services, and abortion will become even more concentrated in large metropolitan areas. Even in the largest metropolitan areas, however, whether women, doctors, nurses, counselors, and the clinics can be protected from violence remains an open question. Even though the murder of Dr Slepian has been condemned by anti-abortion groups, the activists in the anti-abortion movement are likely to continue to target vulnerable women and their health care providers.

The importance of political and legal challenges over abortion and concerns over violence at abortion clinics pale in comparison with the growing shortage of doctors willing to carry out abortions. Provision in many areas is on the borderline now. For example, a clinic in Duluth, Minnesota, which serves women in forty-two counties in Michigan, Wisconsin, and Minnesota, relies on the services of a 78-year-old doctor who flies in every week. There are no abortions carried out in Prince Edward Island, and the only freestanding clinic in New Brunswick has to fly in a doctor from another province to carry out abortions (Makin 1998: D3). Continuation of the status quo will lead to further concentration of abortion services in the largest metropolitan areas of the largest and most cosmopolitan states and provinces and in the hands of an ever-shrinking number of doctors.

Class differences in abortion access will grow. We are returning to the double standard of pre-*Roe* and pre-*Morgentaler* days when women with status, connections, and money could get special permission for legal abortions in hospitals while working-class and poor women either did without or sought abortions in less-than-sanitary conditions from unskilled practitioners. In the US, abortions will become less affordable in those thirty-four states that do not fund abortions for poor women, especially when funding bans are combined with parental consent laws and waiting periods. In Canada, the lack of abortion services outside the largest metropolitan areas and the lack of provincial insurance coverage in some freestanding clinics generate a set of costs among those women who are least likely to have the means to cover them. Abortion is becoming more of an economic good available for those who can afford it rather than a constitutional right assured to all who wish to exercise it.

Intimidation of women seeking advice and services and of doctors and health care workers willing to provide advice and services has escalated into a geography of fear and violence which is no longer isolated and random. The murder of Dr Barnett Slepian following the shooting of four other doctors across Canada has turned anti-abortionist violence into a systematic and trans-border geography. This geography, in conjunction with the geography of diminished medical access, means that many North American women face daunting obstacles in attempting to exercise their constitutional right to have an abortion. Although the right to abortion is theoretically the law of the land in both the United States and Canada, the practice of abortion varies greatly from place to place. The only way out of this untenable and hypocritical situation is to ensure that legal abortion services are widespread in every part of the US and Canada and thoroughly integrated into the practice of reproductive medicine. Only then will a geography of access and choice replace the current geography of inequality and fear.

Acknowledgments

Research on the Canadian content of this chapter carried out by M. W. Rosenberg was supported by a grant from the Social Sciences and Humanities Research Council of Canada (Grant No. 410–98–0658). All opinions expressed are those of the authors and do not in any way represent the views of the Government of Canada.

References

Alan Guttmacher Institute (1998) http://www.agi.org.
Badgley, R. F., Caron, D. F., and Powell, M. G. (1977) *Report of the Committee on the Operation of the Abortion Law*, Ottawa: Minister of Supply and Services Canada.
Bankole, A., Singh, S., and Haas, T. (1998) "Reasons why women have induced abortions: evidence from 27 countries," *International Family Planning Perspectives* 24, 3: 117–27.
Berger, J. (1998) "His beliefs pushed doctor to keep role at abortion clinic," *New York Times*, October 26: 1, 23.
Canadian Abortion Rights Action League (CARAL) (1999) "Canadian abortion clinics," http://www.caral.ca/clinics.htm.

Crane, C. (1998) "Therapeutic landscapes: a case study of feminist health care," unpublished MA thesis, Department of Geography, University of Washington.

Dorczak, A. (1991) "Unborn child abuse: contemplating legal solution," *Canadian Journal of Family Law* 9, 2: 133–56.

Gelb, J. and Palley, M. L. (1987) *Women and Public Policies*, Princeton, NJ: Princeton University Press.

Globe and Mail (1998) "Abortion doctor all too aware of job's dangers," *Globe and Mail*, October 26: A4.

Gober, P. (1994) "Why abortion rates vary: a geographical examination of the supply of and demand for abortion services in the United States in 1988," *Annals of the Association of American Geographers* 84, 2: 230–50.

—— (1997) "The role of access in explaining state abortion rates," *Social Science and Medicine* 44, 7: 1003–16.

Harlap, S., Kost, K., and Forrest, J. D. (1991) *Preventing Pregnancy, Protecting Health: A New Look at Birth Control in the United States*, New York: The Alan Guttmacher Institute.

Henshaw, S. K (1995) "Factors hindering access to abortion services," *Family Planning Perspectives* 27: 54–9, 87.

Henshaw, S. K. and Van Vort, J. (1990) "Abortion services in the United States, 1984 and 1985," *Family Planning Perspectives* 22: 102–8, 142.

—— (1994) "Abortion services in the United States, 1991 and 1992," *Family Planning Perspectives* 26: 100–6, 112.

Herman, D. (1994) "The Christian Right and the politics of morality in Canada," *Parliamentary Affairs* 47, 1: 268–79.

Holcomb, H., Kodras, J., and Brunn, S. (1990) "Women's issues and state legislation: fragmentation and inconsistency," in J. E. Kodras and J. P. Jones III (eds) *Geographical Dimensions of United States Social Policy*, New York: Edward Arnold: 178–99.

Joffe, C. (1995) *Doctors of Conscience*, Boston: Beacon Press.

McConnell, M. L. (1989) "Even by commonsense: Morgentaler, Borowski and the Constitution of Canada," *The Canadian Bar Review* 68: 765–96.

MacKay, H. T. and MacKay, A. P. (1995) "Abortion training in obstetrics and gynecology residency programs in the United States, 1991–1992," *Family Planning Perspectives* 27: 112–17.

McLaren, A. (1981) "Birth control and abortion in Canada, 1870–1920," in S.E.D. Shortt (ed.) *Medicine in Canadian Society: Historical Perspectives*, Montreal: McGill-Queen's University Press: 285–313.

MacLean's Magazine (1998) "The National Magazine/Maclean's Poll," *MacLean's Magazine* 111, 52 (December 28, 1998/January 4, 1999).

Makin, K. (1998) "Abortion battle rages on," *Globe and Mail* January 24: D1, D3.

Matthews, S., Ribar, D., and Wilhelm, M. (1997) "The effects of economic conditions and access to reproductive health services on state abortion rates and birthrates," *Family Planning Perspectives* 29: 52–60.

Meyer, D. S. and Staggenborg, S. (1998) "Countermovement dynamics in federal systems: a comparison of abortion politics in Canada and the United States," *Research in Political Sociology* 8: 209–40.

Mohr, J. C. (1978) *Abortion in America: The Origins and Evolution of National Policy, 1800–1900*, New York: Oxford University Press.

Muldoon, M. (1991) *The Abortion Debate in the United States and Canada: A Source Book*, New York: Garland.

National Abortion Federation (1998) "Incidents of violence and disruption against abortion providers, 1998," http://www.prochoice.org/violence/98vd.html.

National Abortion Rights Action League (NARAL) (1998) "Activity in state legislatures," http://www.naral.org/publications/facts/stateactivity.html.

Petchesky, R. P. (1990) *Abortion and Women's Choice: The State, Sexuality, and Reproductive Freedom*, Boston: Northeastern University Press.

Rahman, A., Katzive, L., and Henshaw, S. K. (1998) "A global review of laws on induced abortion, 1985–1997," *International Family Planning Perspectives* 24, 2: 56–64.

Rosenberg, M. W. (1988) "Linking the geographical, the medical and the political in analyzing health care delivery systems," *Social Science and Medicine* 26, 1: 179–86.

Sarick, L. (1998) "Women face varying rules on abortion," *Globe and Mail* January 29: A4.

Shaffer, M. (1994) "Foetal rights and the regulation of abortion," *McGill Law Journal* 39: 58–100.

Statistics Canada (1997) *Therapeutic Abortions, 1995*, Ottawa: Minister of Industry, Cat. No. 82–219–xpb.

Torres, A. and Forrest, J. D. (1988) "Why do women have abortions?", *Family Planning Perspectives* 20: 169–76.

US Department of Health and Human Services (1998) *Health, United States, 1998* PHS 98–1232, Hyattsville, MD: US Department of Health and Human Services, Centers for Disease Control and Prevention.

US Public Health Service (1972) *Abortion Surveillance*, Atlanta, GA: Centers for Disease Control.

Weir, L. (1994) "Left popular politics in Canadian feminist abortion organizing, 1982–1991," *Feminist Studies* 20, 2: 249–74.

Part II

Providing and gaining access to health care

Local areas and networks

6 Home care restructuring at work

The impact of policy transformation on women's labor

Allison Williams

Introduction

The policies of the welfare state actively shape gender relations by transforming working conditions and employment opportunities for women in the health care workforce. These policies frequently incorporate significant, though implicit, assumptions about gender roles. The ease or difficulty with which women can enter paid work, the way in which the unpaid work of caring for others is treated, and the regulation of marital and family relationships are all central arenas where gender relations are constituted, and these are influenced in significant ways by the nature and extent of state intervention (Orloff 1993).

For decades Canada's national health care system has provided full-time and relatively well-paid jobs for women, while offering essential support services that help alleviate the many contradictory demands on women – the burdens of the "double day." Women not only deliver health and welfare services but also are the chief consumers of these services, although the services they seek and receive are often on behalf of others, such as their aging parents. Cuts in state support for social and health programs, and the restructuring strategies used to achieve budgetary cuts, have critical effects on women's paid work in health care and women's unpaid work in the domestic sphere (McDowell and Pringle 1992). This chapter explores the impacts of funding cuts and restructuring in the Canadian health care system on women's paid work in the home health care sector, a sector dominated by women.

Given that the nature of welfare arrangements and restructuring strategies vary so much across space, a geographical perspective is essential to understanding the effects of restructuring on women health care workers (Pinch 1997). The geographical site selected for investigation is the northern region of Ontario – Canada's most populous province. Northern Ontario is a highly rural region, consisting of approximately 86 percent of the province's total land area but only 10 percent of its population, much of which is resident in small towns dominating the landscape (Beggs 1991). This region has been labelled "medically under serviced" as it has traditionally experienced a shortage of specialty health services and health care resources. Because all provincial home care programs evolved in the southern part of Ontario, and were thereby shaped for and by a well-serviced, densely populated region, the specific cultural and geographic needs of the northern region have yet to be addressed (Williams 1996).

Not-for-profit home care agencies are examined because such agencies have traditionally been funded mainly by public moneys and have, in many cases, operated much like a public service. Compared with their for-profit counterparts, not-for-profit agencies have traditionally provided higher rates of pay and better benefits, and they have a proven reputation for maintaining service standards and quality care. The three primary practitioner groups employed in home care are examined: registered nurses (RNs), registered practical nurses (RPNs), and home support workers (HSWs). The varying effects of restructuring on these occupational groups are assessed through an analysis of changes in the labor process and the consequent time–space relations of practitioners' work. The chapter begins with an overview of health care reform and women's work in the health care industry. I then consider the restructuring of home care in Ontario, highlighting the importance of place in providing a specific socio-political-historical context for restructuring. Next, the research methodology and results are presented, followed by a short discussion of the impacts – all of which are far reaching.

Health care reform: reshaping women's work

Health care reform is defined by the contemporary social, political, and economic milieu in which it is imbedded (Dear *et al.* 1979). Numerous factors – such as a dwindling economy, demographic changes due to a growing dependent aging population, and cost escalation – are motivating countries such as Canada to explore more cost-efficient health care practices (Barnett and Barnett 1997; Hurst 1991; Monk and Cox 1991; Van DeVen 1996). An important component of efforts to control costs is the shift away from institutional health care towards a home-based care system (Lesemann and Martin 1993). In the past two decades, most Western countries have cut spending on institutional care, while expanding the variety and scope of home care services. Thus, many Western countries have experienced a broad shift in the geography of health care, from centralized, hospital-based care to decentralized, home-based care. Despite the expansion of home care, it too has been a target of cost-efficient strategies, including privatization, reducing benefits, limiting access to services, and performance monitoring (ibid.). Under privatization, programs and services formerly provided in the public sector have been transferred to the private and voluntary sector, or defined as the private responsibility of the family. Although some have been hesitant to criticize privatization, arguing that it is simply a change in the form of the welfare state (Laws 1989; Mohan 1995), the impacts of privatization for informal carers and health care workers have often proved to be negative.

The restructuring of health care often entails transformations in the labor process. The labor process defines the dynamic between the work itself, the object upon which work is undertaken, and the instruments of labor (Lee 1991). It describes the nature, mechanisms, and processes of power and control in paid work. The adoption of new labor processes is often governed by finances, although management type, the state of relations between management and labor, and size of organization are also implicated (Massey 1995). The transformations in the labor process caused by health care restructuring can be comprehensively analyzed in terms of the impacts on women's work and the quality and quantity of services delivered. Such transformations are apparent in shifting work structures, work functions, work expectations, and working conditions – all of which affect the quality of work life for formal practitioners, not to mention the quality of care provided to clients. Although working conditions normally refer to the physical surroundings in which an individual works, such as those unduly hazardous or detrimental to health (e.g. excessive noise, air pollution, or excessive heat or cold), they are extended here to include job demands, role characteristics, and organizational characteristics and policies (Brief *et al.* 1981).

The retreat of the welfare state, and corresponding shifts in the labor process, are affecting women in numerous ways (Webster 1985). The restructuring taking place in women's work in the home and in the workplace is intensifying the experience of the double day (Brodie 1994; Luxton and Reiter 1997). Women make up a majority of the health care workforce and therefore bear a disproportionate share of the costs and impacts of restructuring. Class and race interrelate with gender to further disadvantage certain groups of women. Although the broad impacts of restructuring on women have often been discussed, the effects on women's everyday lives are less well understood. These effects are explored in the sections that follow for women's formal caring work in the home care sector in northern Ontario.

Women in home health care

Women predominate in many health care occupations, illustrating the prevalence of gender-based occupational segmentation (Bakshi *et al.* 1995). Such segmentation is a reflection of social structures, cultural values, and attitudes that channel women and men into different types of employment opportunities. Hanson and Pratt (1995) have shown that space and place (i.e. local context) are also clearly implicated in the social construction of occupational segmentation. Among the various explanations of the ways in which women are segmented in the labor force (Kobayashi *et al.* 1994), the traditional division of labor best fits the work situation of home care practitioners. Occupational segmentation begins at home, as women's labor market positions are defined in terms of their household responsibilities. Paid care giving is an outgrowth of women's traditional role; it is the result of sex-role stereotyping which places women in jobs that are extensions of their personal lives (Pines *et al.* 1981). Home care accentuates the merging of public and private, as care is given solely in the home and involves domestic tasks that are typically not performed for a wage (Abel and Nelson 1990). Like most care giving work done in capitalist society, formal care in the home is subordinated and devalued in the marketplace when it is done for a wage.

The subordinate position of home health care practitioners reflects the occupational segregation that is also found within the home health care environment. The three practitioner groups of concern in this research (RNs, RPNs, and HSWs) have comparatively little prestige and status (Butter *et al.* 1985; Fisher 1990), as they are all predominately female and located near the bottom of the health care hierarchy, especially when compared with hospital-based physicians and nurses (Figure 6.1).

Furthermore, there is a division of labor within the home care workforce. The differences between the practitioner groups are reflected in each group's occupational status, level of education, pay, and authority. RNs are higher in the hierarchy (as reflected in their higher levels of pay and authority) than RPNs, who in turn are higher than HSWs. In terms of dual labor market

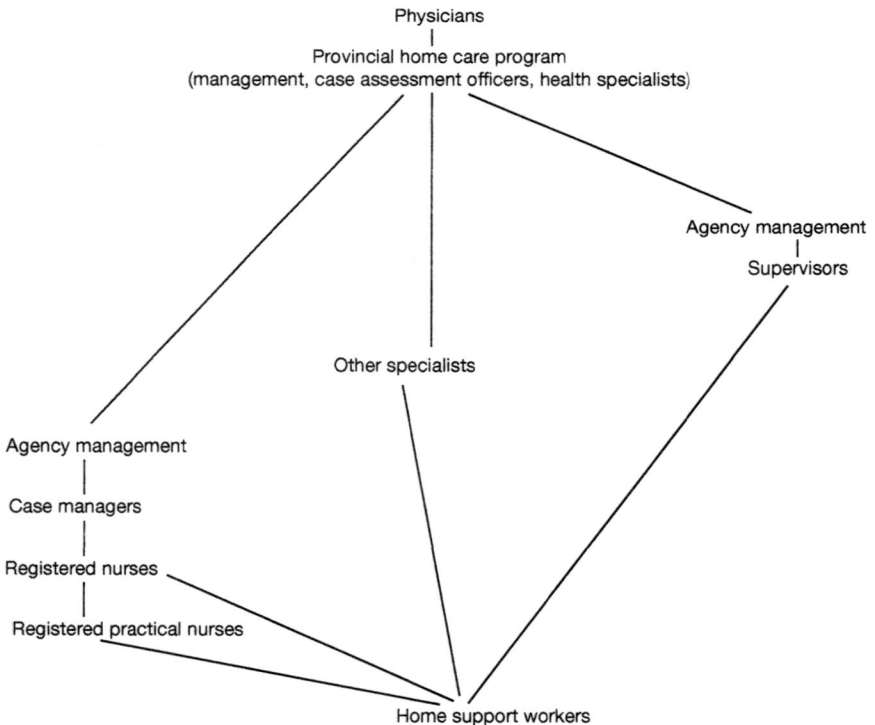

Figure 6.1 The home care occupational hierarchy.

theory, the nurses – RNs and RPNs – make up the primary labor market and the HSWs, the secondary labor market.

RNs and RPNs differ in education and training. RNs either have a university degree or a college certificate acquired from two to three years of education, whereas RPNs have a college certificate after one year of education. Pay for both RNs and RPNs working in home care is relatively competitive in the medical field but less than the equivalent for practitioners working in hospitals (Konka 1995). The majority of RNs and RPNs in the home care sector are unionized. Although RNs and RPNs have traditionally had full-time employment, many are now part of a flexible workforce because of an increase in the number of permanent part-time workers (Armstrong and Armstrong 1990). In contrast to both groups of nurses, HSWs are paid a little above minimum wage with limited benefits (Oriol 1985). HSWs are non-unionized and they have no professional association. They are hired as permanent part-time employees, "constituting a flexible pool of labor, a floating reserve" (Armstrong and Armstrong 1990: 86). Like the other two groups of home care practitioners, HSWs often have demanding schedules, rarely having two days off in a row and often working on weekends.

The differences in the occupational status of the three practitioner groups explain the position of each in the occupational hierarchy. On the basis of previous research that has found a direct relationship between occupational status and job satisfaction, RNs are expected to have the greatest job satisfaction of the three practitioner groups, followed by RPNs, and finally, HSWs (Esland and Salaman 1980). Job stress also varies with status, as low-status occupations are associated with high levels of job stress (Brief *et al.* 1981). Job stress is an important element in job satisfaction – defined as an attitude people experience about their work (ibid.). Stress occurs when people see environmental conditions as threats to their continued well-being (Hudson and Sullivan 1990). Restructuring is challenging these well-known relationships. In keeping with Peck's (1996) argument that labor markets work in different ways in different places, the role of place is highlighted in the examination of the home care labor market in northern Ontario.

The Ontario case

As elsewhere, the three policy determinants strongly influencing home health care policy in Ontario are demographics, economics, and politics. Population aging in Canada means larger numbers of old people, and most significantly, of very old people who typically experience greater physical and cognitive impairments and use a comparatively larger number of health services (Ontario Ministry of Health 1993). This demographic change has motivated the Ontario government to implement a more cost-efficient and cost-effective health care system. Although demographic factors are important, the overriding objective has been to minimize (if not totally erase) the budget deficit. Both the federal and provincial governments in power have prioritized this task and have had success; the federal government has balanced the budget two years ahead of schedule, while the Ontario government plans on balancing the provincial budget by 2000–1, if not earlier. The market-driven structural conditions that are characteristic of Canada's health care reform are evident in the reduction of federal transfer payments to provinces. These cuts, together with deficit-cutting provincial reforms around de-institutionalization and hospital restructuring, have had huge negative impacts on home care – the fastest growing long-term care service in Ontario (White 1994). Despite greater demands for increasingly complex home care services, there is strong pressure to reduce costs. The province has allocated a fixed amount of public funds to the home care sector, so care has had to be rationed. This has clearly impacted the quality of care, as noted by Evans and Wekerle (1997: 3):

> Against a background of economic restructuring, globalisation, and the overriding imperative of deficit reduction, the Canadian "welfare state" is in retreat. This retreat continues a direction that has been apparent since the mid-1970s and one that advanced significantly in the 1980s. However, the 1990s are characterized by a more fundamental challenge to the welfare state that has been fuelled by recent recessions, growing concerns about trade globalisation, the restructuring of the labour market, and a focus on cuts to social spending as the dominant solution to the problem of the deficit. The challenge to the welfare state, however, is not simply a reduction in costs. Canadians are being told that they must scale down the expectations they hold of their governments and accept a significant curtailment in the scope and comprehensiveness of state-provided services. Not only has the quality of care suffered in the home care sector, but also increased demands and diminishing resources have had their toll on formal caregivers – particularly nurses.

Universal public health care is a cornerstone of Canadian society, and most Canadians look upon privatization very skeptically; however in the case of home care, privatization is in full swing throughout the province (Mulligan 1998). The Ontario government has encouraged privatization by opening up home care to the free market, through establishing a competitive tendering process for home care contracts. For many years, the 80/20 rule guaranteed the not-for-profit public home care sector 80 percent of home care funding, leaving the for-profit (private) sector to compete for the remaining 20 percent (Coutts 1996). By canceling this rule, the Ontario government is counting on competition to improve the cost-efficiency of home care. In an attempt to buy time for not-for-profit agencies to become competitive, a four-year Transition Plan has been implemented. This plan slowly decreases the portion of the guaranteed home care volume (hours/visits) that existing service providers had in the past, while increasing the volume that is competitively bid. In year four of the Transition Plan, there is no protected home care volume; it is at this point that not-for-profit agencies are expected to compete fully with for-profit agencies for funding. The not-for-profit agencies have shown some success in this bidding process, although the for-profit service providers are increasingly winning contracts. This is due to the for-profit agencies having a lower rate of unionization, and offering lower wages, minimal benefits, and less control over work life, than the not-for-profit agencies. Service standards have also been questioned. In this increasingly competitive environment, not-for-profit agencies have been carrying out various types of administrative streamlining and labor process change in order to survive. These labor process changes are reflective of what is happening elsewhere in the public sector.

Although not-for-profit home care agencies have had – for the most part – excellent employment practices, they are succumbing to new management programs. They are experiencing closer scrutiny of the services they provide, increasing competition from other service agencies, pressures for fiscal accountability and tighter financial management, and changing demand patterns as knowledgeable customers analyze their health care options (Green *et al.* 1994). As a consequence, the work lives of home care practitioners are increasingly encumbered, as the wages of practitioners make up the bulk of the agency's costs. As will now be discussed, the transformation of the labor process is fundamentally reshaping home care practitioner's lives (Connelly 1995).

Methods

This research employed both qualitative and quantitative methods. The data come from four focus groups and the results of a mail-out questionnaire survey. Respondents were made up of practitioners working in the two largest not-for-profit home care agencies in the province (one agency employing RNs and RPNs, and the other employing HSWs). The focus groups comprised six to ten practitioners (two groups were made up of RNs and RPNs and two groups were made up of HSWs). The semi-directed focus group discussions broadly defined work life issues, which were then explored in greater detail in the questionnaire survey. All the respondents were women, as at the time of data collection, no men were employed in either of the home care agencies concerned. All practitioners employed by the two agencies throughout northern Ontario were asked to participate in the questionnaire survey (n = 1,157), which achieved a 42 percent response rate. No private, for-profit home care agencies – which at the time had comparatively fewer practitioners than the non-profit agencies – were researched. Of the 484 respondents, 70 percent were HSWs, 8 percent RPNs, and 15 percent RNs. To avoid the problems of small samples and to insure reliability, responses from RNs and RPNs were pooled together. Practitioners' assessments of work life were examined using a scale composed of twenty-two items. Each item was a work-related statement with which practitioners expressed their agreement using four standardized response categories: strongly agree (1), moderately agree (2), moderately disagree (3), and strongly disagree (4). The results of the quantitative survey are enhanced using the qualitative data collected in the focus group discussions.

Results

The two practitioner groups differ significantly in education, income, and age (Table 6.1), with nurses (RNs and RPNs) having objectively higher socio-economic status than HSWs. This confirms the expected relationship between occupation and socio-economic status for home care workers (Brown and Scase 1991). It also highlights the diversity among women, even within a relatively narrow employment category (Massey 1995). The HSWs are significantly older than the nurses; younger working-class women tend to be found in higher-status service occupations, while older women are

Table 6.1 Demographic characteristics of questionnaire survey respondents

Characteristic	Practitioner group	
	Nurses % (n = 131)	Home support workers % (n = 353)
EDUCATION		
grade 8 or less	–	8
high school	–	49
community college	68	0
university	23	9
graduate school	5	0
INCOME		
less than $10,000		5
$10–29,999	10	36
$30–49,999	23	35
$50–69,999	32	18
$70–79,999	35	6
MAJOR WAGE EARNER IN FAMILY	31	27
ETHNICITY		
English Canadians	65	55
AGE		
median	39	44
MARITAL AND FAMILY STATUS		
widowed	2	6
married	75	68
have children	80	87
of those who have children, children still at home	91	68

Note
Characteristics in bold are significantly different (p < 0.05) between practitioner groups according to Mann–Whitney U tests.

concentrated in occupations (such as home support) that involve commodified forms of domestic work (Gregson and Lowe 1994: 128). The majority of practitioners in both groups are living the double day – coming home from work to care for children. The average number of children at home for each practitioner group reflects the age differences, as younger nurses are still in their childbearing years, while children of the relatively older HSWs often have left or are leaving home. The greater representation among HSWs of ethnic groups other than English Canadian confirms that class and race interrelate with gender to further disadvantage women. Several HSWs are French Canadian or Aboriginal or represent various other ethnic identities. Only the Italian ethnic group was more strongly represented among nurses due to the long history of Italian-Canadian settlement in northern Ontario (Algoma District Health Council 1996). The lower occupational status characteristic of the HSW group is consistent with the experience of ethnic minorities (Brown and Scase 1991; Littler and Salaman 1984) and immigrant women (Donovan 1989).

Using exploratory factor analysis with oblique rotation, the relationships among the twenty-two work life items were examined (Alan and Duncan 1990). The final rotated solution was restricted to three factors, each with an eigenvalue close to or greater than one. Factor 1 had the largest eigenvalue value (2.94), followed by Factor 2 (1.23) and finally, by Factor 3 (0.76). The three factors accounted for 24 percent of the variance, so their limited explanatory value has to be emphasized. Factors were interpreted based on items with substantial loadings (large absolute +/– values), which reflect the strength of the association between individual items and factors (ibid.). The three factors were identified as follows: Factor 1: working conditions; Factor 2: job stress; and Factor 3: work motivation and support (Table 6.2).

To evaluate differences in assessments of work lives between the two groups, an analysis of variance was carried out comparing the average factor scores for women in each practitioner group. Significant differences were found for two factors, "working conditions" ($p < 0.05$) and "job stress" ($p < 0.01$). The nurses view their working conditions and job stress less favorably than do HSWs. These two factors are discussed below, supported by the representative work life items showing significant differences across practitioner group (Table 6.3).

Factor 1: working conditions

Nurses' mean scores on the "working conditions" factor are significantly ($p < 0.05$) less favorable than those of HSWs, illustrating that nurses are less satisfied with their working conditions than are HSWs. It is the cumulative effect of the differences in the ratings of all items making up the factor "working conditions" that creates this significant difference between the two groups. Mean ratings differ significantly on only one of the five items that load highly on this factor, "hours are flexible and convenient." Nurses have

Table 6.2 Exploratory factor analysis results for work life item loadings on obliquely rotated factors

Item	Oblique rotated loadings		
	Factor 1: working conditions	Factor 2: job stress	Factor 3: motivation and support
f) chances for promotion good	**0.64**	−0.06	0.26
u) respected by community members	**0.50**	0.21	−0.16
d) job security good	**0.44**	−0.05	0.04
k) enjoy commuting between clients	**0.43**	0.06	−0.07
t) hours flexible and convenient	**0.42**	−0.20	−0.06
p) job responsibilities decreasing	0.01	**−0.61**	−0.02
o) job requires resourcefulness	0.06	**0.40**	−0.14
s) work not stressful	0.12	**−0.40**	−0.27
j) enough time to get job done	0.30	**−0.36**	−0.08
v) not supervised too closely	−0.07	−0.11	**−0.56**
i) work personally rewarding	−0.03	0.10	**−0.52**
l) at ease in clients' homes	0.07	0.10	**−0.47**
e) enjoy clients	0.07	0.18	**−0.40**
g) respected by other members of the health care team	0.15	−0.04	**−0.44**
c) good support from and communication with office staff	0.10	**−0.30**	**−0.37**
q) employees chosen fairly when extra work available	−0.00	−0.20	**−0.35**

Note
Factor loadings greater than 0.3 are in bold. Six other work life items not listed here were included in the analysis, but did not show loadings greater than 0.3 for any of the three factors. Items have been somewhat shortened from the original questionnaire.

significantly ($p < 0.05$) lower overall levels of agreement (mean = 2.16) with this statement than HSWs (mean = 1.59). Nurses' comparative lack of flexibility and convenience in work hours may be related to shift work and the number of hours they work. Nurses, who work around the clock, work comparatively more hours per week than HSWs, who work only in daytime. The nurses average twenty-eight hours per week, whereas HSWs average twenty-five hours per week. Forty percent of the nurses work between thirty and thirty-nine hours per week, compared with only 32 percent of HSWs. Only 4 percent of HSWs work forty or more hours per week, whereas 10 percent of nurses do. The difference in hours between the two practitioner groups is also reflected in the number of additional hours that practitioners would like to work, as HSWs wish to work more additional hours than do the nurses.

Casual and part-time nurses are frustrated with their hours, as illustrated in the qualitative data. This group makes up a numerically flexible workforce, which allows the agency to adjust their labor inputs over time to meet

Table 6.3 Differences between groups for working life items

Quality of work life items	HSW means	RN/RPN means	Differences	t-value
a) **work is interesting**	**1.48**	**1.34**	**0.135**	**2.25**
b) pay is good	2.88	2.74	0.143	1.47
c) **good support and communication with office staff (F3)**	**1.90**	**2.32**	**–0.421**	**–3.77**
d) job security good (F1)	2.10	2.28	–0.181	–1.80
e) enjoy clients (F3)	1.24	1.21	0.034	0.61
f) chances for promotion good (F1)	2.97	3.03	–0.058	–0.59
g) respected by other members of health care team (F3)	1.96	1.87	0.084	0.79
h) a lot of freedom to decide how to do the work	2.02	1.97	0.043	0.47
i) **work personally rewarding (F3)**	**1.78**	**1.33**	**0.449**	**4.63**
j) **enough time to get job done (F2)**	**1.85**	**2.29**	**–0.439**	**–5.07**
k) enjoy commuting between clients (F1)	2.07	1.95	0.124	1.21
l) **at ease in clients' homes (F3)**	**1.64**	**1.36**	**0.282**	**3.20**
m) comfortable with medical equipment	1.65	1.63	0.027	0.36
n) benefit package good	2.5	2.64	–0.137	–1.18
o) **job requires resourcefulness (F2)**	**1.56**	**1.21**	**0.351**	**6.72**
p) **job responsibilities decreasing (F2)**	**3.13**	**3.64**	**–0.506**	**6.61**
q) employees chosen fairly when extra work available (F3)	2.26	2.29	–0.034	–0.28
r) **feel well-trained**	**1.66**	**1.82**	**–0.198**	**–2.51**
s) **work not stressful (F2)**	**2.75**	**3.07**	**–0.323**	**–3.65**
t) **hours flexible and convenient (F1)**	**1.59**	**2.16**	**–0.565**	**–6.15**
u) respected by community members (F1)	1.61	1.58	0.028	0.38
v) not supervised too closely (F3)	1.72	1.76	–0.037	–0.44

Note
Items in bold show a significant difference between the mean values for practitioner groups at the 0.05 significance level. Items have been somewhat shortened from the original questionnaire.

fluctuations in output (Pinch 1997). These nurses are dissatisfied with the small number of hours they are working, the lack of control that they feel they have over their work schedule, and the hindrance their work causes to their lifestyle:

> the dissatisfaction . . . unstable work schedule due to my casual status. And I absolutely detest calling in at 11 a.m. in the morning to say "do you have anything for this evening or for tomorrow," and not being able to go and have a day that I can go somewhere because I have to stay around in case they call me.
>
> (RN3, FG2)

In contrast, the HSWs – all of whom are employed part-time – are found to have more control over their work schedules. HSWs are grateful for the flexibility of their work hours, as it enables them to meet their family responsibilities:

> They [management] let me choose my own hours. They're pretty flexible, like. If you want to work just mornings, you can work just mornings. If you want to work full-time, if the clients are there, she'll let you work full-time. Being able to get the days off when you want them, especially when you got smaller kids, like when Wayne was little, he got sick, and I needed to know that I can take the time off and not lose my job.
>
> (HMKa, FG4)

It seems as though HSWs have more of a participatory role in determining their work hours then do nurses. Management will work around HSWs' requests, trying to ensure hours are rearranged, not reallocated. This does not seem to be the case for nurses, who are comparatively more expensive to employ, as the management appears to have become more rigid about work schedules. This confirms that the relations between management and labor are implicated in the adoption of new labor processes, as Massey has suggested (1995).

Differences in the evaluations of the two practitioner groups on Factor 1 may also be due to the reference group(s) that practitioners use when assessing the items making up this factor (Romero 1994). For example, home care nurses may be assessing their working conditions relative to those of hospital nurses or their own managers. They may view their working conditions as less satisfactory than those of comparable health care professionals. In contrast, HSWs may feel satisfied about their work when comparing it with other employment opportunities that are open to them, as stated by one focus group participant:

> It pays more than if you went for waitressing, or cleaning rooms, or whatever. It's above minimum wage, so if you don't have any skills and

you can get into a job like this, then it's great, 'cause you only have your home skills, eh?

(HMKe, FG4)

Using these service occupations as reference groups, HSWs may evaluate their jobs relatively favorably.

Factor 2: job stress

Nurses also assessed the second factor less favorably than did HSWs. The questionnaire data show that the nurses feel significantly more job stress (p = .001). This is evident in the significant differences (p < 0.05) in the ratings of the four main items making up this factor (Table 6.3). These include: "have enough time to get job done," "job responsibilities are decreasing," "work is not stressful," and "job requires resourcefulness." Although ratings of the fifth item, "not supervised too closely", are not statistically significant, nurses are also less satisfied (mean = 1.76) than are HSWs (mean = 1.72).

Nurses (mean = 3.64) show a significantly higher level of disagreement (mean = 3.13) with the item "job responsibilities are decreasing." Recent changes in home care give nurses an enhanced responsibility for complex and technologically demanding job tasks. The transfer of patients from institutional care to home care translates into a larger number of sophisticated skills in the home, as pointed out by an RN:

> when I started ten years ago with [name of agency], the type of call [was] totally different than what we are getting now. We [now] have all kinds of programs that were unheard of ten years ago. We do a lot of high-tech work in the homes . . . we are now perfectly capable of doing it and are doing it. We're doing the IVs, we're doing the dialysis, those kinds of things; we do a lot more in the homes as opposed to educating.

(RNd, FG2)

Such shifts in workload are becoming more frequent across the public sector, as Pinch (1997) has identified in his discussion of functional flexibility. Functional flexibility involves firms extending the range of skills of their workers and may involve breaking down the barriers between different occupations.

Nurses do not always feel confident about their knowledge of these new complex skills. This is particularly the case for RNs who are assigned to overnight "on-call" duty:

> Well you know I find that there's some girls that know all these technical skills and they're doing them everyday and then there's all of us girls,

the RNs that are on night call and have this same big fear of being called out to change a[n IV] pump . . . or something like that and not having a clue of what to do. And we all have to take our turn on night call . . . when I put that beeper on at 11 p.m. 'til 7–8 in the morning, I'm on call; anything can happen and there's tons of anxiety there, and yet I'm not alone.

(RNc, FG1)

The lack of confidence felt by many nurses is blamed on lack of training:

you are all supposed to handle any situation so they have you do a little quickie [training] session and say okay, you can do it, you're okay.

(RNc, FG1)

Dealing with increasing work responsibilities without proper training adds to job stress. Cost is undoubtedly the reason why these nurses are not being given the appropriate training needed to properly manage the new technology and the greater sophistication of patient cases now found in the home.

The increased number of sophisticated work tasks is one of the many challenges requiring nurses' resourcefulness. Nurses (mean = 1.21) see themselves as required to be more inventive and resourceful on the job than HSWs (mean = 1.56). This may be because nurses are trained to work within a well-equipped institutional setting and have to manage without much equipment in the homes.

And work is really challenging . . . you have to be innovative. You don't have the resources that the hospitals have, so you end up doing some really different things; using door knobs to hang things on, that kind of thing.

(RNe, FG2)

In contrast, HSWs are trained to work in a domestic environment, so their work tasks rarely extend beyond the home domain.

As a result of cost pressures, job responsibilities are increasing while time allowances for patient visits are decreasing. The implementation of increasingly constraining time limits has added to practitioners' job stress. The two practitioner groups differed significantly in their attitudes toward the time available to complete a job, as measured by the item "have enough time to get job done." Nurses (mean = 2.29) show a higher level of disagreement than HSWs (mean = 1.85). Nurses have to cope with time constraints more than do HSWs, undoubtedly due to the fact that nurses are more expensive to employ than are HSWs. According to the nurses, cost-saving strategies translate into the intensification of work, defined as increases in labor productivity via managerial and organizational changes (Massey 1995). The intensification of work for nurses has been identified as one of the most important changes affecting the public sector workforce in recent years (Pinch 1997). Time limitations, in addition to increasing job responsibilities of a sophisticated nature, are some of the many factors contributing to practitioners' job stress, as measured by the item "work is not stressful." The significant difference ($p < 0.05$) in practitioners' assessments, with nurses feeling more job stress (mean = 3.07) than HSWs (mean = 2.75), reflects the comparatively greater time–space constraints being experienced by nurses.

Nurses spoke about how rushed they feel with tight schedules. One RN spoke about her reaction to the imposed time constraints:

> they'll [home care agency] give you six patients that are all . . . needy in the afternoon and like they're suppose to spread out for the whole day, but you cannot fit six people in the morning and you know that the last one is going to be chomping at the bit when you walk in the door or you're even afraid to phone them because you don't want to tell them that you can't make it 'til 1 p.m. So you just zip right through lunch and skip all your coffee breaks trying to get these six morning patients in four hours – now that's stress.
>
> (RNe, FG1)

Clearly, the resources of time and space are becoming increasingly limited due to health care reform. The boundaries limiting behavior across time–space, as defined by Hagerstrand (1975), are clearly being stretched. Of the five facets of time–geographic reality defined by Hagerstrand (1975), the one which is being particularly challenged here is the limited capability of human beings to participate in more than one task at once, coupled with the fact that every task has a duration (Giddens 1984). Although home care practitioners may be able to do more than one task at once, they cannot be in more than one place at once.

Driving from one household to another complicates the time–space constraints that practitioners are experiencing as a result of work intensification and enhanced functional flexibility. Although management may wish for time–space convergence or the shrinking of distance in terms of the time needed to move between different locations (Janelle 1969), the time it takes to drive from household A to household B has not changed as a result of reform (speed limits remain unchanged!). An RPN discussed her sense of dissatisfaction with time expectations given the spatial challenges she faces:

> What I'm not satisfied with . . . is the limited time we get; thirteen people in a day and you have half an hour for each person and that includes traveling time and, quite often I'm in about four or five different [geographical] areas in one day, and I could spend ten minutes with each person and still not make up my time.
>
> (RPNa, FG2)

Another RN had a different response to the time-constraints:

> The time limit now – I don't even bother with the time limit; I do my thing and if I go over and I don't care about it and I just get paid for what they're going to pay me anyway; but I do feel good at the end of the day; I don't feel short-changed or anything. I'm not rushing anymore.
>
> (RNc, FG1)

As a result, this latter nurse would work a longer day, beyond the hours for which she is paid. This is a clear case of costs for health care being shifted to home care practitioners as a result of labor process change.

Job stress and poor working conditions are directly related to absenteeism and turnover. Increasing job stress and declining working conditions may also have negative effects on employee retention, as job satisfaction – defined by both working conditions and job stress – is related directly to turnover. Better working conditions would enhance workforce retention (Canadian Nurses Association and Canadian Hospital Association 1990). Job stress has been found to be an important reason why nurses leave the profession (Employment and Immigration Canada 1989; Goldfarb Corporation 1988), and may explain why nurses have been working fewer years than HSWs. Although the difference in age across the two practitioner groups may contribute to the variations evident in job tenure, job stress undoubtedly plays a role. Of HSWs in the sample 40 percent have been working for thirteen years or more, whereas only 28 percent of the nurses have been employed that long. Of the nurses 68 percent have been working for the same home care agency for four years or less, whereas only 57 percent of the HSWs have been employed by the same agency within the previous four years. Nurses are carrying out more complex tasks, working more intensively, and working longer hours than HSWs. The comparatively greater stress experienced by nurses may be one of the factors contributing to their comparatively short job tenure. This is problematic in the medically under-serviced region of northern Ontario, which has difficulty recruiting and retaining health care practitioners.

Conclusion

Health policy reform in Ontario not only has brought about a broad shift in the geography of care, but continues to have adverse effects on home care practitioners. As in most other publicly funded sectors in Ontario, and throughout much of Canada, women are being hard hit by health policy reform. The state has assumed that women will pick up the slack and intensify both their paid work and their unpaid caring duties. This has been evident in the formal caring work of home care practitioners in northern Ontario.

One of the surprising consequences of reform is the differential impact of restructuring on the two practitioner groups. Restructuring is resulting in more severe time–space constraints for nurses than for HSWs. Nurses are being forced to serve more patients in less time (intensification of work) while being given increased responsibility for tasks (functional flexibility). Nurses – the practitioner group that has the highest occupational status in home health care – are experiencing worse working conditions, more job stress, and thereby less job satisfaction than HSWs – the practitioner group with relatively low occupational status. This is unexpected given the often-cited inverse relationship between occupational status and job satisfaction. A similar phenomenon has been observed with physicians in New Zealand (Kearns and Barnett 1992), and with various other groups of health professionals throughout the Western world. Perhaps the higher status occupations are feeling the impacts of restructuring more because they begin with higher expectations and therefore have further to fall. The HSWs are already at the bottom of the human health care hierarchy; consequently, their expectations may be comparatively less than those of their co-workers.

The changing labor process for home care practitioners in Ontario may have serious repercussions for availability of health care resources, particularly for medically under-serviced areas, such as northern Ontario. Job satisfaction for these practitioners is related directly to turnover and is of great importance for maintaining continuity and quality of care. The increased job stress and declining working conditions of practitioners will undoubtedly impact the quality of care provided, in a similar way to that already documented in the case of hospital workers (Armstrong *et al.* 1994). Together with the rationing of care, labor process transformations appear to be negatively impacting the quality of care.

Since the completion of this research, management has begun to replace RNs with RPNs, as a result of RNs being more expensive to employ than RPNs. Thus far RPNs are being hired as part-time workers, further evidence of management implementing numerical flexibility. This strategy has raised questions with regard to the standards of care now in place. RNs in home care, and indeed in all sectors of the health care system, have been demoralized by the changes brought about by reform. The hard-won gains in wages have made RNs comparatively expensive to employ. Canadian RNs have lost confidence in their profession and are leaving to work elsewhere, often in the USA. Consequently, Canada is experiencing a nursing shortage – a problem of great concern in medically under-serviced areas, such as northern Ontario.

The declining opportunities for RNs point to a changing distribution of jobs in Canada. Employment growth has become skewed, so that there are now a few highly skilled, well-compensated jobs, and many unstable, relatively poorly paid jobs (Duffy and Pupo 1992). Job growth is concentrated in the service sector, often in part-time, non-unionized, and lowly paid positions, where the vast majority of workers are women. Advocacy for policy change is necessary if women's position in the labor market is to recover from what has been forced upon it in recent years.

References

Abel, E. K. and Nelson, M. K. (eds) (1990) *Circles of Care: Work and Identity in Women's Lives*, Albany, NY: State University of New York Press.

Alan, B. and Duncan, C. (1990) *Quantitative Analysis for Social Scientists*, New York: Routledge.

Algoma District Health Council (1996) *Multi-Year Plan for Community Long-Term Care Services*, Sault Ste. Marie: Algoma District Health Council.

Armstrong, P. and Armstrong, H. (1990) *Theorizing Women's Work*, Toronto: Garamond Press.

Armstrong, P., Armstrong, H., Choiniere, J., Feldberg, G., and White J. (1994) *Take Care: Warning Signals for Canada's Health System*, Toronto: Garamond Press.

Bakshi, P., Goodwin, M., Painter, J., and Southern, A. (1995) "Gender, race and class in the local welfare state: moving beyond regulation theory in analyzing the transition from Fordism," *Environment and Planning A: Government Policy* 27: 1555–76.

Barnett, P. and Barnett, R. (1997) "A turning tide? Reflections on ideology and health service restructuring in New Zealand," *Health & Place* 3, 1: 55–8.

Beggs, C. (1991) "Retention factors for physiotherapists in an underserviced area: an experience in northern Ontario," *Physiotherapy Canada* 43, 2: 15–21.

Brief, A. P., Schuler, R. S., and Van Sell, M. (1981) *Managing Job Stress*, Boston: Little, Brown.

Brodie, J. (1994) "Shifting the boundaries: gender and the politics of restructuring," in I. Bakker (ed.) *The Strategies of Silence: Gender and Economic Policy*, London: North–South Institute: 46–60.

Brown, P. and Scase, R. (1991) *Poorwork: Disadvantage and the Division of Labor*, Philadelphia, PA: Open University Press.

Butter, I., Carpenter, E., Kay, B., and Simmons, R. (1985) *Sex and Status: Hierarchies in the Health Workforce*, Washington, DC: American Public Health Association.

Canadian Nurses Association and Canadian Hospital Association (1990) *Nurse Retention and Quality of Worklife: A National Perspective*, Ottawa: Canadian Nurses' Association.

Connelly, M. P. (1995) *Gender Matters: Restructuring and Adjustment, South and North. In Gender and Economic Structuring*, Ontario: Centre for Research on Work and Society, Working Paper Series No. 12, York University.

Coutts, J. (1996) "Privatizing care for patients at home: an issue on the boil," *The Globe and Mail* 17 April: A8.

Dear, M., Clark, G., and Clark, S. (1979) "Economic cycles and mental health care policy: an examination of the macro-context for social service planning," *Social Science and Medicine* 13C: 43–53.

Donovan, R. (1989) "Work stress and job satisfaction: a study of home care workers in New York City," *Home Health Care Services Quarterly* 10: 97–114.

Duffy, A. and Pupo, N. (1992) *Part-time Paradox: Connecting Gender, Work and Family*, Toronto: McClelland & Stewart.

Employment and Immigration Canada (1989) *Workers with Family Responsibilities in a Changing Society: Who Cares?*, Ottawa: Employment and Immigration Canada.

Esland, G. and Salaman, G. (1980) *The Politics of Work & Occupations*, Toronto: University of Toronto Press.

Evans, P. M. and Wekerle, G. R. (1997) *Women and the Canadian Welfare State: Challenges and Change*, Toronto: University of Toronto Press.

Fisher, B. (1990) "Alice in the human services: a feminist analysis of women in the caring professions," in E. K. Abel and M. K. Nelson (eds) *Circles of Care: Work and Identity in Women's Lives*, Albany, NY: State University of New York Press: 108–31.

Giddens, A. (1984) *The Constitution of Society: Outline of the Theory of Structuration*, Cambridge: Polity Press.

Goldfarb Corporation (1988) *The Nursing Shortage in Ontario: A Research Report for the Ontario Nurses' Association*, Toronto: Ontario Nurses' Association.

Green, E., Hobbs, L., and Mousseau, J. (1994) "Introducing quality management in the community: the VON experience," *Canadian Journal of Nursing Administration* 7, 1: 62–75.

Gregson, N. and Lowe, M. (1994) *Servicing the Middle Classes*, London: Routledge.

Hagerstrand, T. (1975) "Space, time and human conditions," in A. Karlqvist, L. Lundqvist, and F. Snickars (eds) *Dynamic Allocation of Urban Space*, Farnborough: Saxon House: 3–14.

Hanson, S. and Pratt, G. (1995) *Gender, Work and Space*, London: Routledge.

Hudson, R. and Sullivan, T. A. (1990) *The Social Organization of Work*, Belmont, CA: Wadsworth.

Hurst, J. W. (1991) "Reforming health care in seven European nations," *Health Policy* 24, 5: 7–14.

Janelle, D. (1969) "Spatial reorganization: a model and concept," *Annals of the Association of American Geographers* 59: 348–64.

Kearns, R. and Barnett, J. (1992) "Enter the supermarket: entrepreneurial medical practice in New Zealand," *Environment and Planning C: Government Policy* 10: 267–81.

Kobayashi, A., Peake, L., Benenson, H., and Pickles, K. (1994) "Introduction: placing women and work," in A. Kobayashi (ed.) *Women, Work, and Place*, Montreal, Canada: McGill-Queen's University Press: xi–xiv.

Konka, J. (1995) Director, Home Care Program, Sault Ste Marie: Algoma Health Unit, personal interview.

Laws, G. (1989) "Deinstitutionalization and privatization: community-based residential care facilities in Ontario," in J. L. Scarpaci (ed.) *Health Services Privatization in Industrial Societies*, New Brunswick: Rutgers.

Lee, R. (1991) *The Dictionary of Human Geography*, Oxford: Basil Blackwell.

Lesemann, F. and Martin, C. (eds) (1993) *Home-Based Care, the Elderly, the Family and the Welfare State: An International Comparison*, Ottawa: University of Ottawa Press.

Littler, C. R. and Salaman, G. (1984) *Class at Work*, London: Batsford.

Luxton, M. and Reiter, E. (1997) "Double, double, toil and trouble . . . women's experience of work and family in Canada, 1980–1995," in P. M. Evans and G. R. Wekerle (eds) *Women and the Canadian Welfare State: Challenges and Change*, Toronto: University of Toronto Press: 198–221.

McDowell, L. and Pringle, R. (eds) (1992) *Defining Women: Social Institutions and Gender Divisions*, Cambridge: Polity Press.

Massey, D. (1995) *Spatial Divisions of Labour*, Basingstoke: Macmillan.

Mohan, J. (1995) *A National Health Service? The Restructuring of Health Care in Britain since 1979*, New York: St Martin's Press.

Monk, A. and Cox, C. (1991) *Home Care for the Elderly: An International Perspective*, Westport, CT: Auburn House.

Mulligan, P. (1998) "US health-care model not worth transplanting," *Toronto Star* 9 March.

Ontario Ministry of Health (In-Home Services Branch) (1993) *Program Description: Placement Coordinator Services*, Ontario: Ministry of Health.

Oriol, W. (1985) *The Complex Cube of Long-Term Care*, Washington, DC: American Health Planning Association.

Orloff, A. (1993) "Gender and the social rights of citizenship: the comparative analysis of gender relations and welfare states," *American Sociological Review* 58, 3: 303–28.

Peck, J. (1996) *Work Place: The Social Regulation of Labor Markets*, New York: Guilford.

Pinch, S. (1997) *Worlds of Welfare: Understanding the Changing Geographies of Social Welfare Provision*, London: Routledge.

Pines, A. M., Aronson, E., and Karfrey, D. (1981) *Burnout: From Tedium to Personal Growth*, New York: The Free Press.

Rafuse, J. (1996) "Private-sector share of health spending hits record level," *Canadian Medical Association Journal* 155, 6: 749–50.

Romero, M. (1994) "Chicanas and the changing work experience in domestic service," in W. Giles and S. Arat-Koc (eds) *Maid in the Market*, Halifax, NS: Fernwood Publishing: 48–55.

Van De Ven, W. P. M. (1996) "Market-oriented health care reform: trends and future options," *Social Science and Medicine* 43, 5: 655–66.

Webster, B. (1985) "A woman's issue: the impact of local authority cuts," *Local Government Studies* 11: 19–46.

White, G. (1994) Personal correspondence, Ministry of Health (In-Home Care Branch), Toronto, Ontario.

Williams, A. M. (1996) "The history of home care in Ontario: a geographical analysis," *Social Science and Medicine* 42, 6: 937–48.

7 "Thank God she's not sick"

Health and disciplinary practice among Salvadoran women in northern New Jersey

Caroline Kerner, Adrian J. Bailey, Alison Mountz, Ines Miyares, and Richard A. Wright

Introduction

Public health literature suggests that immigrant Latina women and their children have low rates of health care coverage and utilization in the United States (Chavez *et al.* 1997; Flores and Vega 1998; Guendelman *et al.* 1995; Halfon *et al.* 1997; Zambrana *et al.* 1994). Recent media reports further dramatize this situation in the context of significant declines in rates of benefit receipt for some non-citizens. For example, the share of welfare benefits received by non-citizen households fell at twice the rate for US citizens between 1996 and 1999. In Los Angeles County, applications for public aid by legal immigrants dropped by 71 percent (Brandon 1999).[1]

Scholars agree that poor economic standing, inability to speak English, and a lack of knowledge of rights act as barriers to health care for immigrants (Flores and Vega 1998; Gany and De Bocanegra 1996; Leclere *et al.* 1994; Wilson 1995). Recent changes in immigrant health care patterns, however, have occurred at the same time as a rise in anti-immigrant sentiment and new federal and state legislation that restricts access to services and citizenship in the US (Chavez *et al.* 1997; Hilfinger Messias 1996; Leclere *et al.* 1994). This restricted access to citizenship and residency characterizes a new and growing class of immigrants – those accorded temporary legal status.

We contribute to the discussion of immigrant women's health by focusing on the way health and health care are constructed in an immigrant community that lacks permanent legal rights of residence. In common with a growing number of European nations (Vedsted-Hansen 1994) the United States grants "Temporary Protected Status" (TPS) to a variety of immigrant groups with refugee-like experiences. TPS provides applicants and their families temporary permission to reside and work in the US. Status adjustment claims can also be submitted by those granted TPS. Successful claims are partly contingent upon applicants proving continuous residence in the US, ability to be economically self-sufficient, and good moral character.

Many Salvadorans who arrived in the US in the 1980s are part of a class of immigrants with such temporary status, and still await final decisions on their legal status. We refer to their state of limbo as "permanent temporariness" and argue that it pervades the economic and social dimensions of Salvadoran everyday life. We examine how economic marginality puts routine medical check-ups and preventive medicine out of reach, and how the employment opportunities for Salvadoran men and women restrict access to health insurance and limit information about health opportunities. Drawing on recent work in the geography of health we further consider how permanent temporariness inscribes itself on immigrant bodies through the disciplinary power of the Immigration and Naturalization Service (INS) interview for status adjustment.

We find that Salvadorans seek to make themselves visible and invisible to the INS in very particular ways, and that health and health care behavior have become an arena in which the disciplinary power stemming from the condition of permanent temporariness manifests itself. Overall, we believe Salvadoran women are missing out on opportunities for health care that is affordable and attentive to their needs. We close by raising the long-run implication for society of having a large number of immigrant women not seeking and/or postponing medical care.

Placing the social construction of health and health care

Medical geography theory has advanced in recent years through the synthesis of the new cultural geography with the geography of health. The new cultural geography's study of environmental, individual, and societal factors in landscapes can be applied to understand the formation of "therapeutic landscapes" (Gesler 1992: 736). Gesler defines therapeutic landscapes as terrains in which healing or health-seeking behavior takes place. This cultural approach relates to a socio-ecological model of health, in which "what occurs in a place . . . has profound importance to health" (Kearns 1993: 141). Such a synthetic model is valuable in exploring immigrants' negotiation of health and health care, which is influenced by the social, political, and economic structures that exist in a particular place (Dyck 1992). Factors such as ethnicity, immigrant status, socio-economic status, location of residence, and the political structures in a place all affect the health of individuals, their attitudes toward health and illness, and the actions they take with regard to health and health care. Because of their often marginalized place in US society, immigrants' negotiations of the health care system are influenced by these overlying structures intertwined with value systems drawn from their country of birth.

Isabel Dyck (1992: 243) proposes a research agenda for studying the everyday context of immigrant women's health and asserts that "there is growing evidence that people do define their health, illness, and appropriate responses situationally, and that 'recipes for action' concerning health care will be interpreted in the context of particular places." In other words, health-seeking behavior will vary in space because the immigrant experience tends to be place-specific.

We contribute to this initiative by framing the geographies of immigrant women's health in the context of a broad set of power relations operating in a place. Dorn and Laws (1994: 108) invite medical geographers to enter the discussion of body politics by giving voice to the geographical dimensions of the experiences of deviant bodies, which they define as "bodies that do not conform to social norms." Influenced by Foucault's idea of biopolitics and the "biomedical gaze," Ong (1995: 1244) applies the idea of the deviant body to immigrants' experiences with Western biomedicine in her study of Cambodian immigrants and refugee medicine. She asserts that not only does biomedicine involve the practice of restoring bodies to health, but it also embodies a process of social, economic, and political control of the "biopolitical subjects of the modern welfare state." Ong illustrates how refugees resist this hegemonic force by creating "webs of power" as a counter to top-down forms of social control.

We proceed by examining how such disciplining occurs in particular places. To do this, we draw on recent literature from the geography of health and wellness (Eyles and Woods 1983; Gesler 1992; Kearns 1995). Following Dyck (1992) we see place as both a container of prevailing attitudes toward health and health care use, and a recursive arena in which health is socially constructed and health outcomes affect other social processes such as community activism, transnational linkages, and definition of family. Such a recursive view of space offers one way to better understand the considerable geographic variations we know exist between health practices in different places.

We embrace an epistemology appropriate to a place-based analysis of the social construction of health where multiple sources of economic and symbolic power operate. Dyck (1993) discusses the problem of generalization about culture in exploring geographies of immigrant health. Thus we sought to avoid generalizing the roles of culture in the lives of immigrant women by putting personal testimonies in the broader context of community experience. This resembles the approach of Anderson (1987) who calls for studies of migration and health which reveal not only women's perspectives on health and health care, but also how these perspectives are contextualized in the "macro structure and micro processes" operating in a place. Her case studies of immigrant women's experiences of chronic illness (Anderson 1991; Anderson *et al.* 1991, 1995) involve a qualitative methodology to address this research agenda, providing insight into the social context of immigrant health. Her scholarship also emphasizes that ethnicity alone does not determine how a woman experiences her illness.

Research design

Salvadorans are one of the fastest growing immigrant groups in the United States (Red Nacional 1997). Small Salvadoran communities began appearing in Washington DC in the 1960s and 1970s (Repak 1995). Larger numbers of Salvadorans arrived in Los Angeles and a handful of other large metropolitan areas in the late 1970s and the 1980s following the massive political and economic dislocations associated with civil war in El Salvador. Although rival groups signed a formal Peace Accord in 1992, migrants from El Salvador continue to arrive, and today the US Salvadoran community numbers in excess of 1.3 million persons (Red Nacional 1997). Following Los Angeles, the largest settlements of Salvadorans are located in New York and Washington DC. Within the New York metropolitan area, significant clusters of Salvadorans are found in Long Island (Mahler 1995) and Hudson County, New Jersey. Our research is one of the first to describe health experiences among Salvadorans who comprise the Hudson County community.

To study and understand the nature of health issues in this place we combined data which described the structure of the community and the prevalence of health care behaviors with data that represented the local constructions of health and health care in the Salvadoran community (i.e. a mixed methods approach, see McKendrick 1999; McLafferty 1995). Between the summers of 1997 and 1998 we worked on four fronts. Throughout the fifteen months we carried out expert interviews with leaders of community organizations, health care providers, public health officials, consular officials, and other individuals whose responsibilities extended to the Salvadoran community in New Jersey. These expert interviews helped us hone a semi-structured interview format, and we went on to complete fifty-six of these semi-structured interviews with Salvadoran-born men and women. Following this we conducted in-depth interviews with thirteen Salvadorans in New Jersey before administering a structured intercept survey to 183 Salvadorans in the summer of 1998 (see Mountz *et al.* 2000). The findings we report below derive from all these sources, and have been closely informed by our ongoing associations with the communities we seek to represent.

The Salvadoran community of Hudson County, New Jersey

One reading of Hudson County's Salvadoran community suggests it mirrors many contemporary transnational immigrant populations in the US (see Cordero-Guzman *et al.* 1997). Community leaders told us that approximately 20,000 Salvadorans live in Hudson County, in neighborhoods that vary from inner city, deindustrialized to low- and middle-income suburban. Our intercept survey indicated that about half of the community is married. Many have children still living in El Salvador, and some parents had not seen their children in ten years. Like many Salvadorans in the US, over four-fifths of the community send remittances to El Salvador, typically $100–$300 per month. Wages are earned in a wide variety of occupations, reflective of the diverse northern New Jersey labor market.

Unlike in many other immigrant groups, however, legal status and associated issues frame daily life in the Salvadoran community we studied. Salvadorans originally came to the New York metropolitan area to flee the civil war in El Salvador. Although fewer than 5 percent had been granted asylum by the INS at the end of 1998, as many as 300,000 Salvadorans have obtained temporary residence in the US, as a result of both TPS and a separate lawsuit filed by the American Baptist Churches on behalf of Central American immigrants and settled out of court in 1991 (*American Baptist Churches v. Thornburgh*, 760 F. Supp. 796, N.D. Cal 1991; see Coutin 1998). Members of the latter "ABC settlement" and those with TPS (hereafter referred to collectively as members of the ABC class) do not receive all of the benefits enjoyed by refugees (for example, there is no residential assistance) or immigrants (for example, they cannot come and go freely, or bring family members to the US). However, being part of the ABC class provides Salvadorans *el permiso*, literally, permission to work. At the national level, approximately one-third of Salvadorans are permanent residents, one-third are undocumented, one-quarter were granted temporary residence as members of the ABC class, and the remainder are US citizens or asylum applicants (Red Nacional 1997). We believe that about one-half of the Hudson County Salvadoran community were members of the ABC class when we conducted our study, and we accent their experiences below.

The legal condition of permanent temporariness shapes employment possibilities, transnational family obligations, and the construction of identity. Although members of the ABC class are eligible for formal employment permission, the temporary designation of this status gives employers an upper hand in setting the employment parameters of Salvadorans. For example, one factory worker in the ABC class told us that although her status allows her to work legally, it also leads her to accept an unjust and unsafe employment situation rather than change jobs or demand benefits.

Crucially, for members of the ABC class, a successful application for status adjustment (that is, permanent residence and eligibility for citizenship) turns on the ability to be able (among other things) to articulate to INS good moral character and the potential to be a productive law-abiding citizen. The need to construct a kind of idealized identity means that INS practices become a kind of panoptic that frames individual and community strategies (Coutin 1998; Foucault 1977). Indeed, the Salvadorans we spoke with believed that in order to continue living their lives in the US they must actively construct their identities to mirror an idealized US norm. We argue that the prospect of an INS interview disciplines Salvadorans into making particular economic, geographic, and health choices in support of this constructed identity.

Salvadoran women's health and health care patterns

Semi-structured and in-depth interviews suggested that Salvadorans' main health concerns include catastrophic health events, workplace injuries, asthmatic and respiratory diseases, and fatigue. Pregnancy and childbirth were the health conditions that most often led Salvadoran women to seek medical attention. In common with uprooted populations, community leaders reported direct experience with, or knowledge of, individuals affected by psychological disorders associated with refugee-like experiences. These manifested as substance abuse, child abuse, and domestic violence.

Women respondents mentioned workplace conditions and injuries as sources of health problems. Typical is the experience of this 31-year-old woman who is part of the ABC class and who works in a clothing factory:

> I work in embroidery, doing the same task over and over. This work has ruined my eyes, and now I need to buy glasses. My employer doesn't pay for this. Now I can't even see to drive without them.

This same worker also recounted how she suffers from severe asthma, a condition that first developed in El Salvador, but has been aggravated by her current job conditions. She works for forty hours a week in the summer, but is required to work sixty hours each week during the busier winter season. Her respiratory condition is at its worst in the winter, at the same time when she is forced to work overtime. Her boss threatens to terminate her if she is absent, and thus she explains that often she is "working sick."

During times of medical emergency, our respondents chose fee-for-service doctors located in the local area. This ABC class woman is typical:

> In January, I was coughing up blood. My husband was so nervous that he was shaking. He told me go to the hospital, but I said no, it was too expensive. So I went to a doctor instead.

Many of the doctors' offices are located along Bergenline Avenue, the main commercial strip and focal point for Salvadoran social and economic life in Hudson County, and they occupy storefronts beside restaurants and shops. Indeed, this high concentration of offices hampered the application one local Community Action Center made for the funding of its health program (Phaire, personal communication, 1998). However, the fee structure makes most doctors' offices an expensive option for Salvadorans. For example, of 115 area doctors surveyed in 1994, only three accepted Medicaid.

Nearby community health clinics were rarely, if ever, used by Salvadorans in Hudson County, despite the presence of specialized services and subsidized treatment options in these clinics. This finding is in stark contrast to prior research that reports a tendency for immigrants to use such community health clinics (Chavez *et al.* 1997) in addition to emergency rooms (ibid.; Zambrana *et al.* 1994). Low utilization may be linked to the lower accessibility of these clinics compared with the proximity of fee-for-service providers on Bergenline Avenue. However, local officials told us of their efforts to publicize and legitimize this community resource. For example, at the opening of a new community health center, the mayors of several towns addressed an audience in both Spanish and English, emphasizing the value of public health facilities that serve all residents of Hudson County.

Given this pattern of fee-for-service health care utilization, it is perhaps not surprising that an overwhelming majority of our respondents told us they postpone non-emergency health care and, unless they are covered by health insurance, do not seek preventive health care options. Indeed, fearing the high cost of operations, hospital stays, and medications, some Salvadorans told us they were postponing indefinitely costly medical procedures until such time as they could legally return to El Salvador, where the expense was much less. Others, often with bad experiences of US health care, indicated that they send for medicines from El Salvador to treat health conditions. For example, one uninsured 38-year-old mother who was part of the ABC class now uses medicine from El Salvador because she does not trust US health care after paying for expensive and ineffective treatments for her son's bronchitis. Other communities with legal recourse to transnational migration strategies (for example, Puerto Ricans in New York City) also make use of medicines imported from home areas.

The semi-structured and in-depth interviews also indicated that Salvadoran women were more likely to meet with health providers than were men. Furthermore, women were usually responsible for all interactions with social services, particularly as pregnancy is an avenue into the health system and social services. Social workers in the area also report that women were less likely to be "harassed" by social security and also qualify for more services, so they were more likely to be sent by the household to seek care.

Information as a barrier to health care

Throughout our fieldwork we were struck by the confusion and misinformation that characterized Salvadorans' knowledge of the health system. While the marginalization of the Salvadoran community – linguistically, culturally, and politically – contributes to the prevalence of incorrect information about the resources available to Salvadorans in Hudson County, the disciplining effect of uncertain legal status also frames the individual and collective strategies for sharing potentially helpful information.

Prior research has identified how the lack of Spanish-speaking and Latino staff acts as a barrier to care (Zambrana *et al.* 1994). The language barrier likewise prevents Salvadorans from accessing health resources in Hudson County, and also results in confusion and mistrust during health care encounters. This confusion surrounded health insurance, health care rights, and government assistance. For example, we saw confusion over what insurance covers, who is eligible, and how the process works. In an often-repeated example, two Salvadorans described hospital visits for severe migraines and a sports injury during which they were "given a Tylenol" and then charged several hundred dollars. Similar stories of expensive and useless hospital visits spread easily through the Salvadoran community. Accounts of (negative) experiences with hospitals, social services, or public health centers get generalized to all such institutions, with few distinctions made between them. Salvadorans told us that these accounts were good reasons for avoiding medical treatment and distrusting hospitals and doctors.

Some (mis)understanding of basic rights derives from the inappropriate application of information from one place to another. In this regard, Proposition 187, passed by California voters in 1994 to require publicly funded health care sites to refuse care to illegal immigrants and report them to INS (Ziv and Lo 1995), is an example. One informant regarded Proposition 187 as a part of the US welfare system, which also encompassed all public health and community health centers, including those privately funded. Another informant referred specifically to Proposition 187 in expressing her concerns about access to health care in Hudson County. These examples reflect the perception that a California policy also applied in Hudson County, New Jersey. Moss *et al.* (1996) reported that Proposition 187 represented a specific bias toward, and attack on, Latinas in particular, and exacerbated their feelings of social and economic marginalization.

Salvadorans were also uncertain about the relationship between (federal) social security provisions and the use of community health facilities. One pregnant 28-year-old undocumented Salvadoran woman described a recent experience in a community health clinic in the following way:

> When I went for treatment in the clinic, they sent me to Social Security, who said they have a rule about qualifying, and we don't qualify. So we cannot use *this clinic* anymore. [emphasis added]

Her words indicate a misunderstanding of the relationship between the (institutionally separate) community health clinic and Social Security office. In this instance we believe that the provider at the health center suggested that she go to Social Security to determine if her child would qualify for (federal) assistance. Upon finding out that her child did not qualify under federal guidelines, the woman was reluctant to return to the clinic because she assumed it operated on the same metric. However, she would not have been turned away from the community health center, as here all patients are assessed according to their ability to pay.

What emerged during the fieldwork is the view that, for Salvadorans, health care is a private/individual concern, and not yet a public/community matter. With regard to information sharing, Salvadorans indicated that they do not discuss with friends issues of preventive care, community health resources, insurance coverage, or specific health problems. There was also little indication of networking with co-workers, who are often Spanish-speaking Latino immigrants and another potential source for shared information concerning health insurance and workers' rights.

A Salvadoran father of three and member of the ABC class expressed his frustration at the current lack of access to health care information:

> This is what we want – to learn how to prevent. What we are doing now is the minimum prevention. If we knew more, we would do more, true? Here in this country is all of the information. What is lacking is a contact, to be able to access all of the information there is. To have access to people who know where one can find this information.

Although individual Salvadorans spoke of the importance and gravity of health issues, a clear community consensus on, for example, how to improve health care access, had not yet arisen. The same man explained:

> Here [the community organization] is the only source for information. This is the closest source to us for information. But although there is this fear [about health care and illness], people haven't been coming to meetings. But now [the organization] is working better. For example . . . the program for health, is very important.

While previous literature documents the importance of social networks among immigrants (Lynam 1985) and Central Americans in particular (Leslie 1992), our interviews and observations suggest that permanent temporariness continues to limit the utility of social networks for sharing health information. Salvadorans in general live with a sense of powerlessness regarding their rights in the US. Salvadorans in Hudson County may be in a weak position to make demands for basic benefits because they are only one small group of many Latino immigrants, both undocumented and documented, who live and work in Hudson County.

Legal status and labor market conditions make it unlikely that worker organizations can effect change in the near future. There seem to be many obstacles to such organizing, as amplified in a discussion with a trash collector who had been on the job for one year and had yet to discuss employee benefits with co-workers:

> There are people of different nationalities at this job. I don't speak with them in relation to this. Perhaps when I have more time with the company I will get this. The company is being bought out, and I spoke with one of the new owners, and they told me they have a good medical plan for their workers but I am waiting for that.

Material conditions

Our semi-structured and in-depth interviews revealed how Salvadorans' economic marginalization was bound up with their health concerns. This relationship unfolds in a number of ways. As Salvadoran wages are low and medical expenses are high, many Salvadorans take on long-term medical debt or postpone treatment. Women are especially vulnerable in this regard as they earn less than men (the results of the intercept survey showed that working women earned an average of $287 per week while working men earned an average of $462 per week). One Salvadoran man in the ABC class told us:

> I pay $800 for this apartment, electricity and gas. Every month $800. I earn to survive and pay for this, but if I get sick there is no money. If I have a car it is necessary for my work. Vehicle, rent, food – there is money, but it is hard to save money for a medical problem.

We spoke to Salvadorans currently paying anywhere between $50 and $500 in medical bills each month to cover previously incurred costs of treatment.

Like many immigrants, Salvadorans have low rates of health insurance: 41 percent of the ABC class Salvadorans who completed the intercept survey reported having health insurance, under half the prevailing national level (US Bureau of the Census 1998). There was no difference in rates of health insurance between women and men. These low rates of insurance were linked to the types of work Salvadorans perform, the high rates of turnover in these positions and sectors, and discrimination against Salvadorans on account of their legal status. A 40-year-old Salvadoran woman we spoke with had worked in the same factory for the past four years, and was still awaiting employee health benefits. We also found that turnover was often precipitated by health problems at work, suggestive of a negative spiral of poor health, limited health care, and fewer employment opportunities.

Among those who do have insurance we heard stories of unfavorable coverage provisions. Policies have high deductibles or may not cover pre-existing conditions and non-emergency visits. Typical here is the experience of this middle-aged male Salvadoran worker who was part of the ABC class, who explained that his persistent backache, made worse by heavy lifting on the job, was not covered for treatment:

> They [the employer] don't give me much protection. When someone falls, you get the insurance to go to the hospital. In an emergency, yes. But a problem like this, not a fall on the job, it doesn't cover you. I have had this job for one year, and I don't have anything.

Fear, invisibility, visibility, and identity

Our informants told us repeatedly that fear of contact with institutions remains a strong driver of health care behavior. As the following quote exemplifies, this fear arises in complex ways:

> One thinks "Oh my god, oh my god, please don't get sick, because I cannot pay for the hospital." This is a problem for me. It is mostly an economic problem, but it affects everything, because if I don't pay, I do not have a good reputation in this country. If the institutions here know that I cannot pay, they are going to think of me as a bad person. If I have credit, but I can't pay for the hospital, my credit is damaged. I am a person who works honestly and doesn't do wrong. If I don't pay, it is not because I don't want to, but because I can't. But they do not know the difference. One has to have a good reputation to present to immigration. If I don't pay the hospital, when I go to my interview for immigration, they will not think I am an honorable person here. They will think I am a person who is not working well here. All of this leaves you with a fear, do you understand?

Prior literature indicates that some immigrants provide false social security numbers and information to health care providers and social services to avoid identifying themselves to immigration authorities (Hilfinger Messias 1996). In a San Francisco study, 75 percent of undocumented Salvadoran women cited fear of deportation as the main barrier to seeking health care (Hogeland and Rosen 1990). Salvadoran informants provided new insight into how this fear affects health through the strategies they use to construct identities that are both invisible and visible. Two connected concerns influence how Salvadorans construct an appropriate identity.

First, the use of community resources for receiving health care is explicitly associated with welfare, and looked upon negatively. Thus, in the eyes of community health clinics, Salvadorans are largely invisible. In the eyes of ABC class Salvadorans, those who rely upon public resources – be they other Salvadorans from within the community who may be recently arrived and undocumented, or groups from outside the community (for example, African Americans) – are acting inappropriately. So while many women and their children qualify for social services and assistance for medical expenses, and Hudson County provides an affordable community health network catering to immigrants, ABC class Salvadorans tend to avoid these institutions. Citing American nativism and the negative portrayal of Latino immigrants as undocumented aliens who take advantage of the US welfare system, our respondents told us that their fear of being un-American by using social services has resulted in some families wanting to have children but deciding not to, because of fear of having to go on welfare. In this case, the stereotype of "international welfare migration" is completely reversed. Community leaders also spoke of a generalized distrust of government institutions which stemmed from the conditions of flight many in the ABC class experienced in El Salvador in the early 1980s.

Second, those Salvadorans in the ABC class anticipate their presentation before INS to adjust status, and as such strenuously avoid the use of charity, community health, or any social services, all of which are associated with public aid and being a public burden. However, we also heard from ABC respondents that having a US-born child in the family, and part of the INS application, could strengthen the chance of a successful outcome. We found Salvadorans seeking to make themselves visible to the INS and its disciplinary authority in very particular ways.

Emblematic of those subject to INS disciplinary power, this Salvadoran mother now "feels fear" because she once sought Medicaid benefits for her child:

> We feel fear because we received Medicaid for the child and this could trouble me when I go to immigration for my interview and they tell me that I received public assistance. This is something that will cause us problems. But the little girl has the right to be in a program, true? But if we do not [take advantage of social services for the child], then we sacrifice the little girl's health? But *thank god she is not sick*, for then we would have to PAY a doctor to get her vaccines and check-ups. [emphasis added]

This quote helps us understand how the interactions between Salvadorans and institutions are freighted with hidden disciplinary power that can be traced to legal standing and permanent temporariness. It reinforces the idea that many in the community see poor health as an individual's (or family's) burden, resolved by visiting a doctor's office and paying for the service.

Conclusion

Health and health care have become arenas of social control as Salvadorans with impermanent legal status in the US make themselves invisible and visible in particular ways as US residents and workers. Within the household, women are more likely to seek health care than are men, but neither women nor men who lack health insurance utilize preventive strategies. Indeed, some individuals postpone health interventions until such a time when they can return to El Salvador. There exists confusion about health rights, and health care information is locally based – mostly within walking distance of the home for those who lack access to a car and are unfamiliar with public transportation. Poor health is feared because it involves large, unpredictable outlays of resources, it increases dependency on others, and it undermines ability to work.

We characterize three ways in which disciplinary power affects health. These are: first, through limited information and limited opportunities for activism on health issues; second, through economic marginalization and intense financial pressures that derive from conditions of work in the US and the practice of remitting to support family and kin in El Salvador; third, through fear of institutional contact and construction of an identity that stressed self-reliance, non-dependency on state resources, and connections to the US.

Living in the shadow of the INS interview, current health care behaviors in this particular Salvadoran community may lead to a series of negative public health consequences in the medium and long run. ABC class Salvadorans in the US are especially susceptible to war-related medical insults that are often asymptomatic. For example, Gaffney *et al.* (1997) discuss post-traumatic stress among Salvadoran women, and Locke *et al.* (1996) have described the prevalence of previously undetected chronic illness and mental health problems in Central American women and children who are refugees of war. Health care workers emphasize the importance of the primary care physician in identifying these unique problems, and referring the patients for psychiatric evaluation. As many Hudson County Salvadorans see health care as involving a fee-for-service exchange, and not a long-term patient–doctor relationship, such health issues remain unaddressed.

Our fieldwork suggests that women may be especially at risk. The Salvadoran community largely consists of young adults in their twenties and thirties, and this means that women's age-specific risk of morbidity (and in some cases, mortality) is currently greater than men's (attributable to pregnancy and childbirth). By not having access to a regular source of care women may be putting themselves at risk in the long run. However, as health care is constructed as a private, fee-for-service good, and women earn sixty cents to the male dollar, it seems likely that women's access to primary health care will continue to be restricted.

Furthermore, some Salvadoran women may have a stronger application portfolio as foreign-born mothers of US-born children. But the pressures of constructing an idealized non-dependent identity lend more power to the disciplining force of the INS, prompting women to avoid preventive medicine for themselves, and thus increasing the risks of long-term poor health. We know that women are more likely than men to interact with social services, and saw above how at least one mother is already internalizing the stress of negotiating health care for her family and herself.

Acknowledgments

Grants from the National Science Foundation (SBR-9618317), and the Dickey Center, Rockefeller Center, and Rahr Endowment at Dartmouth College supported this research. The authors thank the editors for their helpful suggestions and remain responsible for the contents of the chapter.

Note

1   However, Fenton *et al.* (1997) conclude that only a small group of patients were likely deterred from using health clinics in low-income California neighborhoods following the passage of Proposition 187 in 1994.

References

Anderson, J. M. (1987) "Migration and health: perspectives on immigrant women," *Sociology of Health and Illness* 9, 4: 410–37.

—— (1991) "Immigrant women speak of chronic illness: the social construction of the devalued self," *Journal of Advanced Nursing* 16: 710–17.

Anderson, J. M., Blue, C., and Lau, A. (1991) "Women's perspectives on chronic illness: ethnicity, ideology, and restructuring of life," *Social Science and Medicine* 33, 2: 101–13.

Anderson, J. M., Wiggins, S., Rajwani, R., Holbrook, A., Blue, C., and Ng, M. (1995) "Living with a chronic illness: Chinese-Canadian and Euro-Canadian women with diabetes – exploring factors that influence management," *Social Science and Medicine* 41, 2: 181–95.

Anderson, L. M., Wood, D. L., and Sherbourne, C. D. (1997) "Maternal acculturation and childhood immunization levels among children in Latino families in Los Angeles," *American Journal of Public Health* 87, 12: 2018–21.

Brandon, K. (1999) "Immigrants worry that taking benefits may hurt chances for residency," *Chicago Tribune* January 6.

Chavez, L. R., Hubbell, A. F., Mishra, S. I., and Burciaga Valdez, R. (1997) "Undocumented Latina immigrants in Orange County, California: a comparative analysis," *International Migration Review* 31, 1: 88–107.

Cordero-Guzman, H. R., Grosfoguel, R., and Smith, R. (1997) "Transnational communities and the political economy of New York City in the 1990's," New York: New School Conference Proceedings (February 21–2).

Coutin, S. B. (1998) "From refugees to immigrants: the legalization strategies of Salvadoran immigrants and activists," *International Migration Review* 32, 4: 901–25.

Dorn, M. and Laws, G. (1994) "Social theory, body politics, and medical geography, extending Kearns's invitation," *Professional Geographer* 46, 1: 106–10.

Dyck, I. (1990) "Context, culture, and client: geography and the Health for All strategy," *The Canadian Geographer* 34, 4: 338–41.

—— (1992) "Health and health care experiences of the immigrant woman: questions of culture, context and gender," in M. V. Hayes, L. T. Foster, and H. S. Foster (eds) *Community, Environment and Health: Geographic Perspectives*, Victoria: University of Victoria Press: 231–56.

—— (1993) "Ethnography: a feminist method?", *The Canadian Geographer* 37, 1: 52–7.

Dyck, I., Lynam, J. M., and Anderson, J. M. (1995) "Women talking: creating knowledge through difference in cross-cultural research," *Women's Studies International Forum* 18, 5/6: 611–26.

Eyles, J. and Woods, K. J. (1983) *The Social Geography of Medicine and Health*, New York: St Martin's Press.

Fenton, J. J., Moss, N., Khalil, H. G., and Asch, S. (1997) "Effect of California's Proposition 187 on the use of primary care clinics," *Western Journal of Medicine* 166, 1: 16–20.

Flores, G. and Vega, L. R. (1998) "Barriers to health care access for Latino children: a review," *Family Medicine* 30, 3: 196–205.

Foucault, M. (1977) *Discipline and Punish*, London: Allen Lane.

Gaffney, K. F., Choi, E., Yi, K., Jones, G. B., Bowman, C., and Tavangar, N. N. (1997) "Stressful events among pregnant Salvadoran women: a cross-cultural comparison," *Journal of Obstetric, Gynecologic, and Neonatal Nursing* 26, 3: 303–10.

Gany, F. and De Bocanegra, H. T. (1996) "Overcoming barriers to improving the health of immigrant women," *Journal of the Medical Women's Association* 51, 4: 155–60.

Gesler, W. M. (1992) "Therapeutic landscapes: medical issues in light of the new cultural geography," *Social Science and Medicine* 34, 7: 735–46.

Guendelman, S., English, P., and Chavez, G. (1995) "Infants of Mexican immigrants: health status of an emerging population," *Medical Care* 33, 1: 41–52.

Halfon, N., Wood, D. L., Valdez, B., Pereyra, M., and Duan, N. (1997) "Medicaid enrollment and health services access by Latino children in inner-city Los Angeles," *Journal of the American Medical Association* 277, 8: 636–41.

Hilfinger Messias, D. K. (1996) "Concept development: exploring undocumentedness," *Scholarly Inquiry for Nursing Practice: An International Journal* 10, 3: 235–51.

Hogeland, C. and Rosen, K. (1990) *Dreams Lost, Dreams Found: Undocumented Women in the Land of Opportunity*, San Francisco: Coalition for Immigrants and Refugee Rights and Services.

Hubbell, F. A., Waitzkin, H., Mishra, S. I., Dombrink, J., and Chavez, J. R. (1991) "Access to medical care for documented and undocumented Latinos in a southern California county," *The Western Journal of Medicine* 154, 4: 414–17.

Kearns, R. A. (1993) "Place and health: towards a reformed medical geography," *Professional Geographer* 45, 2: 139–47.

—— (1995) "Medical geography – making a space for difference," *Progress in Human Geography* 19, 2: 251–9.

Leclere, F. B., Jensen, L., and Biddlecom, A. E. (1994) "Health care utilization, family context, and adaptation among immigrants to the United States," *Journal of Health and Social Behavior* 35: 370–84.

Leslie, L. A. (1992) "The role of informal support networks in the adjustment of Central-American immigrant families," *Journal of Community Psychology* 20, 3: 243–56.

Locke, C. J., Southwick, K., McCloskey, L. A., and Fernandez Esquer, M E. (1996) "The psychological and medical sequelae of war in Central American refugee mothers and children," *Archives of Pediatric and Adolescent Medicine* 150: 822–9.

Lynam, J. M. (1985) "Support networks developed by immigrant women," *Social Science and Medicine* 21, 3: 327–33.

McKendrick, J. H. (1999) "Multi-method research: an introduction to its application in population geography," *The Professional Geographer* 51, 1: 40–50.

McLafferty, S. (1995) "Counting for women," *The Professional Geographer* 47, 4: 436–42.

Mahler, S. (1995) *Salvadorans in Suburbia*, Needham Heights, MA: Allyn & Bacon.

Moss, N., Baumeister, L., and Biewener, J. (1996) "Perspectives of Latina immigrant women on Proposition 187," *Journal of the American Medical Women's Association* 51, 4: 161–5.

Mountz, A., Bailey, A. J., Wright, R. A., and Miyares, I. (2000) "Methodologically becoming: power, knowledge, and politics in the field," unpublished manuscript, University of British Columbia.

Ong, A. (1995) "Making the biopolitical subject: Cambodian immigrants, refugee medicine and cultural citizenship in California," *Social Science and Medicine* 40, 9: 1243–57.

Phaire, Barbara. Personal communication, July 20, 1998.

Red Nacional de Organizaciones Salvadoreñas en los Estados Unidos (1997) *Information Bulletin*, Washington, DC.

Repak, T. A. (1995) *Waiting on Washington: Central American Workers in the Nation's Capital*, Philadelphia, PA: Temple University Press.

US Bureau of the Census (1998) *Current Population Survey (March)*, Washington, DC: Government Printing Office.

Vedsted-Hansen, J. (1994) "The legal conditions of refugees in Denmark," *Journal of Refugee Studies* 7: 249–59.

Wilson, D. (1995) "Women's roles and women's health: the effect of immigration on Latina women," *Women's Health International* 5, 1: 8–13.

Zambrana, R. E., Ell, K., Dorrington, C., Wachsman, L., and Hodge, D. (1994) "The relationship between psychosocial status of immigrant Latino mothers and use of emergency pediatric services," *Health and Social Work* 19, 2: 93–102.

Ziv, T. A. and Lo, B. (1995) "Denial of care to illegal immigrants: Proposition 187 in California," *New England Journal of Medicine* 332: 1095–8.

8   Babies and borderlands

Factors that influence Sonoran
women's decision to seek prenatal
care in southern Arizona

Cynthia Pope

We didn't cross the border, the border crossed us.
(Chicano activist slogan, Martinez 1995)

The US–Mexico border region can be characterized by social contradictions: by islands of wealth situated in a sea of poverty, by a constant flow of people and trucks across the border side by side with some people who have never crossed (Eisele 1999), by newly arrived immigrants and long-established families. An additional contradiction is the intersection at the US–Mexico border of two very different health care paradigms, one system consisting of privatized medical care and the other socialized. Some Mexican women, in spite of having free access to health care in Mexico, seek medical services in the US. It is this final paradox that led me to question the factors that influence or hinder Mexican women's decision to cross the border for prenatal care. I use this medical time frame because crossing the border to have babies who can then potentially become US citizens has been a recent source of contention in popular media, international politics, and scholarly debates (Brimelow 1995; Hinojosa and Schey 1995; Idelson 1995; Martinez 1995; Ocasio 1995; Skolnick 1995).

The purpose of this chapter is to understand the factors that encouraged Mexican women to or prevented them from making a "temporary crossing" of the border into the US for prenatal care services. I define a "temporary crossing" as a crossing of the international border with a duration from several hours to several days and a return to the Mexican side. I conducted forty-two interviews in two locations with Sonoran women who received prenatal care on the US side of the border at some point in their lives. In addition, I interviewed health care administrators, lay health educators (*promotoras*), and grassroots workers and visited the Mexican side of the border several times to examine the conditions under which some of the participants were living. I used the sister cities of Nogales, Arizona, USA and Nogales, Sonora, Mexico (hereafter referred to as "Ambos Nogales" ("both Nogales")) as a case study to understand if the negative images of Mexican women illegally crossing the border to give birth in the US in any way depicted life in what has been described to me as a traditionally harmonious region due to shared culture, history, and, in many cases, relatives on both sides of the Nogales border. Some of the interview responses were consistent with those in previous studies conducted in the border region (such as a reason given for crossing the border being because of more advanced tests and equipment), but many answers dispel common myths about Mexican women who cross the border. The findings indicate that there is great socio-economic diversity within this cohort and that health care providers frame health care access in community terms; they see Ambos Nogales as a singular community with cultural and historical ties that defy the arbitrarily defined political boundary.

Conceptual framework

The process of crossing from Sonora into Arizona for prenatal care must be understood in its socio-political context. Mexican immigration to the US is arguably one of the most contentious issues in the shared history of the two countries (Dillon 1997; Martínez 1994). New immigration laws are being swiftly passed in the US to restrict Mexican immigration, documented and undocumented, into the country (Golden 1996; Hartman 1996; Hinojosa and Schey 1995; Idelson 1995). To this end, the border itself has become increasingly fortified with physical barriers and border patrol personnel to become what Dunn (1996) characterizes as a military zone meant to deter, amongst other things, the (commonly misperceived) practice of Mexican women crossing the border to give birth to children in the US in order to receive government benefits for the family.

Although scholars have extensively studied the daily and seasonal crossing patterns of Mexican male workers (Bustamante and Cornelius 1989; Herzog 1990), few comprehensive studies of this nature have been conducted addressing Mexican female migrants who cross the border on a temporary basis. Even less research has addressed the border region of Arizona and Sonora, an area that has become increasingly important economically and politically as a major crossing point for produce and individuals and the site of a maquila (foreign-owned assembly plants) boom since the passage of NAFTA (Public Citizen 1996). In addition, while the issue of women crossing the international border to have children in the US has been the subject of considerable controversy in the popular press, little research has been conducted in this area until recently (see Woo Morales 1995). These studies and other works show that many times Mexican women cross not solely to deliver children, but also for prenatal care and other preventive services (Eskenazi *et al.* 1993; Guendelman 1991; Guendelman and Jasis 1990; Nichols 1992). Additional research claims that these services are crucial in maintaining the health of family members (BorderLines 1997: 1; Gallagher 1989; Luna Solorzano *et al.* 1993). For example, when a child or family member becomes ill, it is most likely to be the female in the household who will take that individual to the clinic or care for him or her at home (Brydon and Chant 1989; Zepeda Burkowitz 1993). Women's decisions to cross the border and their implications are complex.

While the literature cited is an important starting point to understand why Sonoran women seek health care in Arizona, I argue that newer frameworks informed by a "reformed medical geography" help to place this phenomenon into theoretical and empirical perspective. To understand this phenomenon and interpret its implications, I turn to emerging conceptual viewpoints in medical geography and public health. Medical geography is increasingly being understood as geographies of health, implying a more thorough theoretical understanding of the interrelation between an individual, social and physical environments, and state policies. This move was initiated by Robin Kearns (1993) and debated in the pages of the *Professional Geographer* in 1993, and the qualitative methodological implications of the debate were expanded upon in the same journal in 1999. In the debates, geographers called for an approach that included more social theory than was seen in traditional medical geography and a move to integrate qualitative methodologies. Dorn and Laws (1994) argued the relevance of social theories such as postmodernism and feminism in interpreting experiences of health and health care. With regard to women's access to health care, Dyck (1995) and Young (1999) note how women's health care decisions and experiences are embedded in the opportunities and constraints of their everyday lives.

In addition to health geographers, public health researchers have also recently acknowledged the need to include more social theory and the role of space and place in individuals' lives in order to provide the most effective health care possible (Iñiguez Rojas 1998; Levins 1998). Scholars in both disciplines agree with the need to examine health, disease, and health care access in a holistic manner that includes the impact of social processes such as immigration, poverty, and public health policy, and the role of place in health care issues. In that vein, concepts from feminist geography are useful in framing this study. Some key points that form the nexus of this study are the central role of understanding difference, focus on the community scale, and exposing women's voices and opinions that have generally gone unheard in much immigration and public health literature on the border and in the mass media. The concept of difference in this study will demonstrate that while the US–Mexico border region may be a culturally contiguous area (Heyman 1994; Martínez 1994), women's border-crossing/health-seeking behaviors are determined not solely by culture, but rather by a myriad of factors. In addition, feminist geographers have emphasized methodologies that incorporate the multiple and subjugated voices of women (and other "others") into the creation of the project in order to better understand a phenomenon and its political implications (Monk 1997; Oberhauser *et al.* forthcoming). In that vein, this project's overarching political and academic goals are to reveal opinions and experiences on the border that generally go unheard in the international political scene and in much scholarly literature, and to destabilize our traditional notions of international borders and women's roles in the Arizona–Sonora border area.

Study area

The population of Nogales, Arizona, is over 90 percent Mexican American, while that of Nogales, Sonora, is approximately 95 percent Mestizo, those of European and Indigenous descent (INS 1993). The regions are tied to each other by shared culture, economy, and demography. As is typical of most border cities, many families on the US side of the border in Nogales, Arizona, have relatives on the Mexican side whom they visit frequently, and vice versa (Dwyer 1994; Herzog 1990; Rubin-Kurtzman *et al.* 1996).

Nogales, Arizona, lies in Santa Cruz County and is home to approximately 30,000 people. Nogales, Sonora, as is typical of many border cities, has a larger population than its US sister city. Population estimates range from 107,000 (El Paso Community Foundation 1996) to 400,000 (Mack *et al.* 1996). People are drawn to these Northern Mexican border cities for work in maquilas (foreign-owned assembly plants), in the military, or for other economic opportunities that the border region offers. However, there is also a significant population in Ambos Nogales (the region comprising Nogales, Sonora, and Nogales, Arizona) of families that have lived in the area for several generations (Eisele 1999; Martínez 1994; Pope 1997).

Health care facilities in Ambos Nogales vary in size, technology, and services provided. The major providers in Nogales, Sonora, are the public health centers in various neighborhoods usually operated under IMSS, the Mexican social security organization. Also on the Mexican side are Red Cross and municipal hospitals, and private practitioners. In Nogales, Arizona, Mariposa Community Health Center is the center of preventive health services, although Carondelet Holy Cross Hospital, private doctors, and the monthly St Andrew's Crippled Children's Clinic operated out of an episcopal church are also frequented by patients from both sides of the line. Both Mariposa and Carondelet offer a wide range of preventive medical services as well as insurance programs for patients. They attend to patients from both sides of the border. St Andrew's is a clinic operated one day per month catering to children with acute and chronic medical conditions. The families that attend are almost exclusively from Mexico, and the care given by medical specialists from Southern Arizona is free of charge.

The Arizona–Sonora border region finds itself at the crossroads of two health care paradigms: a socialized health care system in Mexico and a privatized one in the US. The Mexican medical system provides universal health coverage either for a nominal fee or free of charge. It is a fairly integrated system of hospitals, rural clinics, private doctors, and outreach workers (*promotoras*) to provide medical services and education to the populace.[1] Public services and many medicines are provided free of charge or at very low cost (Borrell 1987); however, private doctors are available for a fee for those who want or need that option. The Mexican health system is becoming increasingly privatized and beginning to resemble its northern neighbor. For example, specialists charge for their services, a reason why some Mexican women choose to cross and use the services at St Andrew's Crippled Children's Clinic.

Despite the fact that access to health care in Mexico is intended to be universal as stated in Mexican policy, many women still choose to cross the border even though that decision may involve risks. This decision to cross for a service such as prenatal care that is already provided free of charge in their home country is complicated ard involves many factors. Reasons cited in past studies on health care usage as to why women *do* choose to cross include an existing doctor–patient relationship, referral from a Mexican doctor, or a personal referral from a family member living in the US (Denman Champion and Haro Encinas 1994; Eskenazi *et al.* 1993; Gallagher 1989). Documented reasons for not crossing northward include a fear of immigration officials, lack of financial resources or access to transportation, and a lack of time or patience to deal with border bureaucracy (Brose 1997; Luna Solorzano *et al.* 1993).

Methodology

To elucidate why women cross the border for prenatal care, I used a type of questionnaire that allowed women to respond to questions without being confined to scripted answers. This study was conducted from June, 1996 through February, 1997 by interviewing forty-two Sonoran residents who were either crossing the border for prenatal care at the time of the study or who had crossed in the past during previous pregnancies. I used a thirty-two-question open-ended survey instrument when soliciting information from the women and conducted semi-structured interviews with health care and policy practitioners in Nogales, Arizona, and Tucson, Arizona. The survey with the women elicited demographic and socio-economic information, border-crossing habits, access to the Arizona indigent health system (AHCCCS), cost of services, perception of quality of services on both sides of the border, services offered in Mexico and the US, experience with the US health system, and family and physician networks. The instrument was created with input from a grassroots bi-national NGO director who lives in the Ambos Nogales region, an experienced researcher in border health and culture at the Southwest Border Rural Health Office, a university professor, and a grassroots outreach educator in Ambos Nogales.

The methodology sounds straightforward but in reality highlights some of the difficulties of conducting research in a politically charged atmosphere and as an "outsider." For example, the original methodology of this project included an equal number of interviews with women living in Sonora who crossed the border as with those who did not cross. The study was to be based on the Sonoran side of the border. However, at the time there was increasing tension on the border with the passage of several new anti-immigration laws. Thus, even though I was accompanied to participants' houses by a well-known and respected grassroots organizer, the interviews generated few responses due to distrust of an outsider.

With the advice and permission of a health care administrator, I changed tactics and interviewed women at Mariposa Community Health Center and St Andrew's Crippled Children's Clinic on the northern side of the border. In order to gain the trust of participants and health care workers as well as understand some of the complexities of border life, I volunteered at the clinic during and after the study. While volunteering was useful, the logistics of interviewing did not give me as much time to speak with the participants as I would have liked. The interviews were conducted while women were waiting to see the doctor, so at times the responses were hurried and there was not time to ask follow-up questions.

The challenges in obtaining the information highlight that being an "outsider" (non-Mexican, Spanish-speaking) had both advantages and disadvantages for the outcome of this project. For example, I had to abandon the original methodology on the Sonoran side because of my outsider status. However, when working on the US side, I was able to gain the trust of participants by working as a volunteer in a health clinic. Seeing me as someone who did not have family ties to Mexican culture but who was interested in issues of social justice and health care access helped to create an atmosphere of trust.

Results and discussion

Demography of participants

In this section I note the socio-demographic characteristics of the participants, highlight differences among responses, and then address similarities in responses to suggest why some women cross the border for prenatal medical services. Each of the forty-two women interviewed for this study spoke Spanish as their first language, and the majority (thirty-five) were married. Since I was interested in women who were currently using the US system or had used it *in the past*, there was quite a difference in ages among the women; the participants ranged from 16 to 62 years old, with the majority being in their 20s and 30s. All had been born in Mexico, thirty-four in the state of Sonora. Sixteen had spent their entire life in the border region, while ten came to the border in 1985 or earlier, five between 1986 and 1990, and nine between 1991 and 1997. Four of those nine participants had recently crossed the border without proper documents and were not sure if they were going to stay in the US or return to Mexico. Two respondents were not living in the region and crossed the border only for the monthly St Andrew's Clinic, which provides specialist pediatric services free of charge and caters to those who cannot afford to pay for specialist services in Mexico. The majority of participants had three children or fewer.

Diversity among women

Diversity is an important aspect of this study. While trying to understand why women cross from Sonora into Arizona, I found the differences among answers and participants to be almost as important as the similarities. Some of the responses appear contradictory and need to be analyzed in more detail than this chapter allows, perhaps through another survey. The differences in responses, not just the similarities, may be integral to better understanding women's movement across the US–Mexico border for prenatal health care.

Economic diversity within this cohort demonstrates that not all women living in the border region are poor and without resources, but at the same time, not only the rich cross. Nineteen respondents stated either that they did not know the household income or that it was unstable. For those who knew, the average household incomes ranged from earning less than the Mexican minimum wage (25 Nuevo Pesos per day or about US $3.50 in 1997 when this study was conducted) to more than US $15,000 per year. The majority claimed that they did not work or worked at home tending to the house and children. Eleven of the respondents said they worked outside the home, four as masons, plumbers, or street vendors, and seven in offices. None of the seven worked for a maquila (foreign-owned assembly plant). The ten women with annual household incomes of US $5,000–$15,000 all had husbands working on the northern side of the border. The one participant with an annual household income greater than US $15,000 had a husband who owned a business in Nogales, Arizona. The best correlation between income and border crossing was that women at St Andrew's Clinic had the lowest incomes of the cohort.

Another aspect of diversity concerns the frequency of crossing the border on a temporary basis. Experiences ranged from having crossed the border once in her lifetime (a new patient for prenatal care at Mariposa Health Center) to crossing the border every day. The highest percentage (26 percent) crossed one to three times per week, and 32 percent of respondents said the crossing was specifically to visit family and friends, while 21 percent claimed that it was exclusively for medical care. The remaining responses included crossing for shopping, visiting a relative's workplace, and entertainment purposes (such as restaurants and bars).

Two questions that merit follow-up studies inquired about preference for the US health system over the Mexican one for prenatal care and about the advantages and disadvantages of each country's system. While all forty-two respondents used medical services in Arizona, only twenty-three stated a preference for the US system over the Mexican one. Fourteen were of the opinion that the health system was "better and more effective in general" in Arizona than Sonora. This seems to be a contradiction, though. If there is not a consensus of preference for the US system, then why cross in the first place?

I raise this issue again in response to a question about advantages and disadvantages of both countries' health systems, as they are reflected on the border. The majority of respondents answered that there were no disadvantages to either system or the doctors. However, when the informants did complain, a long wait was cited as a disadvantage of *both* systems, with waits ranging from thirty minutes to over two hours. The response to this question shows that disadvantages of the Mexican system did not incite women to cross, or at least it was not at the forefront of women's minds when this question was asked.

Another apparent contradiction that merits explanation is the fact that almost one-half would not necessarily use Arizona's or another state's medical services in the future, although they were using them at the time for prenatal care. Of the twenty-three who preferred receiving prenatal care in Arizona rather than in Sonora, the majority would choose to attend Mariposa Community Health Center. The next most popular answer was that usage would depend on the situation. When probed further about the "situation," answers included the necessity for future prenatal care, acute traumas, and cancer treatments. The latter two responses were provided by women who themselves or whose family members had been to Tucson, Arizona (approximately 90 km from the international border) for treatment at the University Medical Center.

Another difference which emerges is the distance traveled to the health care center in Arizona. Twenty-four respondents lived over 10 km from the various health centers, and only five lived within walking distance of the clinics or hospital. Defining the border area as a cultural zone extending from Hermosillo in Sonora to Tucson in Arizona, all of the participants live within the border area. However, many of them live sufficiently far away to question what other factors besides geographic proximity would influence a woman to cross the border, especially since many (sixteen) did not have private transportation and could only rely on Mariposa and St Andrew's courtesy transportation once they reached the northern side of the border.

Similarities among women: common reasons for crossing

These diverging responses and contradictions call for broader explanations to help to comprehend why women want to cross the border if they could legally receive prenatal care free of charge on the Mexican side during the time this study was conducted. As in permanent and seasonal migration, social networks play a role in temporary border crossing (Boyd 1989). This first link addresses the importance of personal networks in the border region, more specifically with family in the United States and friends' usage of the Arizona system. This may be the strongest explanation for crossing and it concurs with other studies conducted in various border regions (for example, Denman Champion and Haro Encinas 1994; Eskenazi *et al.* 1993; Guendelman 1991). In this sample, 81 percent of participants have family in the United States, with the majority of family members living in the Southern Arizona region. In addition to relatives in the US, a circle of friends who use the US system may be influential in decisions to cross the border, as they refer friends and relatives to specific doctors or health centers in the US. Attending a health center in Arizona can be combined with visits to families and friends, thereby making the task of crossing the border less onerous than if it were merely crossing for a doctor's appointment.

In addition, having family in the US affects more than the decision to cross the border for prenatal care. Indeed, family in the US can impact the cost of health care for Sonoran women by making some women with low incomes eligible for US state and federal social benefits, such as welfare and indigent health services. In fact, for some respondents access to Arizona's indigent health care program, AHCCCS (Arizona Health Care Cost Containment System, pronounced as "access"), was a motivation to cross in order to receive care from specialists or certain physicians not covered by the Mexican health network and who charge up-front for services. AHCCCS regulations state that recipients must be Arizona residents. However, as I have stated above, some Sonoran women with family in Southern Arizona apply for AHCCCS. In this study four respondents admitted to being enrolled in AHCCCS and using the addresses of relatives in Nogales, Arizona, to meet eligibility requirements. These participants were interviewed at Mariposa Community Health Center. AHCCCS guaranteed free health care on the northern side of the border for both preventive reasons and more acute problems. Some of these participants were considered to have "high risk" pregnancies and thus would have had to consult a costly private physician in Mexico. The other thirty-eight respondents who did not admit to having or seeking AHCCCS privileges could opt for Mariposa's insurance program, which is available to women of all income levels (Bernal 1997) or could attend St Andrew's Clinic for a pediatric specialist. The co-payments at Mariposa range from nothing to 90 percent of the actual cost of the visit depending on the client's annual income. Unlike in AHCCCS, access to the insurance plan or the health center itself is not dependent on any citizenship reviews. Further research calls for understanding in more depth the price differentials between Nogales, Arizona, and Nogales, Sonora, since the Mexican system is becoming more privatized and AHCCCS regulations change frequently (Freeman and Kirkman-Liff 1985).

With regards to the personal networks, it is important to note the role of health care providers in Nogales, Arizona, and their relationship with their patients as an impetus for crossing. Interviews with health care providers and administrators, as well as personal volunteer work in the region, revealed a strong commitment to providing health care access for women regardless of country of residence. Neither practitioners nor clinics ask for a woman's residency status (although the centers require an address). This willingness to treat women without overarching concern for place of residence is indicative of the philosophy that Nogales, Arizona, and Nogales, Sonora, should not be seen as two separate towns but rather "one community with a gate [border wall] cutting through it" (Swinehart 1997), a sentiment which was echoed by other health care practitioners and educators in the region.

In addition to creating economic access for some Sonoran and Arizona women in this study, the doctor–patient network is strengthened by a common language, and in many instances, a common culture. This common language is one of the main reasons why 70 percent of participants had used US services before they became pregnant. Indeed, most of the respondents had been involved with the US health network for more than two years at the time of the interviews. The pediatricians, health care administrators, and grassroots educators with whom I spoke were fluent in or at least comfortable with Spanish, and the majority of their patients were native Spanish speakers (all forty-two women in this study stated Spanish as their primary language). This contradicts other studies conducted in the border area (Guendelman and Jasis 1990; Luna Solorzano *et al.* 1993; Zaid *et al.* 1996) that cite a paucity of Spanish-speaking practitioners as an impediment to temporarily crossing the border for medical services.

This strong personal network may play a role in some of the women in this study crossing the border not only for prenatal care but also to give birth. While it was my initial desire to demonstrate that women are not flooding across the border solely to deliver children in the US hoping to become US citizens themselves, in this sample, several women *did* give birth to children in Southern Arizona. However, the answers prove to be more complicated than the question, exposing yet more intricacies to border crossing for prenatal care in Ambos Nogales.

Of this sample, eighteen participants who sought prenatal care in Arizona gave birth to all of their children in Arizona. Sixteen respondents gave birth exclusively in Sonora, while five delivered some of their children in the US and some in Mexico (the remaining three chose not to answer). One of the explanations for that behavior was that the location of delivery depended on which side of the border the obstetrician's office was located. In addition, some women believed that being able to enroll their children in the Arizona education system was the most important reason to deliver north of the line. In the Ambos Nogales region, it is not unusual for children with US citizenship to attend school in Nogales, Arizona, while living with their parents in Sonora. They and their parents legally cross the international border on a daily basis. Other participants wanted US citizenship for their children (although they did not admit to wanting it for themselves) because some of their relatives lived in Arizona and they wanted to keep the extended family together. None of the women in this cohort who delivered their babies in Arizona stayed in the US to raise their children. Future research is needed to determine in more detail how this type of decision is made with regards to economics, seasonal or permanent migration patterns, or other factors, especially as immigration laws in the US can sometimes change quickly. Specifically, more detailed ethnographic studies could determine why some women chose to deliver one child on one side of the border and other children on the other side.

Immigration status and health care access

No matter how or when one crosses the Nogales border, one cannot escape the intrusion of the border wall. While the North American Free Trade Agreement (NAFTA) has encouraged economic exchange and a loosening of tariffs between Mexico and the US, US immigration policies concentrate on prohibiting Mexicans from entering the US without certain documentation. Three US federal organizations exist to monitor the border wall. These are the Immigration and Naturalization Service (INS), the Customs Agency, and the Border Patrol. It is generally the INS agents who are responsible for granting or prohibiting access to cross from Mexico into the US. This agency processes passport applications and requests for a "mica," a border-crossing card (also referred to in English as a BCC) issued to Sonoran residents living within 25 km of the international border and valid for trips up to 25 km north of the border. The mica is valid for a person's lifetime and is obtained with sufficient paperwork to prove that the applicant will not migrate permanently to the US. In addition to the mica for temporary border crossing, Sonorans can also purchase visas for travels beyond the 25 km limit and can also obtain a special day-long pass, which can only be used in certain circumstances, such as for attending a health clinic.

This study's results indicate that sufficient pull factors of Arizona health care exist to overcome the fear of US officials confiscating documentation such as visas or border-crossing cards. Seven women stated that obtaining the necessary immigration papers and dealing with the border procedures were a negative aspect of using Arizona facilities and consulting Arizona physicians. Ironically, none of the remaining thirty-five participants listed immigration concerns as an impediment to future crossing even though several knew friends who had their documentation confiscated after not being able to pay for emergency room bills on-site at Tucson hospitals. Further questioning should be conducted as to why these participants felt safe crossing the border.

Several women were at various stages in the migration process, although all claimed to be Mexican citizens at the time of the interview. However, after conducting the interviews, their immigration status was difficult to ascertain without doubt. This is one of the hazards in working in a fieldsite as contentious as the US–Mexico border and with a topic as sensitive as border crossing. Some respondents claimed that they were working toward obtaining their green cards (permanent resident status) because of family in Nogales, Arizona, but worried how new US federal and Arizona state laws would affect border crossing and residency applications and, in turn, how this would affect their health care options. Several others claimed they never crossed unless they are granted a special day-long pass. The day-long pass was issued to these women at St Andrew's Clinic and was arranged through an agreement between Nogales INS and the directors of the clinic. Participants attending the other centers (Mariposa Community Health Center and Carondelet Hospital) possessed micas, which allowed them unlimited border crossings and could be confiscated in certain circumstances, such as if they traveled beyond the geographical limits without a visa. In spite of the increasing militarization of the border, the participants stated that the border wall cannot sever historical, social, and economic ties that the two Nogales share. Indeed, all forty-two participants said they would continue to cross, despite the fact that seven had friends who had their micas confiscated.

Conclusion

This study reveals the importance of understanding women's movements for prenatal care in the context of a border space linked by a common culture, thus challenging traditional notions of political geography at the US–Mexico border. It cannot be doubted that the Arizona–Sonora border indeed comprises a region with shared social and historical roots dating back before the current political boundary was drawn in the 1850s. However, some respondents' answers show that it is important to keep in mind the diversity and multiple dimensions of Sonoran women's experiences of crossing the border for health care usage and access within this cultural zone. Relying on current thinking in health geography and public health, I have demonstrated how themes of diversity, difference, and the importance of community-level observation interact with overarching political themes such as international immigration policy to influence or hinder women's northward temporary crossing of the Sonora–Arizona border.

This study highlights some important factors that Sonoran women take into consideration when crossing the border for prenatal services. These include a network of family, friends, and health care professionals; experience with the Arizona health care system; economic concerns; and immigration issues. Understanding the decision to cross the border temporarily is useful in enhancing current knowledge about the practical implications of border crossing as well as knowledge about women's health-seeking behaviors more generally.

In empirical terms, the data collected coincide in some ways with current understanding about health care usage in the borderlands, while also highlighting the diversity of experiences and opinions of clients within the Ambos Nogales area. For example, the finding that women cross the border because of their belief that the tests and equipment are more advanced in the US than in Mexico has been cited in other studies. In addition, personal networks (such as friends, family, and health practitioners) in Southern Arizona facilitated border crossing for some women. Some women also crossed because the medical services were less expensive in Arizona than in Sonora, a reason that has not been cited in other academic studies of this nature. For example, some participants attended St Andrew's Clinic, which is staffed by pediatric specialists whose services would have been prohibitively expensive in Mexico for the women I interviewed. At St Andrew's Clinic the services were offered free of charge. In contrast to findings in other studies, immigration was not a major concern for most women, which is surprising considering the increased vigilance on the part of the US at the Nogales border crossing point. However, this sample consisted of women who make the effort to cross the border. There are many more in Sonora who do not or cannot cross for health care. To aid in further understanding the topic, future research should concentrate on the other side of this study's coin – what factors prohibit women from crossing the border?

This study adds to our knowledge about women's health care usage in an international perspective and to the considerable feminist geography literature examining methodological issues and dilemmas (Jones *et al.* 1997). Concepts from feminist geography can help situate the implications of this study in a broader social context. Current feminist research themes, such as an understanding of difference and the consequent emphasis on the necessity for local scale and qualitative research (or a combination of qualitative and quantitative methods), are salient in this study. This project intends to open up the gendered process of decision making about health care in a highly contentious geographic region and, methodologically, highlights some of the dilemmas and implications of conducting research in different cultural areas. The methodology employed reveals the complexities in deciding to cross the Arizona–Sonora border, thus adding a new dimension to epidemiological studies about availability of health care and its use in the border area. One of the methodological considerations that shaped this study was the difficulty in recruiting participants and the impact that had on the outcome of the project. This aspect of geographic research merits further attention in methodological discussions, as the knowledge to which a researcher does not have access (due to cultural "outsider" status or immigration problems, for example) may be as revealing as the information collected. In addition, this study calls for an even more localized examination of border-crossing patterns. While I worked at the community level in Nogales, Arizona, enough discrepancies existed among locations that an even more localized scale may be useful, for example, conducting research in one center and thus gaining more detailed ethnographic information.

While this study highlights why some Sonoran women cross the border for prenatal care in Southern Arizona, the findings are limited to the subset of women who were willing and able to make the journey. The women who crossed either were economically able to cross, or accessed Arizona's health plan (AHCCCS) which required little or no co-payment, or attended St Andrew's Clinic where all services and some medications are provided free of charge. Due to time and financial constraints I could not interview women who do not cross the border. What they perceive as impediments to crossing and/or why they desire to stay on the Sonoran side of the border demands future research attention.

Note

1   See Solé (1993) for an organized history and description of the Mexican health system, as well as a study of US citizens who cross into Mexico for health care, a phenomenon which is encouraged by lower prices for prescription drugs and some services such as dentistry and cosmetic surgery (Borrell 1987).

References

Bernal, T. (1997) Personal Communication, Administrative Director of Mariposa Community Health Center, Nogales, Arizona.

BorderLines (1997) "Women on the border: needs and opportunities," *BorderLines: Information for Border and Cross-Border Organizers* 5, 4: 1, 4–5.

Borrell, J. (1987) "Psst, you wanna plastic surgeon?", *Time* 15 June: 60.

Boyd, M. (1989) "Family and personal networks in international migration: recent developments and new agendas," *International Migration Review* 23, 3: 638–70.

Brimelow, P. (1995) *Alien Nation*, New York: Random House.

Brose, L. (1997) "Socio-cultural barriers to preventive health care: HPV in Ambos Nogales," unpublished MA thesis, University of Arizona.

Brydon, L. and Chant, S. (1989) *Women in the Third World: Gender Issues in Rural and Urban Areas*, Aldershot: Edward Elgar.

Bustamante, J. S. and Cornelius, W. A. (1989) *Flujos migratorios Mexicanos hacia Estados Unidos*, Mexico City: Comisción sobre el futuro de las relaciones México–Estados Unidos.

Denman Champion, C. A. and Haro Encinas, J. A. (1994) "De la investigación a la acción. La revisión de la atención primaria a la salud en Nogales, Sonora," *Revista de El Colegio de Sonora* 7: 39–72

Dillon, S. (1997) "US–Mexico study sees exaggeration in migration data," *New York Times* 31 August: A1.

Dorn, M. and Laws, G. (1994) "Social theory, body politics, and medical geography: extending Kearns's invitation," *Professional Geographer* 46, 1: 106–10.

Dunn, T. J. (1996) *The Militarization of the US–Mexico Border 1978–1992*, Austin, TX: The Center for Mexican American Studies.

Dwyer, A. (1994) *On the Line: Life on the US–Mexico Border*, London: Latin American Bureau.

Dyck, I. (1995) "Putting chronic illness 'in place.' Women immigrants' accounts of their health care," *Geoforum* 26, 3: 247–60.

Eisele, K. (1999) "Landscapes of solidarity: children's perceptions of life on the US–Mexico border," unpublished MA thesis, University of Arizona.

El Paso Community Foundation (1996) *The Border/La Frontera: The United States/Mexico International Boundary*, El Paso: El Paso Community Foundation.

Eskenazi, B., Guendelman, S., and Elkin, E. P. (1993) "A preliminary study of reproductive outcomes of female *maquiladora* workers in Tijuana, Mexico," *American Journal of Industrial Medicine* 24: 667.

Freeman, H. and Kirkman-Liff, B. (1985) "Health care under AHCCCS: an examination of Arizona's alternative to Medicaid," *Health Services Research* 20, 3: 245–66.

Gallagher, K. (1989) *Use of Prenatal Services: Special Population Needs Assessment*, Tucson, AZ: Southwest Border Rural Health Research Center.

Golden, T. (1996) "In anti-immigrant storm, the pregnant wait," *New York Times*, National Edition, 16 October: A1, A14.

Guendelman, S. (1991) "Health care users residing on the Mexican border," *Medical Care* 29, 5: 419–29.

Guendelman, S. and Jasis, M. (1990) "Measuring Tijuana residents' choice of Mexico or US health care services," *Public Health Reports* 105, 6: 575–83.

Hartman, P. (1996) "Arrests of undocumented up 34 percent," *Tucson Citizen* 14 October: B1.

Herzog, L. (1990) *Where North Meets South: Cities, Space, and Politics on the US–Mexico Border*, Austin, TX: Center for Mexican American Studies, University of Texas at Austin.

Heyman, J. (1994) *Life and Labor on the Border: Working People of Northeastern Sonora, Mexico, 1886–1986*, Tucson: The University of Arizona Press.

Hinojosa, R. and Schey, P. (1995) "The faulty logic of the anti-immigration rhetoric," *NACLA Report on the Americas* 29, 3: 18–23.

Idelson, H. (1995) "House panel bill cracks down on legal and illegal entry," *Congressional Quarterly* 53, 28 (15 July): 2073–5.

Immigration and Naturalization Service (INS) Computer Database (1993) Nogales, Arizona.

Iñiguez Rojas, L. (1998) "Geography and health: themes and perspectives from Latin America," *Cadernos de Saude Publica/Reports in Public Health* 14, 4: 701–12.

Jones, J. P. III, Nast, H., and Roberts, S. (1997) "Introduction," in J. P. Jones III, H. Nast, and S. Roberts (eds) *Thresholds in Feminist Geography*, Lanhan, NJ: Rowman & Littlefield: 21–35.

Kearns, R. A. (1993) "Place and health: towards a reformed medical geography," *Professional Geographer* 45, 2: 139–47.

Levins, R. (1998) "Looking at the whole: toward a social ecology of health," Robert H. Ebert Health of the Future Lecture, Baltimore, MA: The Johns Hopkins University.

Luna Solorzano, M., Gonzalez-Marshall, S., Guernsey de Zapien, J., and Meister, J. (1993) *Cross-Border Referral for Prenatal Care: Development and Evaluation of Referral Networks*, Tucson, AZ: Southwest Border Rural Health Research Center.

Mack, M., Soloff, L., and Enriquez, R. (1996) *Arizona Border Environmental Health Resource Directory*, Phoenix, AZ: Arizona Department of Health Services.

Martínez, O. (1994) *Border People: Life and Society in the US–Mexico Borderlands*, Tucson: The University of Arizona Press.

Martinez, R. (1995) "Fighting 187: the different opposition strategies," *NACLA Report on the Americas* 29, 3: 29–32, 34.

Monk, J. (1997) *Geography: Discipline Analysis*, Women in the Curriculum series, Baltimore, MD: Uptown Press.

Nichols, A. W. (1992) "Health care," in V. K. Pavlakovich and M. A. Worden (eds) *Free Trade: Arizona at the Crossroads, Sixty-First Arizona Town Hall*, Tucson: The University of Arizona Press: 168–81, 207–8.

Oberhauser, A., Mains, S. *et al.* (forthcoming) in *Geography at the Dawn of the 21st Century*, Washington, DC: Association of American Geographers.

Ocasio, L. (1995) "The year of the immigrant as scapegoat," *NACLA Report on the Americas* 29, 2: 14–17.

Pope, C. K. (1997) "Babies and borderlands: factors that influence Sonorans' choice to seek prenatal care in Southern Arizona," unpublished MA thesis, University of Arizona.

Public Citizen's Global Trade Watch (1996) *NAFTA's Broken Promises: The Border Betrayed*, Washington, DC: Public Citizen Publications.

Rubin-Kurtzman, J., Ham-Charde, R., and Van Arsdol, Jr, M. (1996) "Population in trans-border regions: the Southern California–Baja California urban system," *International Migration Review* 30, 4: 1020–45.

Skolnick, A. (1995) "Crossing 'line on the map' in search of hope," *Journal of the American Medical Association* 273, 21: 1646–8.

Solé, C. (1993) "The Mexican health care system," in D. C. Warner and K. Reed (eds) *Health Care Across the Border: The Experience of US Citizens in Mexico*, Austin, TX: Lyndon B. Johnson School of Public Affairs, University of Texas at Austin.

Swinehart, L. A. (1997) Personal Communication, Director of Nursing, Carondelet Holy Cross Hospital, Nogales, Arizona.

Woo Morales, O. (1995) "Las mujeres mexicanas indocumentadas en la migración internacional y la movilidad transfronteriza," in O. Woo Morales (ed.) *Mujeres, migración y maquila*, Mexico City: El Colegio de Mexico.

Young, R. (1999) "Prioritizing family health needs: a time–space analysis of women's health-related behaviors," *Social Science and Medicine* 48: 797–813.

Zaid, A., Fullerton, J., and Moore, T. (1996) "Factors affecting access to prenatal care for US/Mexico border dwelling Hispanic women," *Journal of Nurse-Midwifery* 41, 4: 277–84.

Zepeda Burkowitz, M. (1993) "La mujer como eje de la salud familiar," in I. M. de Castro, E. Araoz Robles, and F. Aguilar Almada (eds) *Mujer: Salud y sexualidad, cultura, y participación social*, Hermosillo, Mexico: El Colegio de Sonora.

9 Differing access to social networks

Rural and urban women in India with reproductive tract infections and sexually transmitted diseases

Suprabha (Sue) Tripathi

Introduction

This chapter focuses on how women in India create and use social networks within gendered spaces to gain information and resolve problems related to reproductive tract infections (RTIs) and sexually transmitted diseases (STDs). In developing countries such as India, rural to urban migration is increasing the spread of STDs among women living in urban and rural areas (ICMR 1990; *Times of India* 2000). It is estimated that eight to ten million people in India, many of them women, will be infected with STDs by the year 2010 (Health Care Media Center India and WHO 1992). In India, women's knowledge of RTIs and STDs and utilization of medical care services reflect their status in society. Rural women are especially vulnerable to RTIs and STDs due to their subordinated social and economic status. Their perceptions of risk and their knowledge and skills in interpreting prevention methods are often inadequate. They frequently are blamed and stigmatized for having an STD and therefore do not obtain treatment. The emphasis of the chapter, therefore, is on rural women, although social networks of both rural and urban women are discussed.

The purpose and hope of this research are to help design intervention and prevention strategies that employ the language, symbols, and graphs women use to describe their diseases. The study creates a new conceptual approach that may help future researchers to understand culturally sensitive issues relevant to the prevention and treatment of STDs. It suggests that it is not sufficient to focus on high-risk groups or high-risk behavior, although these are certainly important, because the spread of STDs through the general population is linked to the status of women. Thus, knowledge of women's health problems and how they arise is important. In the chapter three key concepts – space, place, and health – are used to examine how women create and engender space; perceive RTIs and STDs; have differing access to medical services; and use four systems (kin, belief, traditional, and Western medical systems) to resolve problems related to RTIs and STDs. In exploring links between these, the chapter provides evidence that social networks in India are gendered, primarily due to the opportunities and constraints arising from women's different location from men in the social structure of Indian society. The use of social networks is critical to women with RTIs and STDs, especially among poor rural women, since their access to medical centers for RTIs and STDs is minimal.

Literature review

Although several micro-level studies have documented the different uses of health services by women in India (Das Gupta 1987; Leslie 1991), little community-based research on women's sexual problems in India has been undertaken. Consequently, these problems tend to remain invisible (Bang and Bang 1991). Studies on STDs and AIDS in India in the last decade focused primarily on patterns of sexual transmission of AIDS in urban India (Catterall 1982; Kapur 1982; Jeyasinghe *et al.* 1985; Mathai *et al.* 1990), women and their health problems (Daswani and Britto 1984; Chanana 1987; Meera 1990; Shiva 1992), and women's access to health care (Ramalingaswami 1987). At the turn of the last decade, there was a shift in research from patterns and modes of transmission to issues of sexuality and sexual behavior that included the urban poor and women in rural India (Bang *et al.* 1989; Elias 1991; Bhattacharya and Senapati 1993; George 1993; Grover *et al.* 1993; Nag 1993; Rao *et al.* 1993; Savara and Shreedhar 1993), perceptions and attitudes of rural and urban women on STDs and AIDS (Bang and Bang 1991; Pachauri 1992), and cultural contexts of sexual behavior (Basu 1990; Bang and Bang 1991; Ramachandran 1992; Khan 1993; Pachauri 1993, 1994a). In particular, pioneering work on women's perceptions of STDs in rural India involved research conducted by Bang *et al.* (1989), Bang and Bang (1991, 1994), Patel (1994), SEWA (1994), Narayan *et al.* (1994), and Patel *et al.* (1994). These studies indicated that a majority of women who suffered from one or more sexual problems never sought any treatment since services were insensitive to their needs and were culturally inappropriate (Favin 1990). These findings depict both the magnitude and neglect of women's STDs in rural India.

In addition, primary health care centers in India have meager provision for addressing the problem of STDs in rural areas. While there are 275 STD clinics in urban and rural areas, Jeyasinghe *et al.* (1985) and Mathai *et al.* (1990) report that only a third of all patients in the STD clinics are women. Since most of the STD clinics cannot afford to employ female doctors solely for women patients, many women might delay their visit and therefore treatment of the disease (Gittelsohn *et al.* 1994). Further, due to the stigma associated with STDs the majority of women do not attend these clinics. Consequently, diagnosis and treatment of women's sexual problems as well as documentation of epidemiological trends are very difficult. Moreover, the neglect of women's perspective in the design and implementation of India's health services has resulted in their under-utilization by women. Other factors that play an important role in the differential uses of health services by women are social, economic, and behavioral determinants such as discrimination against women, cost of health care, time cost, and a lack of information that may limit women's understanding of the benefit of health services.

Theoretical perspectives: patriarchy, a spatial framework

In India, social roles are defined largely on gender differentiated types of work, including, for example, the exclusive responsibility of women for childcare and domestic work. This gender division of labor is hierarchical, supported by notions of male superiority and privilege that go beyond sex differences to incorporate ideas about the "naturalness" of women's labor, their sexuality, and their role in human reproduction. The organization of society around such notions and the sustained privileging of men are incorporated in the concept of patriarchy. Yet, in using Western formulations of patriarchy in analysis, some of the special characteristics of Indian society must be kept in mind. Patriarchy in India includes age and caste, as well as gender stratification. Being part of an asymmetrical society with many caste-based occupations, women are viewed and treated primarily as sources of reproduction and labor to be exploited.

In India, gender relations are not identical to those associated with the capitalist mode of production but have beginnings in early kinship societies (Krishnaraj 1992). While men dominate women in all patriarchal societies, older women have special status and power over younger women in India. Paradoxically, there is also a strong notion of female sexuality as threatening to both males and females, and hence, the need for its control (Nadagouda *et al.* 1992). This is achieved through strict segregation of sexes so as to minimize social contact except among close kin. Women have the onus of guarding their honor, which is reinforced through dress (*purdah*), attitudes towards covering their body, restrictions on social interaction, and the division of labor in day-to-day life. Caste, religion, and cultural norms further determine role differentiation between men and women. Caste rules limit individual freedom for men and women through marriage regulation, restrictions on social and economic mobility and choice, and ritualistic norms prescribing purity and pollution. Although seclusion and controls on mobility effectively cut women off from many spheres of knowledge, interaction, and activity, they are able to create their own space and culture, working together as a family unit.

Understanding the roles of women will help in analyzing the demarcation of space by gender, which spheres of activity are dominated by men and women, and how women utilize their networks within their "space" to solve personal problems. In this sharply segregated society, women do many activities together or share them and have opportunities to develop a women's culture (Das 1976). Certain spheres of activity are clearly demarcated as women's (e.g. cooking, cleaning), and although functioning within an overwhelmingly male dominant system women have some power or autonomy.

For instance, while women are less likely to be involved in waged activities a large proportion, especially young women, are cultivators, vendors, and paid/unpaid laborers (Basu 1992). Thus although women are largely confined to maintaining the household, their "external" world is not limited to that of men. In the absence of men, who leave home for the day, women gather together in the fields, shops, streets, and at home in small groups to catch up on each other's lives, discussing the latest scandals, and attending to the myriad tasks that a labor-intensive and financially tight domestic economy demands. This is their space: a space dominated and controlled by women; a space without men. This division of space reflects and influences the sexual division of labor, women's roles, and separation of home life (unpaid labor) from work (paid labor). The interactions between groups of women in different places – at home, in the field, temple/mosque, and shopping center – are central to a woman's social network. These places are nodes of inter-action, a common ground on which to meet. A woman's social network therefore mirrors the beliefs and social customs of Indian society, the social and gender relations, and the segmentation of space. These networks bind women together in space and over time. Through these networks, women are bounded, shaped, and influenced by social relations and in turn, repro-duce and transform their spatial relations. This study was designed to investigate such social networks and how they were used by women in relationship to STDs.

Methodology

This study used qualitative and quantitative methods to map and interpret women's social networks for coping with STDs. Qualitative research methods involved the use of group discussion, key informant interviews, disease narratives, and disease scenarios, although only results from group discussion and key informant interviews are discussed here for purposes of brevity (Table 9.1). The ethnographic information reflected the terms, categories, meanings, and beliefs women had about sexually transmitted diseases. The emphasis was on gathering contextual data in the words and phrases of local people that provided information on the "hows" and "whys" of women's actions. While qualitative methods were used to understand the creation of and basis for women's social relationships, quantitative methods, specifically Q analysis, were used to map women's actual social networks in their search for "treatment." Q analysis provided information about the structures of women's social networks and the key people within those networks.

A survey questionnaire was administered to 172 rural women and 37 urban women who were infected with STDs. The women came from four districts of India: Faridabad, Haryana (rural); Haora, West Bengal (rural); North Arcot-Ambedkar, Tamil Nadu (rural and urban); and Pune, Maharashtra (urban) (Figure 9.1). The districts were chosen to represent the diversity of cultural and demographic conditions in different regions of India.

Table 9.1 Types of qualitative research methods used

Method	Respondents (N = 172 rural + 37urban)	Results
Group discussion for obtaining an overview of women's illnesses including reproductive tract infections and sexually transmitted diseases.	All rural women (172), social workers, block nurses, *dai* (midwife), informal leaders in the community (women), quacks, indigenous health practitioners, local touring medical doctor and assistant	Contextual information, citing common reproductive tract infections and sexually transmitted diseases
Key informant interviews and in-depth interviews for obtaining specialized information regarding women's diseases	Western medical practitioners, women at the STD/AIDS clinic, government hospital, private clinic (90)	Symptoms, causes, and treatment of sexually transmitted diseases

Access to medical records and the presence of STD/AIDS centers were also important factors in the choice of these four study areas. All four districts had at least one STD/AIDS center, government and private hospital. Each study area represented diverse cultural groups, with distinct kin practices which influenced the way women used their social networks to resolve problems related to RTIs and STDs. An additional reason for selecting these districts was to link the findings of this study to constructive programs through various action groups already in existence in these villages, such as in North Arcot-Ambedkar and Pune. The primary languages used to collect data were Hindi, Bengali, Marathi, and Tamil. While the author is fluent in the former two languages, interpreters were required for the translation of Marathi and Tamil into Hindi and/or English. In many cases, social workers, nurses, and accompanying doctors provided help in the translation.

Since state policies did not permit the author to conduct research in rural villages in Pune, urban women were included in the sample for this study area. Urban women were also included in the sample for North Arcot-Ambedkar. In both samples, approximately half of the women were casual sex workers (twenty of a total of thirty-six women in Pune, and seventeen of a total of thirty-eight women in North Arcot-Ambedkar) or prostitutes residing in urban centers. Consequently, their social networks do not reflect the typical networks of women in rural or urban India. This study therefore presents an interesting mix of two diverse social networks, those of casual sex workers and women belonging to other occupational groups within a specific social setting. Although this research provides a better understanding of how the broader social circumstances of women's lives affect their ability to promote their own health and that of their families, it does not aim to provide a comprehensive coverage of research needs for health problems of all poor rural women in India.

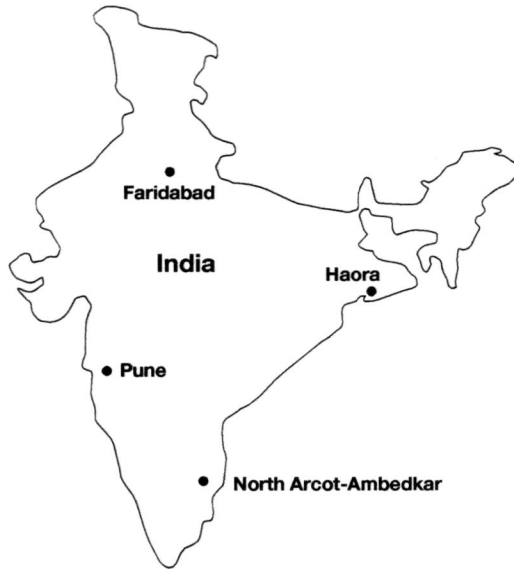

Figure 9.1 Faridabad, Haora, North Arcot-Ambedkar, and Pune districts, India.

Sample procedures and data collection

The hidden nature of STDs and women's limited access to health services made it difficult to identify a representative sample of women with STDs. Random sampling was not possible. Instead, information from health care providers, gained through purposive sampling, was used to select women to participate in the research. Approximately 40 percent of the women in the sample were chosen based on medical records. These were women with STDs who were attending the designated health facilities (hospitals, STD clinics, etc.) located in the four districts and villages. All of the women had been examined at these facilities in the previous six months. An additional group of women, approximately half the sample, was identified based on interviews with local social workers and block nurses who go on tours to villages. These health care providers were invaluable sources of information about women with STDs. They referred women to services and provided generic medicines to women with STDs. The remainder of the sample included women identified by other health providers including medical doctors, registered and unregistered practitioners, and indigenous doctors such as the *vaid*, *hakim*, and homeopath (Leslie 1976). These diverse sampling methods were followed in Faridabad and North Arcot-Ambedkar; however in Pune and Haora the sample was only drawn from STD clinics. Women over 16 years old who had a sexually transmitted disease in the past year or had symptoms of reproductive tract infection (RTI) or STD were included in the study. The questionnaire examined the current and past histories of women's experiences with RTI and

STD. Every possible effort was made to ensure that the individual and her family were not stigmatized, and the consent of each woman was obtained.

Religious and caste composition

The religious composition of women surveyed varied across the four study areas. Excluding those in Haora, the majority of the women in the study were Hindus (65 percent). Minority groups included Muslim *Meos* in Faridabad, Sunnis in Haora, North Arcot-Ambedkar, and Pune (30 percent), and Christian populations in North Arcot-Ambedkar (5 percent). Although *Meos* are Muslims, their characteristics are distinct from those of Sunni Muslims, whose religious practices are in accordance with Muslim customs. *Meos* claim their descent from Hindu ancestry and have distinct Hindu customs such as marriage practices. The presence of Christian populations in North Arcot-Ambedkar is historical and not atypical; it can be attributed to the spread of Christianity during the sixteenth century in the southern state of Tamil Nadu. Pune lies in the "Hindu belt," and had the largest concentration of Hindus in the sample.

In all four regions, the ranking of caste groups was religious, ritual, or secular. The most important criterion in caste ranking was the notion of "highness" or "lowness," grading the population into a hierarchical social order as upper caste (Brahmins, Kshatriyas, and Vaishyas, 25 percent) and lower-caste groups (scheduled castes, 38 percent). The formal ranking of castes was defined primarily in terms of the belief in ritual purity and pollution and rules of social distance between castes. Among Hindus, higher and lower sub-caste groups did not enter into hypergamous relationships, that is, they did not marry "higher" than the other sub-castes within their own caste group. The caste system was codified and adapted to local circumstances and was very distinctive in the villages.

Among the two minority religious groups in Haora and North Arcot-Ambedkar, namely Muslims and Christians, there was a widely held view that caste stratification is characteristic of Hindu social organization only. While rejecting the gradation of social groups on the basis of birth, Muslims and Christians accepted the social segmentation of the caste system as practiced among the Hindus and generally abided by its numerous restrictions. Caste restrictions included maintaining the social distance among ethnic groups, and the practices of endogamy (marriage practices within village) and commensality (practices of pollution and purity). Thus, the social stratification among these minority religious groups had an elusive quality to it since it had no systematic mythological and theological basis. In summary, the sample populations for Haora and North Arcot-Ambedkar were characterized by the presence of alternative religious identities, namely Christian and Islamic religious traditions. These religious traditions intersected with local configurations of power and Hindu principles of caste hierarchy creating a unique cultural context in each place.

Qualitative analysis

Group discussions and key informant interviews indicated how women perceived diseases. The following dominant trends emerged from such discussions.

First, women created a disease hierarchy in all four districts. They identified four diseases as common, recurring, and key RTIs and STDs: white discharge, syphilis, genital sores/warts, and HIV and AIDS. White discharge was viewed as the most common, recurring disease while HIV and AIDS comprised an unknown or deadly disease, depending on the level of information received by women within their social networks. These key diseases were associated with faulty diets, excess heat, body diseases (*ang rog*), general weakness, contraceptive methods, childbirth and abortion, menstruation, poor hygiene, and eating and sleeping habits.

Second, women viewed RTIs and STDs as natural phenomena, a woman's kismet or fate, and associated such diseases with religion, and the physical and social environment. These included witchcraft and the displeasure of deities. In particular, in Faridabad and Haora persistent cultural habits and beliefs about disease often delayed timely treatment. As the illness progressed, the causative agents of disease were associated with spirits, supernatural forces, and local gods and goddesses, especially by lower-caste groups. Upper-caste Hindus adhered to the principles of *dharma* (the moral and cosmological order) to get rid of the disease and rigidly followed prescribed ceremonies to appease the responsible gods/goddesses. In comparison, women in North Arcot-Ambedkar and Pune were more open to the ideas of Western medical practitioners. In all four districts, curative measures often centered on the strict control of diet and home-made remedies such as the intake of fennel seeds with sugar in water, milk, herbs, and other syrups.

Third, women's perception and information about diseases influenced the way women rated sexual diseases. Rating of STDs was linked to the frequency, degree of "pain," perception, and information about diseases. In particular, rural women in Faridabad and Haora rated STDs according to "perceived severity" of the disease, which was not based on scientific classification of diseases. As the frequency of disease increased, so did the perceived threat of the disease. Thus, recurring diseases such as white discharge and genital warts and sores were believed to be more severe than HIV and AIDS. Although traditional beliefs about diseases persisted, women in North Arcot-Ambedkar and Pune ranked diseases according to scientific classifications. In both districts, HIV and AIDS were ranked as most severe, "dangerous" diseases that endangered the lives of people.

Fourth, timely intervention from block nurses, social workers, and local medical doctors aided women with STDs to seek medical help in North Arcot-Ambedkar and Pune. The educational efforts of health personnel and social workers helped in dispelling myths about STDs. Yet, women had misconceptions about STDs. For instance, white discharge, a common RTI, was associated with weakness, backache, and painful menstruation, syphilis with excessive heat and consumption of hot, spicy food, and genital sores and warts with frequent intercourse, eating sweets, and problems related to child-bearing. While the majority of the sample population in North Arcot-Ambedkar and Pune stated that HIV and AIDS could be contracted by sexual transmission, blood transfusion, and infected needles, women in Faridabad believed that HIV and AIDS could also be transmitted through mosquito bites and coughing. Most women in Haora had not heard of the disease.

Fifth, treatments for all sexual diseases were based on women's previous experiences of responding to ill-health. Three main modalities of treatment were prevalent: use of home remedies, visits to traditional practitioners, and visits to Western medical practitioners. Specifically, in Faridabad and Haora, most women resorted to home remedies and traditional medical systems while in North Arcot-Ambedkar and Pune, women primarily used Western medical systems. Particular diets were followed by women to eliminate diseases. Following traditional customs, women felt the need to consume "cold" foods when they had these diseases since they felt such diseases were due to excessive heat in the body. Since shame prevented women from reporting symptoms of the disease to practitioners, home remedies were viewed as the first and, in many cases, the only treatment for common recurring diseases.

Sixth, women related that kinship and marriage patterns dictated their health-seeking behavior. They preferred to establish social relationships with female members of the same age, status, and caste, kin, or religious group. For certain STDs, such as HIV and AIDS, husbands were included in their social networks and were the primary source of contact with the "external" world. Several women felt that they had limited access to health care since most practitioners were male and discussion of STDs was taboo. In addition, their spatial mobility was restricted due to factors such as distance to STD center, stigma, and seclusion of women (*purdah*), which affected the way they sought treatment.

Quantitative analysis: Q analysis

Q analysis was used to map the social networks used by women in gaining information and treatment about STDs and to identify the key members of those networks. This technique involves analyzing the connections between individuals to identify how they structure their world through relationships via the use of symbols, graphs, and simple language (Gould *et al.* 1984). The method is based upon the rigorous definition of sets, the explicit specification of relations between sets, and the hierarchical ordering of elements in sets. In this research, "sets" refer to the four systems – kin, belief, traditional practitioner, and Western medical practitioner – with which women interact in dealing with STDs and RTIs (Figure 9.2). The "elements" of each set are the main people to whom women turn in describing symptoms, gathering information, and seeking medical help. The Q analysis methodology and

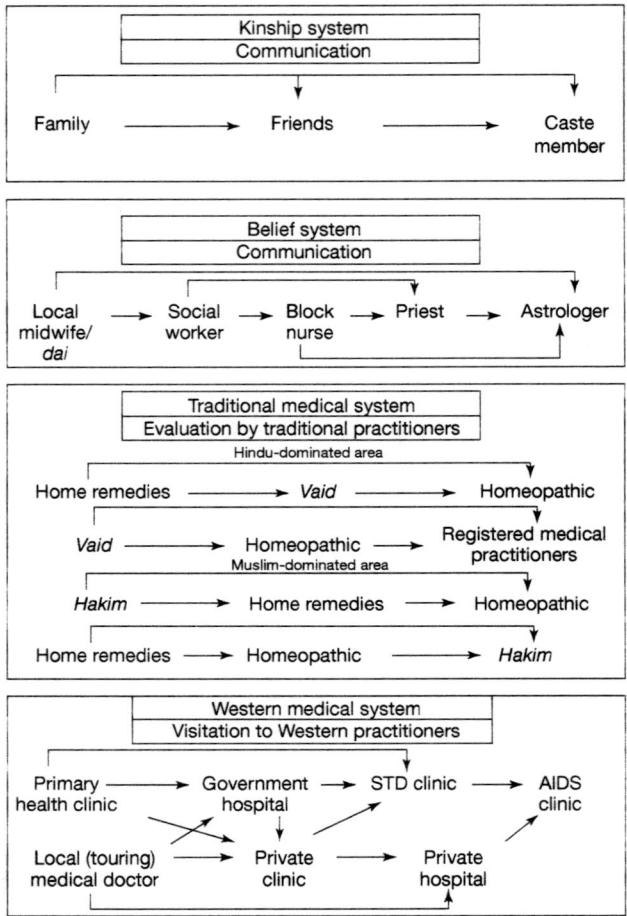

Figure 9.2 Social networks used by women for RTIs and STDs in Faridabad and Haora, India.

results are discussed in more detail in a related publication by the author (Tripathi 2000). In contrast, this chapter highlights general features of women's social networks and their links to place-based differences in culture, patriarchy, and social organization that exist in each of the four study areas.

In Q analysis, the relative importance of a particular system (set) in women's social networks is represented by its sample size which describes the number of times women interacted with members of the system. For example, in Faridabad the kin system had a sample size of 109 (Table 9.2). This means that the women in the Faridabad sample interacted with 109 kin members in addresssing STD/RTI problems. The fact that the sample size (109) is much larger than the total number of women in the Faridabad sample (86) shows the importance of the kin system in women's social networks. The sample size for the belief system was much smaller (21), indicating that it was a less important source of information and support than was the kin system.

Results from Q analysis show that women communicate most often with kin members of the same age, religion, and caste group for common diseases such as white discharge and genital sores and warts, particularly in Faridabad and Haora (Table 9.2). However, in North Arcot-Ambedkar and Pune, women also discuss their disease problem with social workers and occasionally with their mother-in-law. This indicates the open, informal relations women in North Arcot-Ambedkar and Pune have with their kin members and highlights the differences in the kinship structure between the regions. It is not uncommon to find marriages between parallel cousins in North Arcot-Ambedkar, which makes it easier for women to confide in their mother-in-law who could also be their aunt. Such marriages are unheard of and looked down upon in the north and east. Marriages between relatives

Table 9.2 Kin and belief systems used by women for all RTIs and STDs in Faridabad, Haora, North Arcot-Ambedkar, and Pune

Sample size	System	District	Variable X = diseases	Variable Y = members
109	kin	Faridabad	white discharge, chlamydia, viral hepatitis, vulvovaginitis, genital sores, HIV+, syphilis, chancroid	husband, friend, sister-in-law, mother, sister
21	belief		white discharge, gonorrhea, syphilis, genital sores	*dai* (midwife), nurse, priest, social worker, astrologer
61	kin and belief	Haora	white discharge, genital sores, genital warts, vulvovaginitis, genital lesions	husband, friend, mother, sister-in-law, mother-in-law, sister, *dai*
30	kin and belief (non-casual sex workers)	North Arcot-Ambedkar	white discharge, HIV+, genital ulcers, chancroid, syphilis	husband, friend, social worker, mother, mother-in-law
16	kin and belief (casual sex workers)		white discharge, HIV+, genital ulcers, chancroid, syphilis	friend, social worker, casual sex worker agent
13	kin and belief (non-casual sex workers)	Pune	HIV+, white discharge, venereal disease research laboratory, syphilis	husband, friend, mother, *dai*, sister-in-law

are rarely solemnized. The young bride is often far from her natal home and feels insecure about confiding in an unknown authority figure such as the mother-in-law, who is considered the kin member least likely to act as confidante for women in Faridabad and Haora. Among casual sex workers, women also depend on their agent, often regarded as the "mother" of the brothel, to communicate their problem (Table 9.2).

Few women discuss their problems with members of the belief system such as priests, astrologers, quacks, the local *bhagat* (prime devotee of God), and the midwife (*dai*). There is a belief among some Hindus in villages that astrologers can predict the *kismet* (fate) of the infected individual, that the *bhagat* has the power to appease deities, and that the Brahman or priest can diagnose diseases and recommend cures. However, in Faridabad, local midwives are primarily consulted as the severity of the disease increases, for diseases such as gonorrhea and syphilis. Block nurses and social workers are often viewed as members within the kin system and are important nodes of information in women's social networks (Table 9.2).

Traditional practitioners, such as the *vaid*, *hakim*, and homeopath, are more likely to treat women as the severity of the disease increases (Table 9.3). The selection of a practitioner depends primarily on religion and caste affiliation. Hindu women prefer to be evaluated by the *vaid*, Muslims by the *hakim*. Women from the same caste group prefer to visit practitioners belonging to the same or higher-caste group, especially the *vaid*, a Hindu in the upper-caste group. Women also seek help from other sources such as unregistered and registered practitioners. The use of such practitioners is greater in Faridabad and Haora where women's spatial mobility is limited due to the pronounced gendering of space. In particular, women are entrenched in the system of seclusion (*ghunghat/purdah*) which constrains them from seeking help. In addition, women's reproductive health is not viewed as something that needs attention. Women succumb to the dominant religious trends as seen in rural Haora, where Muslim women are dominated by a particular belief system that views women's reproductive health and its multitude problems as inconsequential. Also, "close knit" kin systems and "inward" beliefs that are rigid and relatively less open to change do not help in eliminating misconceptions about diseases.

Although formal and traditional health services are available in all four districts, the use of such services depended on financial and physical availability, level of education, belief, power relations within the family, status of women within the household, and women's perceptions of the threat of sexual diseases. In North Arcot-Ambedkar and Pune, approximately half the sample represents casual sexual workers who frequent formal health service centers. Even more intriguing is the use of such services by women who are not casual sex workers. Visits to the local STD center, and public and private institutions such as NARI and CMC are more common in North Arcot-Ambedkar and Pune, indicating the value these women attach to their reproductive health and to formal health services. In addition, they have higher

Table 9.3 Medical systems used by women for all RTIs and STDs in Faridabad, Haora, North Arcot-Ambedkar, and Pune

Sample size	System	District	Variable X = diseases	Variable Y = members
34	traditional medical	Faridabad	white discharge, vulvovaginitis, syphilis, gonorrhea, chlamydia, viral hepatitis, genital sores	unregistered medical practitioner, registered medical practitioner, *vaid*, homeopath, *hakim*
19	Western medical		white discharge, chlamydia, vulvovaginitis, genital sores, HIV+, viral hepatitis	primary health care center (PHC), STD center, touring medical representative, private hospital
25	traditional medical and Western medical	Haora	white discharge, genital sores	private registered medical practitioner, homeopath, *hakim*, government hospital
27	traditional medical and Western medical (non-casual sex workers)	North Arcot-Ambedkar	white discharge, HIV+, genital ulcers, chancroid, syphilis	STD center, private registered practitioner, private unregistered practitioner, Christian Medical College (CMC), touring medical representative
17	traditional medical and Western medical (casual sex workers)	North Arcot-Ambedkar	white discharge, HIV+, AIDS	STD center, private registered medical practitioner, Christian Medical College
30	traditional medical and Western medical (non-casual sex workers)	Pune	HIV+, white discharge, VDRL + (venereal disease research laboratory, serology for syphilis), syphilis	STD center, *vaid*, private unregistered practitioner, National AIDS Research Institute (NARI), *hakim*, PHC, private hospital
43	kin, traditional medical and Western medical (casual sex workers)	Pune	HIV+, white discharge	friend, STD center, private unregistered practitioner, casual sex worker agent, NARI

levels of education than the women in the other two study areas, and feel less threatened when evaluated by medical doctors. Even among the less fortunate, illiterate women, such as casual sex workers, visits to local STD centers are frequent. Yet, some women disregard their health. For such women, the constraints of other social systems such as *ghunghat/purdah* dominate their health-seeking behavior. The option to choose members within the social network thus depends on women's access to resources, their perceptions about the threat of the disease, and the beliefs and educational level of the women.

Women communicate with, consult, and are evaluated by members within the kin, belief, and traditional systems. Of all four systems, the use of kin members was most dominant in discussions about all diseases. Kin members, who usually belong to the same age, caste, religious, and occupational group, are invariably the first source of contact for most women. Within each system, use of members of the network reflects beliefs about femininity, as well as kinship and marriage structures. For instance, religious norms impede Muslim women in Haora from visiting male practitioners such as *hakims*; casual sex workers do not have access to kin members or traditional male practitioners for fear of ridicule; and rural women in Faridabad are fearful of attending the local STD center because of the stigma attached to STDs. In contrast, although women in North Arcot-Ambedkar and Pune have similar fears and reservations, their concerns about disease and the relatively looser social and cultural constraints in those areas enable them to use members of the Western medical system.

In conclusion, women in rural and urban India have differing knowledge of RTIs and STDs and use social networks differently in dealing with disease. Specifically, women in North Arcot-Ambedkar and Pune, as compared with women in Faridabad and Haora, have greater power in regards to their own health and bodies and exercise considerable decision-making power in conjunction with their husbands. Their ability to work as traders, teachers, and social workers within a dominant patriarchal system reflects the loosening of the strict regimentation of *ghunghat/purdah* in these areas. The system of *ghunghat/purdah* is one form of control within the patriarchal system which varies from place to place reflecting marriage and kinship patterns, differences between genders in power relations, cultural and social values, and women's work in and outside the home.

Conclusion

This chapter blends qualitative and quantitative information to examine the use of various social networks in addressing RTIs and STDs by rural and urban women in diverse regions of India. The qualitative analysis reveals women's perception about RTIs and STDS while the quantitative identifies the actual networks used by women in their health search. The findings emphasize social networks as a key information system for poor rural and urban women who do not have access to information and lack a regular source of health care. These social networks vary regionally and are defined by the social and cultural order specific to each geographic location. Social relations, rooted in place, affect women's actions, ideas, and experiences in coping with STDs.

The use of social networks depends on degree of illness and the social and cultural norms that dictate and shape the behavior of women. Such norms include processes through which a person perceives herself to be ill and chooses and implements strategies to facilitate the restoration of health. These processes are dependent on a large number of factors, such as the physical and social accessibility of traditional and Western medical practitioners, the degree of awareness of an individual towards the presence of health care services, the perception of what these services provide, and the socio-economic status of the individual. For many of the women in this study, poverty and cultural norms create barriers to the use of formal health care services, while social networks provide a means of circumventing these barriers and gaining access to information and treatment.

Looking beyond social networks, the findings of this research reveal that women's empowerment is an essential element for improving women's health in India. Social workers, health educators, block nurses, physicians, and volunteers interviewed during the course of this project emphasized the importance of providing opportunities for women in order to change traditional forms of health-seeking behavior and improve women's access to treatment. Their comments highlight the need for better employment opportunities where women are able to unite and organize themselves around health and social issues, along with improvements in health education and prevention. Changing social attitudes toward sexual diseases is also important. Recommended strategies include establishing HIV prevention training programs run by local *aganwadi* (social workers), involving local women in rural community health programs, enhancing social welfare and family planning programs, and linking family planning with health education. In the long term, any positive change that improves women's status in society will be beneficial, reducing the chances of women being at-risk for sexually transmitted diseases and making it easier for women to seek treatment. In summary, the status of women is crucial for controlling STDs, because it connects the many dimensions of women's lives and the social and spatial networks in which they are embedded.

Acknowledgments

This chapter is part of the author's doctoral dissertation, "Health seeking behavior of rural women in India with sexual diseases and reproductive tract infections." The study was conducted with the support of The National Science Foundation (SBR-9404823) and National Geographic Society (Ref. # 5363–94). The research is a product of the patience and guidance of Dr S. M. Bhardwaj, Professor, Kent State University, OH. Sincere thanks are extended to the Doctoral Dissertation Committee members, Drs Harvey,

Warf, Allensworth, Symons, Ritter, and Tyner. At a personal level, the author appreciates the support and enthusiasm of her parents and husband during her stay in India and during this research.

References

Bang, R. A., Bang, A. T., Baitule, M., Chaudhury, Y., Sarmukaddam, S., and Tale, O. (1989) "High prevalence of gynaecological diseases in rural Indian women," *The Lancet*, 14 January.

Bang, R. A. and Bang, A. T. (1991) "Why women hide them: rural women's viewpoint on reproductive tract infections," *Manushi*, 69: 27–30.

—— (1994) "Women's perceptions of white vaginal discharge: ethnographic data from rural Maharashtra," in J. Gittelsohn, M. Bentley, P. Pelto, M. Nag, S. Pachauri, A. Harrison, and L. Landman (eds) *Listening to Women Talk about their Health: Issues and Evidence from India*, The Ford Foundation, New Delhi: Har-Anand Publications: 79–94.

Basu, A. (1990) "Cultural influences in health care: two regional groups in India," *Studies in Family Planning* 21, 5: 275–86.

—— (1992) *Culture, the Status of Women and Demographic Behavior*, Oxford: Clarendon Press.

Bhardwaj, S. (1980) "Medical pluralism and homeopathy: a geographic perspective," *Social Science and Medicine* 14B: 209–16.

Bhattacharya, S. and Senapati, S. K. (1993) "A pilot study on the sexual practices of the sex worker in a redlight area of Calcutta," paper presented at the Workshop on Sexual Aspects of AIDS/STD Prevention in India, Tata Institute of Social Sciences, Bombay.

Caplan, P. (1985) *Class and Gender in India: Women and their Organizations in a South Indian City*, New York: Tavistock.

Catterall, R. D. (1982) "Sexually transmitted diseases in India and Sri Lanka," *British Journal of Venereal Disease* 58: 338–9.

Chanana, K. (ed.) (1987) *Socialization, Education and Women: Explorations in Gender Identity*, New Delhi: Orient Longman.

Das, V. (1976) "Indian women: work, power and status," in *From Purdah to Modernity*, New Delhi: Vikas Publishers.

Das Gupta, M. (1987) "Selective discrimination against female children in rural Punjab, India," *Population and Development Review* 13: 77–100.

Daswani, M. and Britto, G. A. A. (1984) *Women and Health: A Critical Review of Available Information in India*, Delhi: The Foundation for Research in Community Health.

Elias, C. (1991) *Sexually Transmitted Diseases and Reproductive Health in Women in Developing Countries*, The Population Council, Working Paper, no. 6.

Favin, M. (1990) *Behavioral Determinants of Maternal Health Care: Choices in Developing Countries*, Mothercare Project, Working Paper, no. 2.

George, A. (1993) "Understanding sexuality from the perspective of poor women of Bombay," paper presented at the Workshop on Sexual Aspects of AIDS/STD Prevention in India, Tata Institute of Social Sciences, Bombay.

Gittelsohn, J., Bentley, M., Pelto, P., Nag, M., Pachauri, S., Harrison, A., and Landman, L. (eds) (1994) *Listening to Women Talk about their Health: Issues and Evidence from India*, The Ford Foundation, New Delhi: Har-Anand Publications.

Gould, P., Johnson, J., and Chapman, G. (1984) *The Structure of Television*, London: Pion.

Grover, V., Indrayani, A., and Mullick, S. (1993) "Sexual behavior and use of condoms in a rural population," paper presented at the Workshop on Sexual Aspects of AIDS/STD Prevention in India, Tata Institute of Social Sciences, Bombay.

Health Care Media Center India and World Health Organization (WHO) (1992) *AIDS: The New Challenge*, New Delhi: Health Care Media Center India and WHO.

Indian Council of Medical Research (ICMR) (1990) "HIV infection in women," *ICMR Bulletin* 20, 11: 111–29.

Jeyasinghe, P., Ralilanaiah, T., and Fernandes, S. (1985) "Pattern of sexually trans-mitted diseases in Madurai, India," *Genitourinary Medicine* 61: 399–403.

Kapur, T. R. (1982) "Patterns of sexually transmitted diseases in India," *Indian Journal of Dermatology, Venereology and Leprosy* 58.

Khan, S. (1993) "Cultural contexts of sexual behaviors and identities and their impact upon HIV prevention models," paper presented at the Workshop on Sexual Aspects of AIDS/STD Prevention in India, Tata Institute of Social Sciences, Bombay.

Krishnaraj, M. (1987) "Health – a gender issue in India," in N. Desai and M. Krishnaraj (eds) *Women and Society*, New Delhi: Ajanta Publications.

—— (1992) "Theoretical perspectives and methodology for women's studies," *The Indian Journal of Social Work* 53, 3: 367–84.

Krishnaraj, M. and Chanana, K. (1989) *Gender and the Household Domain: Social and Cultural Dimensions*, New Delhi: Sage Publications.

Leslie, C. (1976) *Asian Medical Systems*, Los Angeles: University of California Press.

—— (1991) *Roles and Rituals for Hindu Women*, Rutherford: Fairleigh Dickenson University Press.

Mathai, R., Prasad, P., Jacob, M., Babu George, P., and Jacob, J. (1990) "HIV seropositivity among patients with STDs in Vellore," *Indian Journal of Medical Research* 91.

Meera, C. (1990) *Indian Women: Health and Productivity*, Women in Develop-ment Working Paper, Series 442, The World Bank, Washington, DC.

Nadagouda, S., Saroja, K., and Rao, A. (1992) "Influence of socio-economic factors on the employed Hindu woman's attitude towards dowry," *The Indian Journal of Social Work* 53: 4.

Nag, M. (1993) "Sexual behavior and AIDS in India: state of the art," paper presented at the Workshop on Sexual Aspects of AIDS/STD Prevention in India, Tata Institute of Social Sciences, Bombay.

Narayan, N., Srinivasa, S., and Prem Rajan, K. C. (1994) "Some experiences in the rapid assessment of women's perceptions of illness in rural and urban areas of Tamil Nadu," in J. Gittelsohn, M. Bentley, P. Pelto, M. Nag, S. Pachauri, A. Harrison, and L. Landman (eds) *Listening to Women Talk about their Health: Issues and Evidence from India*, The Ford Foundation, New Delhi: Har-Anand Publications: 67–78.

National AIDS Control Organization (NACO) (1995) *Country Scenario Update*, Delhi: Ministry of Health and Family Welfare, Government of India.

Pachauri, S. (1992) "Going to scale: NGO initiatives in community health," *Indian Association of Social Science Institutions Quarterly* 2, 2: 57–68.

—— (1993) "Relationship between AIDS and family planning programmes: a ratio-nale for developing integrated reproductive health services," paper presented at the Seminar on AIDS Impact and Prevention in the Developing World: The Contribution of Demography and Social Science, Annecy, France.

—— (1994a) "Women's reproductive health in India: research needs and priorities," in J. Gittelsohn, M. Bentley, P. Pelto, M. Nag, S. Pachauri, A. Harrison, and L. Landman (eds) *Listening to Women Talk about their Health: Issues and Evidence from India*. The Ford Foundation, New Delhi: Har-Anand Publications: 15–39.

—— (1994b) *Reaching India's Poor: Non-Governmental Approaches to Community Health*, New Delhi: Sage Publications.

Patel, B. C., Barge, S., Kolhe, R., and Sadhwani, H. (1994) "Listening to women talk about their reproductive health problems in the urban slums and rural areas of Baroda," in J. Gittelsohn, M. Bentley, P. Pelto, M. Nag, S. Pachauri, A. Harrison, and L. Landman (eds) *Listening to Women Talk about their Health: Issues and Evidence from India*, The Ford Fundation, New Delhi: Har-Anand Publications: 131–44.

Patel, P. (1994) "Illness beliefs and health seeking behavior of the Bhil women of Panchmahal District, Gujarat State," in J. Gittelsohn, M. Bentley, P. Pelto, M. Nag, S. Pachauri, A. Harrison, and L. Landman (eds) *Listening to Women Talk about their Health: Issues and Evidence from India*, The Ford Fundation, New Delhi: Har-Anand Publications: 55–66.

Ramachandran, P. (1992) "Women's vulnerability. AIDS: a symposium on the transmission, prevention and management of the pandemic," *Seminar 96*, August.

Ramalingaswami, P. (1987) "Women's access to health care," *Economic and Political Weekly*, 4 July: 1075–6.

Ramesh, A. and Hyma, B. (1981) "Traditional Indian medical systems as a field of study for medical geographers," *Geographica Medica* 11: 116–40.

Rao, A., Mishra, S. D., and Dey, A. (1993) "A study on sexual behavior patterns of truck drivers and helpers," paper presented at the Workshop on Sexual Aspects of AIDS/STD Prevention in India, Tata Institute of Social Sciences, Bombay.

Savara, M. and Shreedhar, C. R. (1993) "Sexual behavior patterns amongst men and women in Maharashtra: results of a survey," paper presented at the Workshop on Sexual Aspects of AIDS/STD Prevention in India, Tata Institute of Social Sciences, Bombay.

Shiva, M. (1992) "Women and health," in A. Mukhopadhyay and A. Goyal (eds) *State of India's Health*, New Delhi: Voluntary Health Association of India: 265–301.

Society for Education, Welfare and Action (SEWA) (1994) "Beliefs and behavior regarding diet during pregnancy in a rural area in Gujarat, Western India," in J. Gittelsohn, M. Bentley, P. Pelto, M. Nag, S. Pachauri, A. Harrison, and L. Landman (eds) (1994) *Listening to Women Talk about their Health: Issues and Evidence from India*, The Ford Foundation, New Delhi: Har-Anand Publications: 95–115.

Times of India (2000) "AIDS in India," 4 February, New Delhi.

Tripathi, S. (2000) "Health seeking behavior: Q structures of rural and urban women in India with sexually transmitted diseases and reproductive tract infections," *Professional Geographer* 32, 2: 218–32.

World Health Organization (1992) "Global programme on AIDS: current and future dimensions of the HIV/AIDS pandemic," *WHO/GPA/RES/SFI/92.1*, Geneva: Global Program on AIDS.

10 Walking the talk

Research partnerships in women's business in Australia

Lenore Manderson, Maureen Kirk, and Elizabeth Hoban

Introduction

The poor health of Indigenous Australians is a continuing scandal in contemporary Australia. While the infant mortality rate reduced significantly from the early 1970s, overall death rates are still almost four times higher for Indigenous Australians than for other Australians and only 4 percent of Indigenous Australians are aged 60 or older (compared with 15 percent of all Australians). The primary causes of death are heart disease, accidents and injuries, and respiratory diseases. Morbidity rates and hospitalization rates as well as mortality rates are higher among Indigenous than other Australians for a wide number of conditions including diabetes, respiratory diseases, complications of pregnancy, and diseases of the circulatory system (Harrison 1991: 154; Saggers and Gray 1991; Thomson 1991: 55). This chapter draws on our research with one disease that is particularly prevalent among Indigenous women: cervical cancer.

Mortality rates for cervical cancer among Indigenous women are four times those of non-Indigenous women Australia-wide (Jelfs 1995) (around 4.5 percent as compared with 1.1 percent in non-Indigenous women). In the northeast state of Queensland – where the research reported in this chapter was conducted – Indigenous women are ten times more likely than other women to die from cervical cancer (Queensland 1994). These rates may be associated with a high rate of sexually transmissible infections from early ages and lack of services for sexual health. But more generally, lack of access to health services and the lack of choice of services for diagnosis, treatment, follow-up, and care, for any health problem, result in delay in treatment seeking and poor adherence to therapeutic programs. In this chapter, we describe our study of barriers to the diagnosis and management of cervical cancer among Indigenous women in remote, rural, and urban areas of Queensland. A significant component of this chapter is concerned with the methods we used to work with women in communities diversely distributed across the state. Our ability to work with community women, by establishing research partnerships and networks at various levels, sites, and points of the project, was critical to our conduct of the study and our confidence in its findings. This chapter is therefore concerned with field ethics and reciprocity. Hence the title of this chapter: "Walking the talk." It is, as we shall illustrate, an expression that is an injunction to white Australian researchers participating in the reconciliation process.

The second focus of this chapter is the significance of place and space in women's use of health services. This influences women's readiness to participate in screening and to seek care. Indigenous affiliation with place is a familiar story, but the familiarity obscures the specific sensitivities associated with "women's business" – that is, women's health – and women's ability to participate in health programs without "shame," embarrassment, compromise, or fear. As we illustrate, the significance of place in ensuring access to care is not one of measurable distance but, rather, of social and functional distance and cultural safety (Dyck and Kearns 1995; Ramsden 1991). Women in urban centers do not necessarily enjoy better access to services, despite the numeric concentration of mainstream services in city areas of the state. Rather, Indigenous women throughout the state face logistical and personal difficulties presenting to their service of choice.

We conclude by exploring the implications of acknowledging the importance of "walking the talk," "women's business," and the importance of place – and the links between these acknowledgments and cultural safety in order to improve the delivery of health care to women.

The policy background of consultation

Australia's history of violent colonization, the oppression and lack of enfranchisement of its Indigenous populations, and the continuing failure of the state to redress this history has influenced Indigenous attitudes towards research and to white researchers in particular. Historically, much health research conducted with Indigenous Australians – both mainland Aboriginal populations and Torres Strait Island people – has been curiosity driven, without sustainable outcomes in terms of changes in government policy, programs, or health status. As a result, communities and individuals have been consistently uninterested in and often antagonistic to participating in or facilitating health or other research, or to being research subjects. They have, in addition, been critical of their lack of influence in determining research agendas, identifying appropriate approaches, collecting and maintaining data bases, and interpreting findings, and have expressed concern about their lack of ownership of their data. Yet various groups, including peak Indigenous bodies representing multiple organizations and special units of state and federal government departments of health, also acknowledge the need for research to collect information to develop new policies and programs, and hence to better deliver appropriate health and other services.

These contradictory attitudes towards research – a deep suspicion of the motives for research yet the urgent need for more – have found partial resolution at a federal government level. Specifically, consultations between

Indigenous Australians and the National Health and Medical Research Council (NHMRC) resulted in the development of policy and procedural guidelines to ensure that research practice honors the principle of community determination, ensures community involvement in formulating research questions and collecting data (biomedical and/or social), and ensures feedback and benefits to the community (NHMRC 1991; Rowse 1992). The NHMRC guidelines also acknowledge the ethical failures of academics in the past, and request that researchers negotiate their research topics with Indigenous participants and involve them in translating and executing the research protocol. Indigenous communities are also expected to play a role in controlling, interpreting, and disseminating information. This approach does not preclude scholarly inquiry. It does insist that researchers obtain the informed consent of Indigenous participants, that this is demonstrated, and that research findings are reported back to participants in a manner regarded as appropriate by the community. In gaining access to and informed consent from communities and individuals for research purposes, it is imperative too to demonstrate the utility of the research to the communities who might participate in a research project

Our interest in conducting research on cervical cancer reflects partnerships between the state government's department of health (specifically, the Women's Cancer Screening Service), academics, and the Indigenous women who facilitated and contributed to this work. The study of barriers to and appropriate delivery systems for cancer screening in Indigenous communities was conducted in response to the disproportionately high incidence of cervical cancer among Indigenous women, as noted above, but particularly also anecdotal evidence of its prevalence in very young women.

The study aimed to identify barriers to screening; review models of health service delivery to Indigenous women in Queensland and in other Australian states; make recommendations regarding appropriate strategies to provide educational and clinical services; and develop guidelines for a code of best practice in the delivery of health care services. The project therefore had practical outcomes that were intended to improve services for Indigenous women. However, these practical outcomes would not have been possible had the research been conducted without Indigenous consultation and involvement. The constant communication among all participants in the study – that is, among government sponsors of the research, the academics involved, and Indigenous women – ensured both ownership of and commitment to act on its findings.

Defining the parameters of the study

The research protocol was developed on the initiative of Maureen Kirk, and followed her preliminary consultations with Indigenous women over a period of eighteen months. During this period the research team (Manderson, Kirk, Hoban, and Anne Dunne) met infrequently but persistently with the

Women's Cancer Screening Service to explore possible funding of the work. By the time we were awarded the tender to conduct the research, we had a well-established network of contacts throughout the state, as a result of Maureen's personal and work-related links and as a result of other research we were conducting with Indigenous women. This established network allowed us relatively prompt commencement of the research proper – in contrast with other projects where lack of lead time prior to funding carried substantial penalties thereafter (Kelaher *et al.* 1998).

The conceptualization of the study was powerfully influenced by Kirk's unique role as the Aboriginal and Torres Strait Islander Cancer Support person at the Royal Women's Hospital (RWH) in the state capital, Brisbane. This position gave her continuing opportunities to discuss issues with women who were referred to the hospital from throughout the state for diagnosis and/or treatment of cancer. She was also able to consult informally during this period with women from various geographically disparate communities whose seniority and status allowed them to speak, to some degree, on behalf of other women from their own communities, to provide an indication to Kirk of their support for the project to proceed. Kirk's own experience as an Indigenous woman who had survived breast cancer was also a significant factor in identifying the issues that we thought might be relevant to explore within the study.

Queensland is a large state (1,727,200 square km), sparsely populated (about 3.5 million). Around 45 percent of the total population lives in the southeast corner of the state, in Brisbane and its coastal environs. However, 91 percent of the Indigenous community live elsewhere in the state in areas with limited access to regular primary care and no local tertiary medical services (Australian Bureau of Statistics 1996). In general, specialist medical services are concentrated in Brisbane and Indigenous and white women are referred to the Royal Women's Hospital for treatment for various cancers.

Defining "community" is problematic (Kelaher *et al.* 1998). Indigenous communities differ often dramatically as a result of "tribe" and kinship affiliation, community history (although often rival clans are forced to co-exist as a result of violent colonial policies), differences in local perceptions of community and culture, land ownership and political authority, and health status and determinants of health. These differences reflect broad historical, political, and economic differences, and specific micro-differences such as access to power, clean water and sanitation, education, and employment. Identification by geographic residence – as rural, remote, and urban – acknowledges certain proximate and infrastructural issues that potentially affect health status, but this categorization has limitations. Certain rural residential communities, for instance, exist on the basis of long-term historical affiliation to the area, acknowledged in both men's and women's stories of place, origin, and environment. Other groups in rural areas came to live in their communities within living memory, the survivors of those from numerous language groups who were dispossessed of their own country and shepherded together on to tightly controlled "reserves" (Hunter 1993). Thus women may have little shared history with their neighbors, may be newcomers, or may be living in their own country. This is as true for urban as for rural women. Some urban women are traditional owners of the land on which the cities are built. Others moved there to find work, or grew up in white foster homes when they were taken from their mothers by white authorities (Australia 1997).

"Urban" as a means of defining residence is also problematic: population density sits imperfectly on the boundaries of administrative units, and as we discuss further below, population density is not always matched by density of or access to services. Further, acknowledgment of the differences of communities, and not treating Indigenous people as a single population (too often subsumed by the acronym ATSI (Aborigines and Torres Strait Islanders)), established our own sensitivity to Australian social and political history – an essential component of operationalizing "cultural safety" (Ramsden 1991).

The differences among communities throughout the state underlined for us the difficulty in treating Indigenous women as a single group, or as is conventional, on the basis of two broad cultural and phenotypic groups (mainland Aboriginal or Torres Strait Islander). Consultations with women reinforced for us the importance that we travel to various areas throughout the state to meet with women in their own environments. It was also emphasized to us that, prior to collecting information, we should consult with various Indigenous organizations including health councils and community health services, youth services, housing services, and women's groups. Meeting with community groups whose members had already expressed interest in collaboration enabled us to establish a reference group of Indigenous women who met intermittently during the study. We also set up liaison groups in various urban, rural, and remote areas for more regular consultation on an individual basis and, through teleconferences, were able to clarify a modus operandi for the collection of baseline data, and developed protocols for data collection acceptable to the communities.

Consent to conduct the research was provided by the peak community consultative bodies of individual communities as well as our own reference group. Formal letters were sent to the proposed participating communities to complement the informal verbal consent obtained through consultation. In addition, consent was established, either verbally or through signing a consent form, with all individuals who were interviewed. It was also made clear that communities and individuals had the right to withdraw their participation, reclaim any data collected at any stage of the research project, and maintain ownership of data collected from their community. The expectation from community consultation was that we understood the discretion required regarding women's business – that is, matters specifically related to women's reproductive and sexual health – and that this would be reflected in our collection and handling of information. The information that we collected and our interpretations of it were verified via a final stage of research consultation in all communities where we had conducted focus groups and interviews. On this basis, the final report of the research was finalized and approved by the reference group (Kirk *et al.* 1998a). Subsequently, we prepared plain language summary community reports for remote, rural, and urban communities (Kirk *et al.* 1998b, 1998c, 1998d), and distributed these as widely as possible.

Methods

For analytic purposes, we included women from rural, remote, and urban communities to allow us to explore logistical difficulties and the different structural and cultural factors that reflected the heterogeneity of Indigenous women in the state and that we hypothesized might influence the acceptability of different kinds of programs. Practically, we recruited women from four major geographic/cultural areas, in order to capture variations in the distribution of services and possible differences in knowledge of cervical cancer, screening, and health promotion in distinct areas. These were coastal north Queensland and the Torres Strait Islands, including regional cities and remote areas (Cairns, Bamaga, Thursday Island, and five other island communities), far northwest Queensland (the remote towns and adjacent settlements of Mt Isa and Cloncurry, and their coastal referral center, Townsville), rural southwest Queensland (Toowoomba, Roma, and Cherborg), and urban southeast Queensland (Brisbane and Stradbroke Island). The project team[1] spent approximately four weeks in each area.

Ethnographic methods were used. They included focus group discussions (313 community women, 106 health workers), in-depth interviews (40 community men and women, 73 health workers), and case histories (10 women with a history of cervical cancer or currently undergoing treatment). These data were complemented by clinical data and observations of screening sessions and follow-up procedures (11). All focus groups and taped interviews were transcribed. Women were advised in a given community of the anticipated visit of the research team, with timing arranged to avoid ceremonial, holiday, sporting, and work commitments, funerals, and weather disruptions (the latter important because some areas are inaccessible in "the wet," i.e. the rainy season). Focus groups usually involved eight to ten women and were stratified by age into young (largely unmarried) women, middle-aged women, and "grandmothers." The ages of women in these categories tended to be younger than would be the case for Anglo-Australian women, since typically women are sexually active and have children from an early age, and are often grandmothers by the age of 40. We were not strict in other respects, however, but encouraged anyone willing to participate in a focus group to attend. Focus groups worked particularly well with young women who felt especially shy ("shame") talking about sex and revealing considerable gaps in knowledge. In-depth interviews were usually conducted with women who had experiences of abnormal smears or cervical cancer, or had strong views about women's business and the provision of health care.

Topics in the focus groups and interviews were wide ranging. We were interested in Indigenous concepts of health and illness, including how people perceived differences between their own understandings of health and those of others (*whitefellas*). We explored how Indigenous concepts of health affected women's interpretations of physical signs and symptoms, tests, results, and treatment. We were interested too in women's familiarity with government screening programs that were developed in order to identify women's health problems (e.g. the "Well Women's Health Check"). We discussed the roles of different health providers and preferences of gender and association of providers, as we were interested to know whether choice of provider might influence women's acceptance and attendance at health checks, Pap smear follow-up, recall, and return visits. Specifically, we explored what women thought prevention meant, what they understood by terms such as "abnormal" and "cancer," and why they thought Pap smears were performed.

We explored too women's views of "culturally safe" protocols to deliver "women's health" programs in their communities. These included issues of the environment (i.e. where Pap smears were provided), privacy and confidentiality, shame, time issues (convenience or inconvenience of appointments, hurried manner of health worker), possible considerations of Indigenous protocols in delivering women's health programs, health workers' use of technical terms, issues of "duty of care," and the role of "sisterhood" and the "silent stress" associated with supporting "sisters." At the same time, during individual interviews we let women tell their own stories, and those of their families and communities. These were important to hear because of the ways in which the history of racist neglect and violence has affected Indigenous/white relations. Women's stories were often painful for them to recall and recount: too often, they were stories of forced separation of children from parents, husbands from wives, of violence and racism, extraordinary poverty, incarceration, unnecessary deaths. Women also told of rape, domestic violence, and sexual abuse, including from health practitioners. While this kind of history feeds into women's specific use of health services (particularly gynecological), the more general history of genocide underpins all interactions.

Technically, data were analyzed thematically using a simple word processor and search functions rather than a qualitative data manager. This was for practical reasons. Field notes were written up, and focus group discussions and interviews were transcribed at night. Team members had different levels of skill and familiarity with computers, and the fastest and simplest method was therefore to use a word processor. Notes were kept and recorded on a continuing basis, so that the analysis was iterative; the research team traveled together and shared accommodation, and spent each night debriefing and talking through the issues as they emerged. Travel was broken up to allow extended periods in Brisbane, which enabled further debriefing and counseling. This was critical: the stories of unnecessary early death and family crises – inevitable dimensions of some cancer research – were deeply distressing; but the stories of neglect, lack of care, brutality, violence, and sexual abuse were also pervasive and left us deeply troubled and in pain.

As noted above, we reported regularly to the reference group via tele-conference and through face-to-face meetings, and consulted in person and by phone also with liaison groups. In general, meetings were arranged by telephone well in advance, and an agenda and summary of our work – providing the basis for discussion – would be sent by fax in advance of the meeting. We would provide a lengthy verbal summary of our activities and then work point by point through the various key issues that emerged. Since reports followed extensive research, there was little disagreement in interpretation. Of greatest value was the way in which women discussed the findings to identify commonalities and discontinuities, and in so doing, they frequently identified for us new areas of inquiry. Disagreement on interpretation was resolved by discussion; the emphasis in such meetings was on finding the points of consensus.

In the remainder of the chapter, we summarize the findings that emphasize the geographical aspects of women's perspectives of care and the delivery of services. This is not a cheap gesture to the theme of this volume. As we have already indicated, the size of the state, the distribution of its population and services, the history and politics of contemporary Indigenous settlements, and Indigenous meanings of space and place, all point to the value of a cultural geographic as well as anthropological lens.

Cervical cancer screening services for Indigenous women

Under the auspices of the women's cancer screening service of the state government, a number of programs provide for the needs of Aboriginal and Torres Strait Islander women. Three of these are fixed point delivery services in urban areas or regional centers (in Brisbane, Cairns, and Rockhampton), coordinated by the Aboriginal and Islander Community Health Service (AICHS). These programs also provide mobile services within their areas of operation. They ensure that preventive services and clinical care are available to women who are incarcerated, transient, or homeless, or who are geograph-ically isolated or have limited mobility – including those in urban areas without access to regular public transport and those who have small children and find travel difficult. AICHS provides women's health education sessions in homes and conducts workshops for community organizations and education institutions. In general, however, these services have a curative focus and have little emphasis on women's health promotion and education. There are, in addition, two other mobile services – Mobile Women's Health

Nurse (MWHN) Program and the Royal Australian College of General Practice (RACGP) Cervical Cancer Screening – which provide cervical cancer screening and other health services for rural and remote women.

These programs reach only a proportion of the women. Other women have the choice of presenting to a hospital outpatient department or general practice (of family physicians), which offer Pap smear consultations at women's request. In some cases they have access to a dedicated women's health service. Hospitals are unpopular because of their association with terminal illness and death, and women's personal experiences of racism, and statistically they are the least likely places for Indigenous women to attend for cervical screening. However, for some women there is no alternative, or no other free service, and so they may present here. Some women present to their general practitioner for cervical cancer screening. However, in many remote and rural areas there are only male practitioners, and not all are comfortable about providing care to women, either for racist reasons or because of their own perceptions of "culturally appropriate" behavior. One woman recounted her experience of care after delivery and the repair of "a huge tear in my cervix": "When the doctor came around, he stood at the end of the bed and talked about me and never even looked at my cervix. He didn't want to touch me" (remote woman). Women therefore may travel long distances to see a female practitioner or delay screening until a mobile women's health nurse arrives. Women in urban areas also go to great lengths to find a women's health practitioner whom they trust and respect.

Less commonly, women have access to dedicated women's health practitioners trained in women's health and employed in either a general or a women's health program. These practitioners are trained to deliver information, education, counseling, and clinical services including sexual and reproductive health, fertility and contraception, sexually transmitted diseases, cervical cancer screening, and breast screening, and offer a full Well Women's Check every two years, as per health service protocols. Most dedicated practitioners in the state are non-Indigenous and are located in city centers. However, the number of Indigenous women receiving cervical screening from dedicated women's health practitioners is increasing throughout the state in response to women's expressed needs and acceptance of the programs, and the provision of mobile services has improved women's access to female practitioners and their choice of practitioner.

Few nurse practitioners are employed in the urban and regional centers other than with dedicated women's health services such as Family Planning. Nurse practitioners provide cervical cancer screening and women's health education and promotion. In rural and remote communities and towns without female general practitioners, MWHNs provide a regular and broad range of women's health services for all women, who would otherwise have limited or no access to a female practitioner; they usually visit each area on rotation every 6–12 weeks.

Health services that focus on Indigenous women's health, e.g. Aboriginal Community Controlled Organizations, function within certain hours and have no appointment times. In remote areas, Women's Health Programs tend to determine clinic times to suit busy and fixed work schedules, e.g. MWHNs have immense distances to travel between towns and communities and must be rigid about their work schedules. This is a barrier to women accessing the service, where personal, ceremonial, or other circumstances may intervene and inhibit their use of services at a scheduled time. Despite women's health practitioners' commitment to flexibility and the provision of undisturbed time with women, they need to balance time spent in each community against both the logistical constraints and personal capacity to deliver an increasing number of services. This is complicated when consultations go over the allocated time or when women turn up late. Women's health practitioners such as MWHNs work very long days and spend many hours and hundreds of kilometers traveling between communities, and some services run well into the evenings to allow working women to attend. Prearranged appointment times and time limits on consultations have their advantages as many women want to be able to plan their day to arrange child care or have the appointment slot into their work or community commitments.

An additional layer in the provision of health care for Indigenous Australians is Aboriginal health workers (AHWs), predominantly generalist paramedics. Most choose not to perform Pap smears because of kin relationships,[2] limited or no training in women's health, and no legal indemnity.

Many women have histories of sexual abuse, and for this reason were particularly wary of gynecological examination:

> I was a ward of the state as a kid and I was constantly subjected to strips from nurses and doctors who came through to check me for a Ward of the State. That is a very humiliating experience, to be poked and prodded constantly. I just don't like doctors, I can't get rid of this feeling of them invading my body.

Women tell stories of others being raped by health workers when they have presented for Pap smears and such stories are powerful in discouraging presentation. Women also fear breaches in privacy, particularly when social and professional relationships overlap as is the case in most small communities; when this occurred, women were lost to cervical cancer screening for years, or might never return to the health service again.

AHWs' role in women's health includes health education, health promotion, community liaison, the crucial provision of transport for town-based services, and follow-up and recall of women with abnormal Pap smears. In a few cases, trained women AHWs are also able to provide extended support to women and accompany them during treatment. In addition, some AHWs who lack formal training may perform smears under the supervision of nurse practitioners or medical practitioners, primarily in remote communities where women do not have access to female practitioners and do not wish to see a male. However, AHWs may not undertake smears in government hospitals, none are employed by dedicated women's health services such as MWHN services or Family Planning, and very few work in partnership with women's health practitioners.

Women select their practitioner on the basis of gender, and the attitude and mannerisms of the practitioner, and frequently choose a different practitioner for women's business than for their family's health needs. Women in all areas regularly spoke of "never knowing how you will be treated," and would defer screening until a relationship with their practitioner of choice had been established. Length of time a practitioner spends in the community or town influences a woman's trust and respect, and this was a major issue in remote areas where there was a high turnover of practitioners.

The environment of the clinic

Consultation rooms are often located in public hospital outpatient departments. These areas are usually not designated for women's health consultations, precluding privacy and inhibiting modesty and cultural safety.[3] Moreover, it is common for toilets to be attached to patient waiting areas, requiring women to walk through these public areas with urine samples. Where Pap smear clinics share common facilities such as waiting areas and consultation rooms with sexual health programs, the purpose of women's visits to the service are often regarded with suspicion. In addition, consultation rooms in hospital outpatient departments do not always have optimal acoustics, resulting in breaches of privacy concerning the purpose of the visit and creating the potential to generate gossip in the community and nurture distrust in the health service. When women's services operate in such unfavorable conditions and venues, privacy and confidentiality are very difficult to maintain, despite the practitioner's best intentions.

Finding an alternative appropriate, accessible venue for women's health programs is difficult for remote and rural MWHN services. There are examples of a kitchen and a portable room being used for consultation. In one community, the women's health service had to operate in a building next to the Land Council Office and men sat on the front verandah, watching women as they walked by, entered the building, and attended the health service. Men's presence in the consultation area – as passers-by, patients, or staff – heightens women's concern for cultural safety and modesty. In this context, the notion of cultural safety by women is used to indicate the need for discretion in relation to sexual and reproductive health, although these core values have added substance where individual women or members of their family have been subject to sexual abuse.

As already noted, consultation rooms do not ensure privacy. Windows were found to be uncovered, screens may be inadequate or left open when Pap smears are conducted, and doors may have a broken lock or no lock at all. Hygiene is also questionable; in this study, we noted dirty linen and used speculums openly displayed when we were in the consultation rooms; and practitioners are frequently required to take dirty instruments from one building to another, or transport them over long distances before they can be sterilized.

In general medical practices, the environment is not considered particularly important, and practitioners have limited appreciation of the cultural, emotional, or psychological needs of Indigenous women presenting for cervical cancer screening. In contrast, dedicated women's health practitioners emphasize the importance of the environment and may go to great lengths to make the waiting area and consultation room private, comfortable, relaxed, and culturally safe. Some practitioners have involved especially young community women, in decorating, painting, and making screens and curtains for the women's areas. This responds to Indigenous women's own stated needs; they require that the environment where women's business is delivered be warm, friendly, and welcoming. Women feel that the first point of contact determines the atmosphere and environment of the visit, and influences their decision to return.

Women also emphasized the importance of consultation time being undisturbed. Women frequently spoke of telephone interruptions and one woman was abandoned midway through a Pap smear procedure while the practitioner answered a non-urgent telephone call. Other women spoke of other health personnel and secretarial staff entering the consultation room through an unlocked room midway through a private consultation or Pap smear procedure. Women interpreted these interruptions as behavior disrespectful of women's privacy and cultural integrity. If dedicated, undisturbed time is not available, women may refuse to return to the health service or where possible, may seek out an alternative health service or practitioner. This latter option is rarely available to women in remote areas.

Follow-up and recall of abnormal Pap smears

Not all practitioners maintain a manual or computerized follow-up system, nor are they aware of how to organize one. Several public hospitals also lacked a recall and reminder system, or the system had lapsed after repeated attempts to develop and maintain a register. In our research, we found very few examples of towns or communities where a central recall and follow-up system operated for the whole population. Manual recall and follow-up systems, using a register, diary, or card system, are the most common method of following up abnormal smears and reminding women when their next Pap smear is due. In addition, some women's health practitioners have developed their own computerized programs for cervical cancer screening data, which have the potential to improve the efficiency of follow-up and recall.

Health services with a follow-up and recall system are checked regularly. Some services use quarterly information supplied by select state pathology services to check their own data. Maintenance of recall and follow-up systems is generally the responsibility of the women's health practitioner, and some AHWs and registered nurses share this responsibility. However, most AHWs have minimal or no contact with Pap smear results nor with the maintenance of recall and reminder systems. Routine Pap smear reminder letters may be sent to all women who are registered on a health service manual or computerized system at the instigation of the practitioner who maintains the recall and follow-up system. Most general practitioners place the onus on women to follow up their own Pap smear result, requiring them either to telephone or to return for a consultation to obtain their results. Most dedicated women's health services inform women of their normal Pap smear result by letter and a copy of the result may accompany the letter.

Practitioners and health services that do not have a follow-up and recall system in place rely on women to return for their Pap smear result. If they do not return, then they may be informed on subsequent visits to the practice or hospital, or may never be informed of the abnormal Pap smear result. Various methods of follow-up are used. The practitioner may telephone the woman and explain the result and necessary treatment, or send a letter requesting the woman to return to discuss the result. Practitioners or generalist AHWs may visit women in their home and ask them to visit the health service to discuss their results, or give women a letter asking them to return. However, it is not always possible to locate women who have abnormal Pap smear results, as many women are itinerant, mobile, or hide for fear of receiving their result. Women with abnormal Pap smears are referred either directly to a specialist gynecologist or to their general practitioner who then arranges the referral.

The high turnover of health practitioners in rural and remote areas means that hospital Pap smear registers frequently lapse or they are poorly maintained. As a result, women are not offered opportunistic cervical cancer screening or informed of abnormal results. Limited access or denial of access to patient histories is problematic, and women's health programs that terminated with cessation of funding have a legacy of abandoned follow-up and recall systems. Many MWHNs stated that they are obliged to pursue gynecology results themselves, so that they can continue to provide follow-up care of the patient. In this study, we identified women who had never been informed of abnormal smear results or failed to receive advice sent by mail or by personal delivery. One woman who had a Pap smear in September 1996 had still not been followed-up for abnormal pathology twelve months later. Other women were informed but chose not to act on this advice because of fear that the abnormal smear result meant cancer and death, failure to understand the seriousness of the results, or lack of money, transport, or child care to allow the woman to return to the health service.

Notions of cultural safety emerged again in our discussions with women in regard to appropriate mode of advice. Women felt that arrangements for follow-up should be determined at the time of the smear. All women wanted to be informed of their Pap smear results personally or by letter, but personally in the event of an abnormal result; the least preferred option was telephone. The fear of cancer is so far-reaching that women felt it important to have someone sit down with them to explain the results and treatment options. However, women feel shame when they are given their results verbally in a public place, in case someone overhears the information, and even a visit to a woman's home has the potential to create suspicion if the practitioner is also a sexual health practitioner. While some women consider a letter to be a good option, in communities where STD rates are very high, a letter from the women's or sexual health practitioner may also cause shame for women. Further, there are problems associated with recall and follow-up letters. These include illiteracy among women whose first language is not English, lack of privacy of mailboxes, and letters being opened and read by others. Finally, as noted above, there are examples where women have run away or hidden from AHWs, to avoid receiving results, for fear of being told they have cervical cancer. Other women hide or leave their community once they have been informed of an abnormal result, and refuse to discuss their treatment options.

Pathways for the treatment of abnormal Pap smears

All women with abnormal Pap smears are referred to a specialist gynecologist for assessment and most Indigenous women attend a public hospital for their treatment. The referral centers are not evenly dispersed geographically, and women often must travel vast distances to attend their gynecological appointments. In remote and rural areas, women are referred to specialist gynecologists working with the Flying Remote Obstetric and Gynecology Services (FROG) which operates out of referral centers such as Cairns, Mt Isa, and Roma. These services are regular, with referral visits four to six times per year. There are two methods of delivering this mobile specialist gynecologist service. One is the use of a fixed model of service delivery utilizing local established hospitals with static facilities; remote women are referred to these hospitals and the government-run Patient Transport Scheme (PTS) is used to cover the women's transport costs. In contrast, the FROGs in the far north of Queensland use portable equipment and are more flexible about the type of referral centers out of which they operate. Indigenous women living in remote communities and islands also utilize the PTS to access the FROG. The economic burden on PTS in areas where women must travel to a fixed gynecological referral center is significant, and women's health practitioners and specialist gynecologists acknowledge that travel and economic and social factors are major reasons why women do not attend gynecological appointments. Specialist gynecologists perceive the economic advantages in taking the gynecology services to women in remote areas, instead of having them traveling to the fixed referral center utilizing the PTS.

Women in remote mainland communities and the outer Torres Strait Islands experience many logistical and related problems leaving their communities to access a FROG service; for example, bad weather, long delays on unprotected airstrips, long distances to travel to connect with local airlines and ferries, and nervousness and distrust of light planes. Women face difficulties on arrival at the referral centers: no money to pay for a taxi to and from the ferry or plane, no money for food while away from home, no family members to stay with while at the referral center, and worry that their children are safe and are being taken to school. We lack details of the emotional and social burdens on women of leaving their communities for specialist consultations and procedures. However, we know that they are significant in terms of women's compliance for other aspects of their health, e.g. with respect to birthing (Fitzpatrick 1995) and the management of end-stage renal disease (Bennett *et al.* 1995). Dedicated women's health practitioners and AHWs spoke of their need to support women before the appointment, and of accompanying women during the gynecological procedure upon request. Women's distrust of hospitals magnifies their anxiety over their gynecological problem.

Treatment regimes are delivered in tertiary level hospitals and may take up to two months. This necessitates that women are away from their families and communities for long periods of time and oncology specialists acknowledge that this creates enormous problems for them and their families. There are no palliative care services or trained staff in rural and remote communities or towns, and very few Indigenous palliative care staff in Queensland, and non-Indigenous palliative care staff in rural and remote areas have heavy workloads and are required to travel long distances to visit patients. Family members are obliged to care for the women in their terminal stages of cancer with minimal support or assistance from health staff or community services. These limited mainstream services do not meet the emotional, spiritual, and cultural needs of all Indigenous women with cervical cancer.

A substantial number of women leave during the course of treatment or before the treatment even begins. No Indigenous woman (or man) chooses to die away from their community,[4] and if they do, then the cost of bringing their body back to the community (if they live away from the referring hospital) has to be incurred by the family. Women who believe they are going to die during treatment may consequently choose to stay in their communities and not accept treatment, or may return home before completing treatment to be cared for by their family. One woman recounted her reaction to diagnosis with cervical cancer: "I felt numb. I didn't want to talk about it . . . I just remembered, if I was going to die, I wanted to be buried at home."

Conclusion

The issues that emerged from this study drew our attention to the significance of lack of access, racism, inappropriate staff, problems in provisions of services, logistical difficulties, poor quality and choice of services. All these represent barriers to women's participation in screening. Women have had little opportunity to register their dissatisfaction, however, as they are not involved in a voluntary or remunerated capacity in women's health programs in Queensland. Nor are there reference groups or steering committees to advise on program design, planning, implementation, or evaluation processes, nor mechanisms for women to contribute routinely to programs. Health practitioners argue that long-term changes to Indigenous health will not occur if government authorities continue to impose their own health schedules and health priorities on Indigenous women; and they spoke of the importance of women being equal partners in health programs. Women in turn expressed their own wish to be so involved: "I think the whole community is responsible for our health, and it is a combined effort, not just health workers" (rural woman).

We began this chapter by drawing attention to the need for research partnerships. The need for partnerships – for community ownership, involvement, and control – pertains equally in service provision, and this applies regardless of location, structure, or size of community. Throughout the state, presently the Western health model predominates. Doctors, nurses, and health service managers control and provide care; women are the recipients of care. All program goals and objectives are set by the program staff or management committee, often in conjunction with the funding body (usually the state or federal government) with little or no attention to community women's priorities. These priorities, as expressed in this study, were diabetes, drug and alcohol problems, teenage pregnancies, domestic violence, and sexual abuse. Women never mentioned cervical cancer or breast cancer as priorities, despite the high cervical cancer mortality rates.

These are not "culturally" informed notions of health priorities or disease patterns: they represent the health problems that most severely impact on and have highest visibility in Aboriginal and Torres Strait Island communities today. The health issues for Indigenous Australians are not primarily ones of cultural difference between the consumers and providers of the health care system, although recognizing the differences that occur is important in ensuring a culturally safe and appropriate environment for consumers. But for Indigenous Australians as for other Indigenous peoples, cultural safety has wider reference: it encompasses an acknowledgment of how cultural difference historically legitimized economic, political, judicial, and social systems that have produced the contemporary patterns of morbidity and mortality. As discussed in this chapter, these factors in turn underpin the uneasy relations that exist between government departments and Indigenous communities, and between academics and the communities. Creating partnership – both in research and in service provision – involves acknowledging the disempowerment of the communities historically and presently, and the ways in which the history of racism saturates everyday life in contemporary Australia. Thus moving towards reconciliation involves several tasks in public health and clinical services: acknowledging the historical production of illness and disease in Indigenous communities, recognizing and responding to community health priorities, and concurrently, providing services that enhance people's sense of personal safety and care.

Notes

1 Elizabeth Hoban, Maureen Kirk, and Anne Dunne, who was involved in the conception of the project and in data collection.
2 Kinship relations influence use of services for men as well as women, particularly services where assurance of confidentiality is critical such as in sexual health (Mulvey and Manderson 1995).
3 Cultural safety as defined in 1988 by the Hui Waimanawa, Christchurch requires that the validity of (Maori) cultural values be recognized, especially as they relate to their perceptions of health, their tapu, and the holistic nature of their being (Ramsden 1991).
4 See Bennett *et al.* (1995) and Willis (1995, 1999) for a discussion of attitudes to dying away from home and the implications of this for patients with end-stage renal disease and other terminal illnesses.

References

Aboriginal Coordinating Council (1995) *Consultation Protocol: How to Consult Appropriately and Effectively with Aboriginal or Torres Strait Islander Communities*, Brisbane: Queensland Health.

Australia, National Inquiry into the Separation of Aboriginal and Torres Strait Islander Children from their Families (1997) *Bringing Them Home: Report of the National Inquiry into the Separation of Aboriginal and Torres Strait Islander Children from their Families (Commissioner, Ronald Wilson)*, Sydney: Human Rights and Equal Opportunity Commission.

Australian Bureau of Statistics Census of Population and Housing (1996) Selected Social and Housing Characteristics for Statistical Local Area, Queensland, 2015.3, Canberra: Australian Government Publishing Service.

Bennett, E., Manderson, L., Kelly, B., and Hardie, I. (1995) "Dialysis and renal transplantation among Aboriginal and Torres Strait Islanders in north Queensland," *Australian Journal of Public Health* 19, 6: 610–15.

Dyck, I. and Kearns, R. (1995) "Transforming the relations of research: towards culturally safe geographies of health and healing," *Health and Place* 1, 3: 137–47.

Fitzpatrick, J. (1995) "Obstetric health services in far north Queensland," *Australian Journal of Public Health* 19, 6: 580–8.

Franklin, M. A. and White, I. (1991). "The history and politics of Aboriginal health," in J. Reid and P. Trompf (eds) *The Health of Aboriginal Australia*, Sydney: Harcourt Brace Jovanovich: 1–36.

Harrison, L. (1991) "Food, nutrition and growth in Aboriginal communities," in J. Reid and P. Trompf (eds) *The Health of Aboriginal Australia*, Sydney: Harcourt Brace Jovanovich: 123–72.

Hunter, E. (1993) *Aboriginal Health and History*, Melbourne and Cambridge: Cambridge University Press.

Jelfs, P. (1995) *Cervical Cancer in Australia. Australian Institute of Health and Welfare Cancer Series* No. 3, Commonwealth Department of Human Services and Health, Canberra: Australian Government Publishing Service.

Kelaher, M., Baigrie, N., Manderson, L., Moore, L., Shannon, C., and Williams, G. (1998) "Community perceptions of health, illness and care: identifying issues for Indigenous communities," *Women & Health* 28, 1: 41–62.

Kirk, M., Hoban, E., Dunne, A., and Manderson, L. (1998a) *Barriers to and Appropriate Delivery Systems for Cervical Cancer Screening in Indigenous Communities in Queensland: Final Report*, Brisbane: Government Press.

—— (1998b) *Cancer Screening among Indigenous Women in Remote Queensland Communities*, Brisbane: Government Press.

—— (1998c) *Cancer Screening among Indigenous Women in Rural Queensland Communities*, Brisbane: Government Press.

—— (1998d) *Cancer Screening among Indigenous Women in Urban Queensland Communities*, Brisbane: Government Press.

Mulvey, G. and Manderson, L. (1995) "Contact tracing and sexually transmitted disease on the Anungu Pitjitjantjara lands," *Australian Journal of Public Health* 19, 6: 596–602.

NHMRC (National Health and Medical Research Council) (1991) "Guidelines on ethical matters in Aboriginal and Torres Strait Islander health research," approved by the 111th Session of the National Health and Medical Research Council, Brisbane, June 1991, Canberra: Australian Government Publishing Service.

Queensland, Department of Health (1994) Unpublished statistics, Brisbane: Epidemiology and Health Information Branch.

Ramsden, I. (1991) *Kawa Whakaruruhau: Cultural Safety in Nursing Education in Aotearoa*, Wellington: Nursing Council of New Zealand.

Rowse, T. (1992) *Remote Possibilities: The Aboriginal Domain and the Administrative Imagination*, Darwin: North Australian Research Unit.

Saggers, S. and Gray, D. (1991) *Aboriginal Health and Society: The Traditional and Contemporary Aboriginal Struggle for Better Health*, Sydney: Allen & Unwin.

Thomson, N. (1991) "A review of Aboriginal health status," in J. Reid and P. Trompf (eds) *The Health of Aboriginal Australia*, Sydney: Harcourt Brace Jovanovich: 37–79.

Willis, J. (1995) "Do high-technology treatments for renal disease benefit Aboriginal patients in central Australia," *Australian Journal of Public Health* 19, 6: 603–9.

—— (1999) "Dying in country: implications of culture in the delivery of palliative care in Indigenous Australian communities," *Anthropology and Medicine* 6, 3: 423–35.

Part III

Embodied health and illness, perceptions, and place

11 "The baby is turning"

Child-bearing in Wanigela, Oro Province, Papua New Guinea

Yvonne Underhill-Sem

Introduction

In advancing new readings on child-bearing in the third world,[1] tensions between dealing with bodies that are simultaneously "real" and socially constructed (Longhurst 1997) are constantly negotiated. Closely related are the tensions between the modernist presumptions that continue to underlie fertility analysis (Greenhalgh 1996) and subsequently inform national population policies (Basu 1997), and the dynamics of various approaches found in emancipatory feminist scholarship concerned with reproduction (e.g. Ginsberg and Rapp 1995). Furthermore, tensions surrounding the representation of women, especially of women from the third world, are ever present. Negotiating these interwoven tensions is not easy but there are still too many women dying during childbirth in Papua New Guinea specifically, and the third world more generally, for me to avoid some involvement, albeit from an abstract conceptual position.

In this chapter my aim is to ensure that the "missing visual text" (Haraway 1997: 52) of women in Wanigela, Papua New Guinea, can be recognized while still leaving room for governments to deal with the bodies that bleed – too often – to death. My intention is to work towards making connections between the ways in which women talk, or remain silent, about child-bearing and pregnancy and representations of fertility in standard demographic analysis. After a brief introduction to Wanigela in Papua New Guinea, I examine the partialities of fertility represented both demographically and ethnographically. I then examine more carefully the ways in which my understandings of fertility remain incomplete. Finally, I suggest some ways of negotiating the epistemological incompatibilities of non-discursive understanding of child-bearing and pregnancy, and pragmatic population policies.

Guiding my own unapologetic emancipatory intentions is Iris Marion Young's concept of pragmatic theorizing – that is, "categorizing, explaining, developing accounts and arguments that are tied to specific practical and political problems" (Young 1994: 192). The practical and political problem I am concerned with is how national population policies might begin to incorporate new concepts to represent the complexities that are embedded in issues concerning fertility, reproduction, and child-bearing in local communities. In the international arena, critical analysis of the implementation of the International Conference on Population and Development (ICPD) Program of Action held in Cairo recognized the need for conceptual clarity to advance the intentions of the meeting. The major policy shift at this meeting was "away from demographically driven approaches towards policies grounded in concerns for human rights, social well-being and gender equity, with particular emphasis on reproductive health and rights" (Correa 1999: 5). In addition to the concepts of gender, women's empowerment, and male responsibility, which are integral parts of reproductive health and rights advocacy, I would add that the taken-for-granted concept of fertility also requires conceptual clarification.

The main threads

Although the reasons for maternal deaths in the third world are various and overlapping, dominant population and development discourses, including studies undertaken as geographies (e.g. Maudood 1993), attend only to the material, mostly "demographic", and Western medical expression of these events. Thus concerns settle on the need to have both improved economic conditions and a better supply of modern contraceptives. The proliferation of development projects focusing on expanding educational opportunities for women and providing access to credit and improved reproductive health services is the response to these types of policies. Such strategies are not remarkable in the 1990s and it is not my intention to undermine their purpose. Policies of this type continue to warrant expansion because it takes time for some of the insights from the successes and failures of twenty-five years of development to be successfully transformed into action. This is particularly important because of a growing concern that, in the political economic context of the late 1990s, independent governments, including Papua New Guinea, were reneging on their social welfare responsibilities and increasingly adopting neo-liberal economic advice to privatize human welfare services.

My concern is that despite the existence of "sound" or "good" research, emancipatory policy decisions are unlikely without imagining new ways of talking about population and finding new concepts to talk with. To do this it is necessary to unsettle the dominance of positivist/modernist representations of, in this case, child-bearing bodies so that those who may still refuse the possibility of imagination, such as many demographers and population geographers, can at least see that the seemingly natural event of child-bearing is also socially constructed and hence problematic (Alcoff 1996).

By positioning my work and myself in this way, contingent coalitions, which deal with both material and discursive representations of child-bearing bodies, can be made. The possibilities of establishing such coalitions, between different people, places, and over time, rest on politically strategic expressions of sameness which are also cognizant of the fluid constituencies that constitute such coalitions. Allegiances will inevitably change and therefore coalitions will always be shifting. So, although I recognize the differences and unequal power relations between me and the women I lived and worked with in Wanigela, Oro Province, Papua New Guinea, in the complex material and discursive worlds we live in, who is to say which differences are more important, where, when, and to whom? As Audrey Kobayashi (1994) writes, I am as much a part of "my" subjects' project as they are of mine and so following Linda McDowell I attempt to write myself, as well as research participants, into my research practice rather than "hanker after some idealised equality between us" (1992: 409).

Of sites and situations

Papua New Guinea is an independent, sparsely populated country in the Western Pacific divided administratively into nineteen provinces. Although the extractive mineral sector dominates the national economy, 80 percent of the estimated 4 million Papua New Guineans live in rural villages and derive their main livelihoods from subsistence agriculture. A particularly notable feature of Papua New Guinea is that over seven hundred different languages are spoken. This reflects the continued existence of many, small, fragmented, isolated but self-sufficient societies that comprise the modern state (Waiko 1993). Because of the physical and social isolation of many societies, complex trading relationships, and with them trading languages, have developed over many generations to connect these societies. In the recent history of the country, more and different kinds of goods and ideas join these flows.

Wanigela is a collection of twelve settlements in Oro Province. Over a period of about a week in 1995 I counted about[2] 1,500 people living in the greater Wanigela area which stretches from coastal mangroves, over hot grasslands, and up into tropical rainforest on fertile volcanic soils. Three local languages, Ubir, Oyan, and Onjob, are known as well as some English and Papua New Guinea pidgin. The former was introduced by Anglican missionaries at the end of the nineteenth century (see Barker 1987) and the latter through increasing contact with people from other language groups in Papua New Guinea. Subsistence life in Wanigela revolves around slash-and-burn and rotational agriculture, supplemented by hunting and fishing. A relatively small-scale logging operation was active for eighteen months beginning in 1996 but other cash-earning opportunities are limited to garden produce sold at a local market, remittances from relatives living in town, and the irregular sale of some cash crops such as copra and cocoa. With no motorized transport in the area, it took me about four hours to walk between the most distant ends of the settlements in Wanigela with some gardens being further afield.

As a relative by marriage, I have visited Wanigela many times since the mid-1980s. Being contingently "from the place," it is difficult to define precisely when "my research" began and when it will end. However, being also from, at least, two other places (the Cook Islands and New Zealand), I was always checking the portability of the taken-for-granted concepts I used (Katz 1991). My Western tertiary education and that of my husband, with whom I was associated,[3] as well as my having a regular paid job, having lived in other countries, and having "soft skin,"[4] placed me in a position of privilege "in the field." Attaining higher education, writing "books," and knowing something about places and things outside Oro gave me a more attentive audience than my story-telling skills deserved. However, people in Wanigela also told each other that I was "really" (*om dura*) interested in learning about the place as a *tambu* (in-law) and consequently I was told many more stories than I can retell or could record with my audio tape recorder or my trusty solar-powered laptop computer.

Although I had some fluency in one of the local languages, I was accompanied on almost all my interviews,[5] for both the form-filling census as well as the audio-recorded maternity histories, by at least one research assistant and sometimes two. Kena[6] was a young widow with four children and Sorty was an unmarried woman with one child. Both were part of my "extended family" so my relationship with each was mobile and multi-dimensional. Their assistance in accompanying me was also multi-dimensional. They updated me on the situation of the people and families we were about to visit (for instance, recent deaths, sensitive issues concerning the paternity and maternity of children, and relations between "our families" and the ones we were going to interview); eased the language difficulties I had when words, phrases, and concepts with which I was unfamiliar crept into conversations; provided the accompaniment that a "privileged" member of the community was due; assisted in carrying the obligatory gifts of food that people we visited insisted we take home; and provided daily friendship. Despite great care, some people undoubtedly felt compelled or obliged to talk to us for various reasons. Some reasons included the fact that we had walked for a long time in the rain or heat to interview them, or that our families were closely related kin, or that one of us had had a particular conversation with someone in the family we hoped to interview. However, it is left to the situated nature of my subsequent ethnographic representations to work with this "reality" which I use to contextualize demographic representations.

The partialities of fertility analysis

The analysis of fertility in the third world is most often undertaken using standard demographic tools and concepts modified to work with data that are compromised by different systems and practices of data collection. Despite the often-questionable data available for analysis, increasingly sophisticated multivariate statistical techniques have been developed so that "fertility" patterns and trends can be compared across time and place. Because of the statistical need to aggregate data to obtain "valid results," fertility analysis is generated for regional or national level analysis, and in this way it constitutes the basis of what is known about "fertility." It is this representation of fertility that finds its way into population policies. However, as anthropological demographers David Kertzer and Tom Fricke (1997: 1) explain, "by emphasising particular types of methodological development within a relatively closed sphere of pragmatic issues, demography has fashioned the self-image of a discipline whose practitioners are able to apply their standard toolkits to the explanation of demographic behaviour anywhere in the world." For instance, demographers John Bongaarts and Griffith Feeney (1998) have developed a "tempo adjusted total fertility rate" to further refine the more commonly used total fertility rate, which itself is problematic where data are not collected in a particular way. In defending the expected criticisms that such a measure is "excessively hypothetical" they note that "there is a good dose of hypothetical in the conventional total fertility rate . . . and we see the difference as one of degree rather than one of kind" (Bongaarts and Feeney 1998: 286). If similar efforts went into refining representations of fertility from non-demographic perspectives, the possibilities of population policies driven by non-demographic concerns would be more advanced.

It has only been recently that population geographies have begun to engage with the challenges posed by new theoretical debates broadly characterized as "post-structuralist" or "post-colonial" perspectives (Findlay and Li 1999; Graham 1999; Sporton 1999; Underhill-Sem 1999). In the burgeoning field of anthropological demography, this engagement is more advanced (see Basu 1997; Greenhalgh 1996; Kertzer and Fricke 1997; Obermeyer 1997; Scheper-Hughes 1997). In addition to scholarly challenges, anthropological demographers are concerned about how policy-makers might begin to think differently about intervening in population processes that improve human welfare in the third world. For instance, Nancy Scheper-Hughes (1997) captures the complexity of fertility in the *favelas* of northeast Brazil by focusing on infant and child mortality. Where vital statistics are non-existent in poverty-filled places such as these *favelas*, "demography without numbers" means accounting, not for births, but for the "angels," the babies and infants who routinely die and are buried in hastily constructed cardboard boxes. Scheper-Hughes takes a critical interpretive approach by asking what is hidden from view in official statistics and what this tells us about the "collective invisibility of certain groups and classes of people – women and small children in particular?" (1997: 220). In a similar manner, I ask the same questions about what is hidden from view in my demographic and ethnographic representations of fertility in Wanigela.

Exploring the gaps of fertility analysis, what exists but is not yet known, with the analytical tools currently in hand, invites a closer look at taken-for-granted concepts. For instance, take the concept of "the age of a person" or the time elapsed since a person was born. This concept is deceptive in many societies that value oral over written communication. In such situations, demographers and other population "specialists," including many geographers and anthropologists, have developed a range of methods to estimate a person's age. Few ask the question – why is age such an important marker? I suggest that the answer – because it is a biologically essential feature of all humans – reveals the embeddedness of naturalizing impulses in population studies. These naturalizing impulses converge with interventionist governance urges to represent people, and especially women, by numbers and the occurrence of events, by rates. Without such urges, people might be represented by their stories or by their form in various visual texts.

In Wanigela, it is difficult to represent fertility by rates. Not only is the necessary type of data not readily available because, aside from sample surveys such as the one I did, the only written procedures for recording births are incomplete baptism records. There is also no regularity about collecting this information and indeed in some places there is active resistance because of the association of such recording with the demeaning colonial practice of lining people up in groups behind the "head" of the household to count them. However, this is not to say that there are no representations of life and death of individuals. Rather, this occurs in a different way, mostly in the process of negotiating land claims or clarifying clan relationships in marriages. In these representations, the socially constructed, mostly relational, concepts such as "maternity," "paternity," or "relationship to siblings" have as much importance as biological parentage or the chronological age of the individuals concerned. For instance, because clan membership is determined through both biological and social relationships, discussions relating to exchanges of cultural resources, such as when a couple marry, are often extended and complex because of the need to carefully track previous allegiances. The stories that inform these discussions are also represented differently according to the situated knowledge of different people, so there is never a complete alignment of stories although agreements are still reached.

This is messy business, this local historical and contextually situated material, which might invite accusations of relativism and irrelevance. However the partialities of all knowledge producing techniques are never-ending. Consistent with longstanding arguments in the social sciences, Haraway has recently pointed to the combination of both statistical analysis and ethnography "as critical feminist technologies for producing convincing representations of the reproduction of inequality" (1997: 22). While ethnographic techniques have been recognized as part of the methodological "toolbox" for feminist analysis for some time now, only recently have statistical representations found a place in emancipatory scholarship (Haraway 1997; Harding 1995). Rather than "throw it out," it can be used in other ways because "fruitful encounters depend on a particular kind of move – a *tropos* or 'turn'" (Haraway 1992: 67). In the following section I look at how child-bearing in Wanigela is represented both demographically and ethnographically and examine ways of "turning" these insights into information that can inform population policy.

"Children-ever-born": demographic representations of fertility

From a village-wide house-to-house census I collected information about the date of birth, sex, and date of death (where applicable) for all children born to all women aged fifteen years or more who were living in Wanigela at the time. To ensure complete fertility histories I used a number of techniques. I began by recording names for every birth. Where babies died before they were named, they were recorded as "Baby." I also checked whether a woman had used any "modern family planning" techniques after each baby. I also probed for the reason for gaps longer than two years between children. Finally, I worked with kinship links by asking individuals about their siblings and where names came from.

From these data, a summary fertility measure of children-ever-born could be calculated. In general,[7] this analysis showed that women in Wanigela have high fertility and few use modern contraceptives. This is not quite a "natural fertility" population as the population geographer Robert Woods (1979) defines it because there is a history of "birth control" practices in Wanigela although the effectiveness of these practices is difficult to assess. During the period of my household census, I recorded 329 women, aged fifteen and over, who together produced a total of 1,359 live babies, which is expressed as an average of 4.1 births per woman. Compared with 2.65 for all women and 3.37 for currently married women in Papua New Guinea (National Statistics Office 1997: 39), it can be concluded that fertility in Wanigela is higher than the national average.

If only surviving children are related to the women who have actually given birth (mothers), the average number of surviving children per mother falls to 3.8, compared with 3.01 as the national average. Most of the difference between averages for children-ever-born and surviving children occurs for women at older ages, especially those over thirty-five years of age. This indicates that infant and child mortality is higher for older women. Although this is logical since older women are exposed to the possibility of a child dying for a longer time, this analysis may also be understood as representing higher infant mortality in the past. However without further comparative analysis of different age cohorts in Wanigela, nothing more can be said about this possibility.

This is not a surprising result but only becomes meaningful when used comparatively across time and space. Clearly there are other dimensions of fertility missing from this analysis and perhaps more sophisticated demographic techniques could distill more refined rates and produce more carefully qualified results so that the lives, and deaths, of Wanigela women and their children are better represented. Even if this happened, and aside from questions of "for whom" and "for what purposes" would this knowledge be used, there are still some interesting gaps.

Missing from the numbers story

The gaps I am most concerned about are conceptual not methodological ones. However, I touch briefly on one methodological gap to show how it becomes an opening for further conceptual clarification. My own partial assessment of the methodological shortcomings of this survey, especially the coverage and completeness of responses, is that I accounted for "almost all" of the births to those women who were living in Wanigela in 1995–6. This included a number of births where pregnancy was unexpected, unwanted, or unsanctioned as when paternity was questionable or unacceptable, or when the baby died shortly after birth. In demographic terms, however, fertility refers to all conceptions, not just those resulting in a birth, so in a complete analysis all miscarriages and abortions would need to be captured. This is a methodological and a conceptual problem where precise definitions need to account for "diverse social practices through which people create people" as Lynn Morgan found in her study of the "unborn" in the Andes (Morgan 1997: 348). In all my interviews in Wanigela, only one woman, who had trained as a nurse and therefore was familiar with Western medical discourses, spoke, in English, about having had a miscarriage. This is an important issue that requires conceptual clarification before any method-ological improvements, such as more careful interviewing, would be meaningful.

A more interesting conceptual gap, however, concerns how we capture members of the community whose bodies are marked by social definitions that are not consistent with the broad "social" definition I was working with. I did not think there would be a conceptual difficulty in counting all the women in Wanigela although I was expecting problems with assigning women, especially older women, to age groups. However, one omission highlighted the error in my assumption about the overlap of social and natural definitions of women, and following the well-known concept of falsification, one omission can unsettle the whole argument.

Despite the reliability of my research assistants' knowledge of this commu-nity, we missed out a woman, Della, born in 1972 who was said to be *kokok* (Ubir), *longlong* (Pidgin), or intellectually "compromised." I was eventually told she was in her late teens and despite passing her house many times, and even stopping there for a drink a couple of times, I never saw or heard about her. Her name only came up when I was checking names in a kinship story. When asked, both my research assistants exclaimed, "Oh yes, we forgot her." When pressed further, they just said they never see her so they forgot. It was unusual to claim that not seeing a person was the reason for forgetting someone. Indeed there were many people who had not been seen for many years, including the deceased, but were still remembered. There were even other people who were *kokok* and part of village stories. There were also at least two other unrelated people in Wanigela in the 1980s, a man born in 1965, who wandered around barely clad, and a woman born in 1932 who wandered around wearing as many clothes as she could, to whom people also referred as *kokok*.

Clearly, Della had limited social relationships with people in the village. However, the reasons why she was not considered either a member of the community or a woman who has not had children and is never likely to, is related to the process by which bodies are also socially constituted, and therefore variable (Grosz 1994). Missing one young intellectually compromised woman in a small place like Wanigela may not be a major problem for fertility analysis. Furthermore, it may seem a simple case of making sure interviewers directly inquire about the existence of intellectually compromised women. But this highlights a larger problem of the inevitability of omissions of women whose social relationships exclude them from consideration and in the process define their bodies as not needing to be counted. In other places where women like Della, and others omitted on different grounds, constitute a larger number, their omission from calculations of fertility may be more critical.

Abstracting numbers from tables generated by a statistical computer program (SPSS PC) and estimating the number of children ever born per mother is the simplest form of fertility analysis to be generated from survey data like my own. But it is clear that this does not represent the full story. The "demographic facts" of high fertility and little use of modern contraceptives do not account for other discourses surrounding childbirth, which are the focus of the next section.

Stories told and stories heard: ethnographic attitudes

Ethnographic approaches, such as collecting kinship stories and in-depth interviewing after a period of living in an area, provide other ways of enriching demographic representations. Many stories are told, heard, and created in ethnographies which Cindi Katz calls "self-conscious projects of representation, interpretation and invention" (1992: 496). Dealing with issues of interpretation is thus a critical part of any ethnographic representation so in this chapter I adopt Haraway's concept of an "ethnographic attitude." Haraway argues that this attitude can be used in any kind of inquiry because it is "a mode of practice and theoretical attention, a way of remaining mindful and accountable" (1997: 39).

In this chapter, where I am working towards making connections between discursive constructions of child-bearing and pregnancy and representations of fertility in standard demographic analysis, I have many recorded stories and conversations to draw from. However, throughout these recordings I had a sense of frustration that women were not forthcoming about the details of their deliveries despite my considerable but gentle probing. Time and again, I asked, in both Ubir and English, variations of "What was the birth like?", "What was 'it' [the delivery] like?", "How did you deliver the baby?", "Who was in the room with you?", "What was [name of husband, mother, etc.] doing?", "How were they helping you?". Most responses were "It was hard," "It was a little bit hard," or "It was okay."

My frustration led me to take an opportunity, late one afternoon, to ask two women to describe a birth using Ubir terms. I was hoping to find out what the appropriate phrases were and hence to improve my probing. Pem, born in 1959, was a school teacher with five children, and Cres, her widowed mother, born 1926, looked after Pem's children. By paying particular attention to the words used and the words avoided, I began to see the process of birthing quite differently.

Pem and Cres began by telling me that women note the timing of their menstrual periods with reference to three moon shapes: the New Moon (C-shape), the Half Moon (D-shape), and the Full Moon (O-shape). When a woman missed her period she would say "The baby will come after nine moons" and at about the time of her period. When the month comes they would wait for the moon to reach the same shape at which time it would be said that "en roke egat" (your moon has come). Unlike Western medical estimates that focus on a date, this method of estimating time provides considerable flexibility in preparing for the birth of a child. More importantly, and consistent with other ways of marking time in communities which rely on subsistence gardening, it leaves room for women to interpret the changes in their own bodies and anticipate events.

In the early months of pregnancy, when a woman has missed her period but before her stomach begins to swell, a woman might say, "Yau ainafort" (I am pregnant). However, this was rarely said unless the woman was ill. Many women talked about continuing with their regular work and over-looking pregnancy-related physical discomforts to the extent that no one mentioned such things as morning sickness. Feeling tired was common and when it was noticed that a woman was sleeping more, this was taken as a signal for the more common speculative phrase, "ainafort?" (she's pregnant?). When a swelling stomach is noticeable, then it was said "en jever en yan" (that woman has a stomach). The term *yan* refers to the physical stomach of all bodies so that if, for instance, a child has a sore stomach it would be said "fifi en yan ebaban." However, when used in reference to a married woman of an age to have children, it referred to her pregnant state.

Despite the care that Pem and Cres took in getting the details right, I never heard these phrases used to describe pregnant women. Instead the common reference was whether a woman was "staying" or not (*usisiyar o ambin*). Little more was said immediately after it was known that she was not "staying" except what month she would give birth (*roke aifanai uneib*). This cast the whole process of sexual relations and conceptions in a different light. Instead of mapping out pregnancy, for my information only, in a more or less linear and predictable fashion, the use of the phrase "staying" implies pregnancy, as the opposite state, is active. The action of pregnancy is attributed to both the unborn child and its mother and is associated with the idea that anything can happen. A better way to capture this in English might be the phrase "Are you getting pregnant?" which includes acknowledging sexual activity. More importantly, there are many possible responses and outcomes. In this way, trying to find a normative account of pregnancy is unsurprisingly futile.

Even during the description of the actual birth, there was little that I recognized from previous interviews and conversations. Pem and Cres told me that when the first pains begin, a woman would say "yau kau egigiar" (my back is paining). This is also a phrase that could be used for all bodies but had a specific meaning in reference to a pregnant woman, and signaled the impending arrival of birth. When pains became more intense, it was said "fifi irutabir" (the child has turned). In the past it was understood that the child was lying upright, so "a child turning" refers to it putting its head down and readying itself to be born. During this time, the movements of the child are understood as the baby stretching its limbs (*fifi ebi aiyob*). When the baby has "engaged," a woman's stomach is ready (*jever yan ikisiser*). The first show of blood, "tara egat" (blood is coming) was another signal of an impending birth. When the water breaks, it is the baby's house that is broken (*fifi en goai itasab*) which signals the time to tie a rope to the ceiling for the woman to hold as the baby is born.

Of all these phrases, the only one that was common in my interviews was the one referring to the "baby's house" (placenta) where it was often said that to hasten the birth of the "baby's house," the mother would sip water or have her stomach massaged in strong downward strokes. All the other Ubir phrases were used in contexts other than pregnancy or birthing, such as when someone had a wound bleeding profusely it would be said "tara egat." My frustration at not being able to re-present women's experiences of childbirth was not eased by my conversation with Pem and Cres, although I had secured a descriptive account from reliable sources.

Silences in ethnographic representations

It was not until I unexpectedly assisted with the birth of one of my nieces by the light of a small hurricane lamp and a two-cell flashlight, that the basis of my frustration eased. Because, once I had been involved in a birth, the need to describe it no longer existed but, more importantly, neither was there an audience. Prior to this, the closest I had ever come to knowing about the details of a birth was silent but intense eye contact with a sister-in-law when we met again after the birth, in different countries, of our first babies. I then recalled other times when it was known that a woman was in the process of giving birth, but no questions were asked about how she was and how the birth was progressing. This was quite unlike other situations where the detail of an illness, such as the rapid demise of one woman who died from a huge ulcer on her buttock, or an accident, as when a young man was gouged by a wild pig while hunting, was often retold in many ways and with much detail.

As I mentioned earlier, there were differences between me and the women I talked to in Wanigela but, even among my very close friends and family in Wanigela, this was not a topic we discussed in the detail I wanted to record as per other ethnographies on birth (e.g. Jordan 1993). But this silence was not a result of a repugnance of discussing bodily matters or prudity, because this happened for other conditions. Rather, it was through a protective respect for a situation that occurred regularly and extensively and hence where potential dangers for the mother and child are frequent. And the greatest respect that can be given is to relegate something to silence, but not of course from memory. I was unable to identify other situations where knowledge about child-bearing was exchanged or shared. During the interviews, I often probed to find out, in detail, what mothers had "told" or would tell their daughters about childbirth. No one was forthcoming. I recalled intimate conversation I had with friends but although we shared our feelings, never did we discuss the details of childbirth. Eventually I stopped probing. Partly this was because I reluctantly accepted that I was never going to obtain such information. But I also came to appreciate the potency of this information – it really was too delicate to handle. So, just like name avoidance taboos, where the names of certain relations are never spoken, I began to recognize the tremendous respect attributed to the details of childbirth.

Conclusion – how to deal with a baby that turns

How is it possible, then, to relate non-discursive understandings of child-bearing and pregnancy to representations of fertility in standard demographic analysis? There is clearly a great deal missing but how can this knowledge of missing things contribute to pragmatic population policy? What are some of the ways of negotiating the incompatible epistemologies and still advance the debates?

First, the partialities of authoritative accounts and discourses could be recognized. For instance, many women consider their extended years child-bearing and child-rearing with pride not shame. In one interview a woman nursing her twelfth and last child said she and her husband had raised all their children to be healthy but they had only agreed to stop because the latest delivery was "kafakai wawanin" (a bit hard). Previous deliveries were "basit" (okay). She began taking oral contraceptives. Having raised all of her children safely, she proudly said she had no regrets and she could see no reason why her daughters could not do the same.

Second, the birth, or death, of a child could be contexualized to bring out stories of multiple, often contradictory, and always complex power relations between different groups and individuals in Wanigela. For instance, I was interested in the reasons given for early childhood deaths, of which there were a number. I tried the process of triangulation – that is asking a number of people about a particular child or baby who died. Rarely did I hear the same story about how or why the child died. Each child born has its own connections to the individuals with whom I spoke and each of these relationships had its own politics. For instance, in one case the mother quietly avoided discussing why her third-born child died except to keep repeating, "He was sick." Clearly there was still pain associated with this event which had taken place eighteen years earlier. Yet the child's maternal grandmother was equally clear that it was because the child's father was wrongly pre-occupied with land disputes at the time that his family had been the successful target of sorcery. The child's paternal relative and neighbor, a devout Christian, who spoke of the inevitability of God's will, offered yet another angle. It is not surprising that Western religious dogmas, local cultural expectations, and understandings of sorcery are brought into this picture. Such complex relations of power exist and individuals in this community negotiate them constantly.

Finally, working with an ethnographic attitude does not change the calculations and estimates made by demographers. However, it is likely to make us think again about why particular problems are interesting, why particular questions, words, or phrases are articulated, and what value is given to the contributions of other groups of people involved. As Erica Schoenberger writes, "And your answers to these new kinds of questions might plausibly affect the trajectory of scientific enquiry that you follow" (1998: 2). Indeed, the hope is that they will.

So, how can it be done practically? The maternity histories that I collected provided me with an opportunity to contextualize the demographic data I had already collected. I thought it was going to be a simple case of juxtaposing numeric representation with the voices of the women I heard. But this was difficult because the two sets of "data" have different epistemological bases. Furthermore, fertility analysis is largely responsive to government needs (Greenhalgh 1990), with all the complicity this implies for funding fertility research. But then an ethnographic context does not tell us everything either. As I have shown about talking and not talking about child-bearing in Wanigela, the unsaid is not the unknown, but the differently known.

Informed by critical social theory, my project engages directly with ways of knowing that do not necessarily conform to Western ideas of rationality and objectivity. Thus it requires readers as well as listeners[8] to consider the real material body that bleeds and births as well as how women experience and think about the physicality of their daily life as well as what is not said. In this way, Linda McDowell's (1991) "baby" that is constantly threatened with being thrown out with the bathwater instead "turns" yet another way.

Notes

1   This is a contestable concept whose meaning has been addressed more fully than I intend to here (e.g. Escobar 1992). For the purposes of this chapter, I adopt the popular definition that refers to "countries" of the economic south in Asia, Africa,

Latin America, and Oceania. However, my use of small case indicates my discomfort with it as a proper noun.

2   I say "about" purposely because this was a count of names. Not only did I not sight everyone but there were also some people who were not even named such as the intellectually compromised girl mentioned in this chapter.

3   To the extent that I was most often known as "Graham Awan" (Graham's Wife). To those who did not know my family well, and to most small children, I was known as "Yai/Jever Bariau" (European Auntie or Lady). Other nicknames were probably used but I am unaware of them.

4   This was a distinctive part of my difference and so I was constantly reminded to take care when walking through overgrown paths, working in gardens, or in the hot sun.

5   Which included standard demographic questions such as year and place of birth, questions about kinship links, such as name of clan and siblings; and for the women, questions about the birth, and death, of all children they had ever given birth to.

6   All names used in this paper are pseudonyms.

7   Here I use the term "in general" but note Haraway's clarification: "fundamentally there is no way to make a *general* statement outside the never-finished work of articulating the partial worlds of *situated* knowledges" (Haraway 1997: 46, author's emphasis).

8   Because in Wanigela, as in much of the Pacific, oral expression is the primary mode of communication.

References

Alcoff, L. M. (1996) "Feminist theory and social science: new knowledges, new epistemologies," in N. Duncan (ed.) *Body Space*, London: Routledge: 13–27.

Barker, J. (1987) "Cheerful pragmatists: Anglican missionaries among the Maisin of Collingwood Bay, Northeastern Papua, 1898–1920," *The Journal of Pacific History* 22, 2: 66–81.

Basu, A. M. (1997) "The politicization of fertility to achieve non-demographic objectives," *Population Studies* 51: 5–18.

Bongaarts J. and Feeney, G. (1998) "On the quantum and tempo of fertility," *Population and Development Review* 24, 2: 271–91.

Correa, S. (1999) *Implementing ICPD: Moving Forward in the Eye of the Storm*, Fiji: DAWN.

Escobar, A. (1992) "Imagining a post-development era? Critical thought, development and social movements," *Social Text* 31/32: 20–56.

Findley, A. and Li, F. L. N. (1999) "Methodological issues in researching migration," *Professional Geographer* 51, 1: 50–9.

Ginsberg, F. D. and Rapp, R. (ed.) (1995) *Conceiving the New World Order: The Global Politics of Reproduction*, Berkeley: University of California Press.

Graham, E. (1999) "Breaking out: the opportunties and challenges of multi-method research in population geography," *Professional Geographer* 51, 1: 76–89.

Greenhalgh, S. (1990) "Towards a political economy of fertility: anthropological contributions," *Population and Development Review* 16, 1: 85–105.

—— (1996) "The social construction of population science: an intellectual, institutional and political history of twentieth-century demography," *Society for the Comparative Study of Society and History* 38, 1: 26–66.

Grosz, E. (1994) *Volatile Bodies: Towards a Corporeal Feminism*, St Leonards: Allen & Unwin.

Haraway, D. J. (1992) "Otherworldly conversations: terran, topics; local terms," *Science and Culture* 14: 64–98.

—— (1997) "The virtual speculum in the new world order," *Feminist Review* 55: 22–72.

Harding, S. (1995) "'Strong objectivity': a response to the new objectivity question," *Synthese* 104, 3: 331–49.

Johnson, L. C. (1994) "What future for feminist geography?," *Gender, Place, Culture* 1, 1: 103–12.

Jordan, B. (1993) *Birth in Four Cultures: A Cross Cultural Investigation of Childbirth in Yucatan, Holland, Sweden and the United States*, 4th edn, Prospect Heights, IL: Waveland.

Katz, C. (1991) "Sow what you know: the struggles for social reproduction in rural Sudan," *Annals of the Association of American Geographers* 8, 3: 488–514.

—— (1992) "All the world is staged: intellectuals and the projects of ethnography," *Environment and Planning D: Society and Space* 10: 495–510.

Katz, C. and Monk, J (1993) *Full Circles: Geographies of Women over the Life Course*, London: Routledge.

Kertzer, D. I. and Fricke, T. (eds) (1997) *Anthropological Demography: Towards a New Synthesis*, Chicago: University of Chicago Press.

Kobayashi, A. (1994) "Coloring the field: 'race' and the politics of fieldwork," *Professional Geographer* 46, 1: 73–80.

Longhurst, R. (1997) "(Dis)embodied geographies," *Progress in Human Geography* 21, 4: 486–501.

McDowell, L. (1992) "Doing gender: feminism, feminists and research methods in human geography," *Transaction of the Institute of British Geographers* 17: 399–416.

—— (1991) "The baby and the bath water: diversity, deconstruction and feminist theory in geography," *Geoforum* 22, 2: 123–33.

Maudood, E. K. (1993) "Gender relations in rural Bangladesh: aspects of differential norms about fertility, mortality and health practices," in J. H. Momsen and V. Kinnaird (eds) *Different Places, Different Voices: Gender and Development in Africa, Asia and Latin America*, London: Routledge: 80–92.

Morgan, L. M. (1997) "Imagining the unborn in the Ecuadorian Andes," *Feminist Studies* 23, 2: 323–50.

National Statistics Office (1997) *Papua New Guinea Demographic and Health Survey 1996: National Report*, National Statistics Office: Port Moresby.

Obermeyer, C. M. (1997) "Qualitative methods: a key to better understanding of demographic behaviour," *Population and Development Review* 23, 4: 813–18.

Scheper-Hughes, N. (1997) "Demography without numbers," in D. Kertzer and T. Fricke (eds) *Anthropological Demography: Towards a New Synthesis*, Chicago: University of Chicago Press: 201–22.

Schoenberger, E. (1998) "Discourse and practice in human geography," *Progress in Human Geography* 22, 1: 1–14.

Sporton, D. (1999) "Mixing methods in fertility research," *Professional Geographer* 51, 1: 68–76.

Tsing, A. L. (1993) *In the Realm of the Diamond Queen*, Princeton, NJ: Princeton University Press.

Underhill-Sem, Y. (1999) "Of social construction, politics and biology: population geographies in the Pacific," *Asia Pacific Viewpoint* 40, 1: 19–32.

Waiko, J. D. (1993) *A Short History of Papua New Guinea*, Melbourne: Oxford University Press.

Woods, R. I. (1979) *Population Analysis in Geography*, London: Longman.

Young, I. M. (1994) "Gender as seriality: thinking about women as a social collective," *Signs: Journal of Women and Culture in Society* 19, 3: 187–215.

12 Fear and trembling in the mall

Women, agoraphobia, and body boundaries[1]

Joyce Davidson

Anxiety is a feminine weakness in which freedom faints.

(Kierkegaard 1980: 60)

Agora – Gk. Hist. An assembly; a place of assembly, esp. a market place.
(*Shorter Oxford English Dictionary*)

For Kierkegaard, anxiety is a temptress that "disquiets" and "ensnares" the unwary individual, a "feminine weakness" that "is reflected more in Eve than in Adam" (Kierkegaard 1980: 64). Anxiety is a product of woman's more "sensuous" nature, the "immediacy" and openness she exhibits to the felt experiences of her bodily being and to her worldly surroundings (1980: 65). And yet, despite, or perhaps because of, its close relation to sex and sexuality, Kierkegaard recognizes anxiety's essential ambiguity. It presages both the possibility of freedom and of the "fall." "[T]he greatness of anxiety is a prophecy of the greatness of the perfection," (1980: 64) but for the finite and bounded individual freedom's infinite possibilities carry untold risks.

Kierkegaard's misogyny will not allow him to follow his logic to its own conclusion; woman's sensuous proclivities do not, it seems, signify her greater potential for freedom.[2] And perhaps this is just as well, for there is nothing liberating in the disorientating and disabling repercussions of anxiety for those many women who suffer its almost constant presence. Initially at least, Kierkegaard also seems mistaken in assuming that anxiety *per se* is gender specific since studies reveal no appreciable difference between men and women in the incidence of disorders associated with intense anxiety. However, anxiety takes many forms and there are clear signs of sex differences in the manners in which it finds expression. In particular agoraphobia, the fear of public places, does indeed appear to be a predominantly feminine "weakness." In a review of twelve different agoraphobia studies, Clum and Knowles (1991) found that women accounted for 89 percent of sufferers, a figure comparable to those suffering from anorexia nervosa. But, while there has been considerable interest in anorexia among feminists and social scientists concerned to explain its gendered distribution, the same cannot be said for agoraphobia. (See, for example, Bordo (1995) and Battersby (1998). Battersby (1998:46) claims that 90 percent of anorexics are women.) And, although there has been no shortage of *clinical* research into agoraphobia and related anxiety disorders, these have as yet attracted relatively little attention outside their medical and psychological contexts (see McNally (1994: vii), who details the exponential growth of academic papers on the subject published in medical journals in recent years).[3] This chapter forms part of an on-going project that seeks to remedy these shortcomings. Based on in-depth interviews with women attending self-help groups for agoraphobics in Central Scotland, it focuses on sufferers' descriptions of the effects that the disorder has on their experience of embodied identity in relation to place and the consequent disruption to the geography of their lives.[4] Here, I intend to draw (illustratively) on those "psychological" works of Kierkegaard,[5] suggesting that his understanding of anxiety can help us articulate something of the inherently *spatialized* nature of agoraphobia. Kierkegaard can thus aid understanding of sufferers' accounts of their anxious experience of contemporary spaces.

Each of the self-help groups from which interviewees were drawn was composed mainly, and often exclusively, of women, reflecting the gendered nature of the disorder in the population at large. The sufferers whom I interviewed might be described as self-selecting, in that they responded to a request made by me through a "gatekeeper" – the organizer of the group they attended. As a result, my sample could not be described as *representative* of women who suffer from agoraphobia. They tended to be long-term members of the self-help groups, and to be "coping" with their disorder well enough to be comfortable talking about it at length. Without exception, the women who presented themselves were loquacious and articulate in their attempts to convey just how much the disorder has impacted on every aspect of their lives. All were *accustomed* to talking about agoraphobia; at times, they may even have been relaying aspects of a narrative that had already been constructed as they struggled over time to make sense of a life fragmented by their agoraphobic experiences.

There was some variation in the ages of the respondents attending self-help groups; the youngest interviewee, whom I've called Susan, was thirty-three, and Fran, at eighty-two, was the oldest. The ages of the remaining six ranged from the early forties to the mid-sixties. All were married, though one was separated from her husband, and all had children. There is no representation of ethnic minorities; all of the respondents were white. However, their class backgrounds and current social status were diverse, and some of the women commented that the phobia may be the only thing they have in common: "We're all so different, but we all get on so well" (Fiona).

Despite their erstwhile differences it does appear that respondents share significant overlaps in the *spatial* and *temporal* phenomenology of their experiences of agoraphobia. Although the intensity of aversion to different places varies between individuals, sufferers all tended to have the most intense and debilitating difficulties in relation to those spaces of consumption of which the shopping mall is the apotheosis. (In practice few agoraphobics would dare to go near a fully-fledged "mall" since for most sufferers, a small-scale shopping center or supermarket presents a completely terrifying prospect, and even the corner shop may be completely out of bounds.)

The respondents were also alike in being "long-term" sufferers. This too is not unusual since agoraphobia is frequently a chronic condition, a constant and continuing struggle fought over the boundaries of the sufferer's confinement. Most respondents did not believe that they could ever be fully "cured" of agoraphobia; they merely learn to cope with, to borrow another phrase from Kierkegaard, a despair which seems to be a "sickness unto death" (Kierkegaard 1989: 47). "Being phobic is a bit like being an alcoholic. I don't think you're ever completely cured" (Chris).

The nature of agoraphobia

Despite the common misconception that agoraphobia is simply a fear of "open" spaces, it is actually characterized by a complex cluster of phobias connected specifically with public places. These fears may include experiences of vertigo and, ironically, claustrophobia, as Lynn explains: "Agoraphobia doesn't really mean to say that you're afraid of the, sort of, open spaces. You can't actually go into like cinemas and that. It's got a claustrophobic effect, as well, you know."[6] In another respondent's words, "I never agreed with the definition of agoraphobia anyway. I'm fine in an open space. As long as there's no a whole lot o' people there I'm fine" (Carron).

In most cases, the avoidance behavior that characterizes agoraphobia (and sets it apart from simple panic disorder[7]) begins after the occurrence of a panic attack in a public place, such as a busy street or shop. It is likely that initially the individual will not *know* that what she experienced was a panic attack, only that the episode was so utterly horrific that under no circumstances does she want to go through it again:

> Oh god, oh no, I can't breathe, I definitely can't breathe, I'm going to die in a minute, I'm going to collapse and there's no' a soul here to help me . . . it's so irrational it's unbelievable . . . your mind works so fast, your heart's beating, you feel sick, your legs don't want to work, it's . . . it's horrendous.
>
> (Susan)

The sufferer then becomes anxious that by placing herself in a similar situation she may be subject to another attack, and consequently, she steers clear of public places. Ann, herself a long-term sufferer now helping to run her local self-help group, explains:

That's what makes a lot of people agoraphobic, cause they've taken a panic attack when they've been out, and then they're scared to go out . . . they will avoid that street again, or they'll not go out because immediately they get their coat on to go out the next day, they think, "well now what happens if that happens again?"

(Ann)

At first it seems that the sufferer can *place* their fear, locate the roots of their panic at a particular point. But the roots quickly branch out to infiltrate different places. In the early stages, this unpredictability of the panic attack may in fact be one of its most terrifying features:

Often they come completely out of the blue. A lot of people who come [to the group] say "I was just perfectly fine, and I was walking down the road, and then, all of a sudden, you know, the pounding and the racing heart, and the sweating."

(Ann)

As the subject becomes increasingly agoraphobic, she finds she can take little about the geography of her life for granted. Her mental map is necessarily fluid, the boundaries between safe and unsafe space unstable. In the early stages, it must be constantly reconfigured to signify the newly perilous no-go areas, and over time, becomes increasingly restrictive. The subject finds that the limits of her everyday world retreat to a diminishingly small area around her home until eventually no place is considered risk free. The safest, or indeed the *only*, course of action available is simply not to go out at all. "Some people are completely house-bound you know, with agoraphobia . . . I mean I was never completely house-bound, but I did feel the world was getting smaller" (Ann).

Sufferers often find it difficult to articulate their reasons for being house-bound; they cannot say why exactly the world beyond their front door is so threatening, and this can make their condition opaque and puzzling to the non-phobic observer:

I just stopped goin' out, because . . . it's . . . I don't know why . . . Just a feeling I got, I thought there was something out there . . . [shudders] that . . . you know, I felt safe within the house. I think I was running away fae life, you know?

(Lynn)

Another woman, Susan, commented, "For two and a half years I never went over the door . . . no matter how much you wanted to [go outside] you genuinely couldn't because the fear was stronger than anything else."

In most instances it seems clear that staying within the home is basically an attempt to avoid the physical and mental pain of the panic attack. (Fiona, in fact, *defines* agoraphobia as "just where people don't go out because they're frightened they'll have a panic attack.") The experience leaves the sufferer feeling entirely dislocated, uprooted (disembedded) from the context which gives meaning to her surroundings. Faced with this potential threat to the grounds on which her identity is based, the subject feels a need for safe, familiar space that will feel least alien in the event of a crisis; they long for the "relative" comfort provided by their own four walls.

The phenomenology of fear

Agoraphobia does not only result in a gendered "geography of exclusion" which confines women to their homes but is, in many ways, a form of anxiety best expressed in a spatial terminology.[8] Marilyn Silverman, amongst others, has noted that "[s]patial metaphors are well suited to capture the phenomenology of the particular form of panic that occurs when the most fundamental sense of existence and connection is at stake" (Silverman in Bordo *et al.* 1998: 89–90). I would go further. The relationship between space and agoraphobia is not merely metaphorical. Accounts of agoraphobic anxiety suggest that it seems to be spatially *mediated*: agoraphobia is in *essence* an im/mediately spatial affair. The non-locatable fear which typifies agoraphobia, that oppressive, yet inherently intangible "something in the air," is a quality of the dynamic relationship between *self and space, person and place*. For the agoraphobic, anxiety becomes *all-encompassing*, affecting those spaces in, of, and around the self.

It is interesting to note that agoraphobia, a term coined by Westphal in 1871, had earlier been referred to by Benedikt as *platzschwindel* – literally "dizziness in public places" (Mathews *et al.* 1981: 1). "Dizziness" is, if anything, too mild a term for the intensely disorientating personal experience of the sufferer as she seems to "lose touch" with her surroundings, to be standing on the edge of an abyss. The sufferer feels isolated from all external assistance, sucked into a vacuum that threatens to engulf her very being:

> When you have this you feel you're on your own, you feel . . . nobody else has got it, you're in this situation, and it's just like a situation you'll never get out of, *a black hole that you'll never get out of*.
>
> (Ann, emphasis added)

An everyday situation can suddenly lose its familiarity as she is caught in a vortex that spins her out of control. "Suddenly the stage disappears. *The floor drops out*. The players and set vanish or persist as unfamiliar figures in another script in which you have no part" (Silverman in Bordo *et al.* 1998: 90, emphasis added). In such circumstances the sufferer longs for something solid to grab hold of. Susan Bordo describes her own agoraphobic experience thus: "I was stranded on the edge of an enormous [iceberg], rising high out of the sea, *perched, precarious, desperate for walls to plant my hands against*" (Bordo in Bordo *et al.* 1998: 80, emphasis added).

For Kierkegaard too "[a]nxiety may be compared with dizziness" (1980: 61). He (*sic*) whose eye happens to look down into the yawning abyss becomes dizzy (ibid.). "But what," Kierkegaard asks, "is the reason for this" dizziness? *Where does this feeling come from?* The source of the anxiety is not easily *located*. "It is just as much in his [*sic*] own eyes as in the abyss, for suppose he had not looked down?" The "abyss" is not a geographic feature of the landscape of one's everyday life so much as a rift in its fabric. Nor is anxiety simply an "internal" reflex to specific external stimuli. Rather anxiety is evoked by an existential challenge to what for most of us, most of the time, is a well-defined presumption of our concrete self-identity. "I couldn't control it when I was out there. You know, really, you honestly believe you are *on the brink* of death" (Susan, emphasis added).

Agoraphobic anxiety seemingly threatens the dissolution of the self. When it surfaces it erodes the boundary between "inside" and "outside" in such a way that the individual seems, quite literally, "lost." She no longer knows *where* she is, both in the sense that her surroundings have become unfamiliar and threatening and in the sense that she cannot *locate or delimit* her own identity: she feels "spaced-out." Agoraphobia induces a crisis in the "boundary" between self and space that throws the reality of both into doubt. In Bordo's words (1998: 74):

> [e]ach of us [herself and her sisters] has suffered, each in her own way, from a certain heightened consciousness of space and place and our body's relation to them: spells of anxiety that could involve the feeling of losing one's place in space and time.

This phenomenon has been recognized in the clinical literature as "derealization" and/or depersonalization, and involves disturbing and sometimes bizarre changes in one's feelings of embodiment (Chambless and Goldstein 1982; Marks 1987). Roger Caillois (quoted in Grosz 1994: 47) refers to this problematization of the individual's boundaries as "depersonalization by assimilation to space." According to Isaac Marks, "[d]uring depersonalization one feels temporarily strange, unreal, *disembodied*, cut off or far away from immediate surroundings" (Marks 1987: 342, emphasis added).

Susan articulates how frightening this disruption in the sufferers' spatial phenomenology is, and how, in the aftermath, the agoraphobic's world will, quite literally, never be the same again:

> [Y]ou try and make your way back home. And here's another weird thing, you get nearer and nearer to your house, but *your house feels like it's getting further and further away from you*, like tunnel, sort of, vision, and you get so freaked that you actually start physically running. I mean

I've ran down that road with my five year old practically scraping along the ground, because I've been in such a distressed state.

(Susan, emphasis added)

Agoraphobia can be said to create a *garbled* geography, where that "closest in," the body,[9] is no longer safely delimited from the outside world. Public space becomes corrosive to the subject's boundaries;[10] she incorporates the surrounding confusion, and fears that she is "losing her grip" on reality: "I actually thought I was, I was losing my mind, you know. I thought something's definitely wrong" (Lynn). "Well, to begin with, I thought I was going off my head. I really, really thought I was going off my head" (Maggie).

Fear and panic in the face of public space are then the *defining* features of agoraphobia. It disrupts our unconscious sense of ourselves, throwing the relation we have with our bodies, our *selves*, into question.[11] Following the onset of "fear and trembling" as a way of life, there is a loss of *trust* in the integrity of the body; the subject fears being betrayed by it, and is constantly on the look out for breaches of bodily boundaries which might be visible to others. These include, for example, minor discrepancies such as blushing, trembling, or sweating, in addition to more extreme examples, such as screaming out loud, or the loss of bowel or bladder control, manifestations of their fear on the surface of their bodies which would be thoroughly humiliating.[12] The intensely *embodied* nature of these "emotional" states necessitates a reconfiguration of the subject's conception of themselves. The disorder seems to initiate a sense of *separateness* from one's body, not just momentarily, as in the fleeting depersonalization of the panic attack but in the more general sense of creating a constant anxiety which hovers over the question of our bodily and mental identity.

Carron expresses her sense of separateness from her mind whilst at the same time acknowledging the very oddness of the idea that they could ever be separate (she remarks that "normal" people would find her comment strange):

I got up this morning and I thought, "Och I'm no' going to the [self-help] group . . . yeah I'm goin' . . . no I'm not." And it's like that, *the mind changes* all the time. And then when it comes to it, you think, I'm going to have to get my jacket on quick and rush out before it changes again. [laughs] You've got to keep a sense of humor.

(Carron, emphasis added)

In many ways, she experiences her self as less coherent and consistent than she was. She can't rely on herself to be anywhere at a certain time, as she actually doesn't know until the last instant whether or not she will be able to manage the transition between home and not-home. Her ability to negotiate that threshold requires her being in step with her body, and distanced from her anxiety, but whether she can do it or not almost feels like potluck.

Precisely because something seems to have gone wrong agoraphobia forces our bodily and mental states to the forefront of our attention; we are no longer "at one with" our body, and our relationship with it is no longer unconscious or unproblematic. From a phenomenological position it is unsurprising that anxiety should manifest itself both "bodily" and "mentally" since phenomenological theorists such as Merleau-Ponty assume a model of identity which regards the body *as* the self, the "self expressed" (Merleau-Ponty 1962). But, given the ease with which we normally "take for granted" our status as clearly defined individuals, as solid bodies which contain (and also constitute) our personalities, it comes as something of a shock to realize that, in Elizabeth Grosz's terms, we might inhabit "volatile bodies." For Grosz (1994: 79), mind and body alike are not static or impervious to our surroundings but labile and at least semi-permeable:

> The limits or borders of the body image are not fixed by nature or confined to the anatomical "container," the skin. The body image is extremely fluid and dynamic; its borders, edges and contours are "osmotic" – they have the remarkable power of incorporating and expelling outside and inside in an ongoing exchange.

When the ability to subconsciously regulate these processes of incorporation and expelling slips from our control then our very existence as a bounded self is thrown into doubt. "I was startled awake one day to realize that *I was almost entirely gone.* What woke me was my body, whose very being in the world suddenly shifted and changed everything" (Bordo *et al.* 1998: 80, emphasis added). The difference between the sufferer and normalcy is epitomized in Bordo's account of agoraphobia: "Being outside, which when I was agoraphobic had left me feeling substanceless, a medium through which body, breath and world would rush, squeezing my heart and dotting my vision, now gave me definition, body, focused my gaze" (ibid.: 83).

Agoraphobia seems to express an anxiety about one's ability to regulate and control the dialectic between permanence and impermanence, permeability and imperviousness. Interestingly, Kierkegaard's phenomenal psychology also recognizes a similar requirement for balance in a self which has to be seen not as a "given," atomic, and autonomous individuality but as a "process of becoming" (1989: 60), a "project that occurs in time" (Hannay's Introduction in ibid.: 23). "A human being is," he says, "a synthesis of the infinite and the finite, of the temporal and the eternal, of freedom and necessity" (Kierkegaard 1989: 43).

For Kierkegaard, "[p]ersonhood is a synthesis of possibility and necessity. Its manner is therefore like breathing (respiration)" (1989: 70). And like breathing it usually continues unnoticed and unremarked unless problematized. The fear is that once panic has drawn the agoraphobic's attention to the unstable morphology of the self then she becomes focused wholly on the infinite realm of possibilities. "I think people with this disorder are very, very selfish. You don't mean to be selfish, but you're constantly tuned into your body, your self, all about you, all the time" (Susan).

Kierkegaard invokes a spatial metonymics that echoes women's accounts of agoraphobic anxiety. For when the self looks "down into its own possibility" (1980: 61) its anxiety increases; "phantasms succeed one another with such speed that it seems as though everything were possible, and this is the very moment the individual himself [*sic*] has finally become nothing but an atmospheric illusion" (1989: 66). The world begins to spin and the individual must grab "hold of finiteness to support itself" (1980: 61). Whilst Kierkegaard believes that our freedom to act as individuals depends upon imagination – "the medium of infinitization," (1989: 60) – the danger is that:

> when emotion becomes fantastic in this way, the self is simply more and more *volatilized* and eventually becomes a kind of *abstract sensitivity* which inhumanly belongs to no human . . . the person whose emotions have become fantastic . . . *becomes infinitized . . . he [sic] loses himself more and more.*
>
> (1989: 61, emphasis added)

This sensitivity to the infinite, the unbounded, is abstract precisely because it seems to have nothing solid to latch on to; "the object of anxiety is a nothing"(Kierkegaard 1980: 77). And yet precisely because that anxiety is non-locatable it attains a terrible reality. "It's fear of *fear*. It's fear of what . . . this feeling that's gonnae come. It absolutely petrifies you, and you just don't want to face . . . because it's a terrible feeling" (Carron). This "nothing" is the abyss above which the self, made conscious of its possibilities, balances fearing to look down lest it should fall and be annihilated. Ironically, this nothing is also the open landscape against which the self can choose to define its own existence. It is for this reason that Kierkegaard claims "*anxiety is the dizziness of freedom*" (Kierkegaard 1980: 61, emphasis added).

Consumer/consuming culture

> The biggest danger, that of losing oneself, can pass off in the world as quietly as if it were nothing; every other loss, an arm, a leg, five dollars, a wife, etc. is bound to be noticed.
>
> (Kierkegaard 1989: 1)

For Kierkegaard there are two ways of losing oneself: the first in the swirling maelstrom of the imagination's unbounded possibilities, the second by never becoming aware of oneself at all, for example, by focusing one's attention on *being someone else*. The former is, for Kierkegaard, preferable since it is more reflexive; at least the sufferer has become aware of the pliant morphology of their existence, of freedom's possibilities and dangers. In the second case, the individual may often appear untroubled, though this is a result of their having suppressed their own potential by continually misrecognizing who or what they might be. This he refers to as an impotent *"consumption of the self"* (1989: 48). The fact that the person seems untroubled is according to Kierkegaard merely a sign of "a sickness that . . . hasn't yet declared itself" (1989: 50).

Interestingly, the subject who ventures into the mall risks *losing herself* in both ways. On the one hand, faced with so many disparate versions of what the self is or could be, she directs herself towards something she is not; she is compelled to seek an identity behind the idealized images modeled in window displays and advertisements. But, even if she resists the imperative to consume subjectivities, to be an "identity shopper,"[13] she must still negotiate those avenues of corrosive space which seek to break down her resistance to buy, to manipulate her values and emotions and to forget herself in the momentary pleasures of satisfying desires manufactured by others.

Spaces of consumption present grave dangers to the identities of phobic and non-phobic subjects alike. They are assemblages of numerous and overlaid attempts at sensory stimulation, which can render the atmosphere excruciatingly intense. Clearly, the charged space is *intended* to have a certain impact on the subject. "[T]he mall presents a *dizzying* spectacle of attractions and diversions" (Crawford 1991: 3, emphasis added). Mike Featherstone refers to shopping centers' use of "dream-like illusions and spectacles, eclecticism and mixed codes, which induce the public to flow past a multiplicity of cultural vocabularies which provide no opportunity for distanciation (de-distanciation) and encourage a sense of immediacy, instantiation, emotional de-control and childlike wonder" (Featherstone 1996: 103). For the agoraphobic, however, these same geographic effects are resonant of terror rather than wonder; they are more nightmare than dream.

Despite the occasional pool or fountain intended to soothe shoppers' frayed nerves those "captains of consciousness" (Goss 1992: 173) who plan the shopping experience co-ordinate a consumptive assault on our senses designed to make the visitor "shop 'till they drop." They are concerned to create an atmosphere as conducive to consumption as possible; the subject should not be distracted from their purpose by, for example, unnecessary exits, and should be left to decide only between which *particular* consumer goods to buy. In this theater of consumption the subject is discouraged from any free-style performance. They are expected instead to perform their role in a ballet choreographed by others, to sweep up and down the aisles, "go with the flow" of the consumer chorus, and exit stage left only when they have filed past the greatest combination of spectacularly arrayed "goods" possible.

Such spaces are extraordinarily problematic for agoraphobics who derive comfort from the knowledge that they are free to move as they please, and *leave* if they need to. This requires careful positioning relative to an escape route at all times. Spaces of consumption, whether shopping mall or supermarket, do not allow for easy enactment of this defense. Even if one succeeds in negotiating the lines of goods it is still necessary to stand in line and present one's purchases at the till before reaching the exit – "there's a queue in the shop and you think, I must get out of here, I just can't stand in that queue" (Ann).[14] Control seems wrested from her at all levels and, for the subject of uncertain boundaries, shopping is a risky business, best avoided. Avoidance may however be particularly difficult for those with roles as "wife" and "mother." In this case shopping is not only a practical necessity but a moral "duty" inextricably linked with her gendered identity. The inability to perform this duty may be perceived as a disturbing personal failure and initiate serious and debilitating doubts about her self worth. "One thing I will say, it destroys your confidence. It *takes* your confidence, I mean it really does, it knocks it right out you . . . it really screws you up" (Susan). "You feel like a wee ball of nothing. You wonder what you're on the planet for, when you can't do *any* of the things you *should* be doing" (Carron). And, since it is still culturally coded as a feminine pastime,[15] shopping is top of respondents' lists of "things you should be doing."[16]

This part of the sufferer's "job," which requires her to go outside the home, is singularly the most difficult activity for her even to contemplate. Susan Bordo describes a panic attack in a crowded supermarket, when everything feels alien and frightening to her, "the noise, the crying children, the pushing and shoving" (Bordo *et al.* 1998: 34). When it comes to shopping, for example for food, or clothes, or even birthday presents for the kids, the agoraphobic woman has a real problem on her hands, one that almost certainly requires some ingenuity, and outside help, to cope with:

> So then I sort of, if I was going to the shops I would wait for my husband so that he would come with me, you know I found all these different ways. Or I would get somebody else to go to the shops for me, so that basically I didn't have to go to the shops.
>
> (Susan)

Other interviewees recount a similar kind of dependence on various friends and family members. Fran, for example, describes her mother as having to "stand in for her"; in Lynn's case "the kids had to go to the wee shop across the road," or her sister (who also had some experience of panic episodes) would help out. Eventually, Lynn's sister started to encourage her to leave the house herself ("you can't live the rest of your life looking at four walls"), first to visit her at home, two bus stops away, then to go on shopping trips together. "The first day I got the bus down to her, I was hyperventilating when I got off the bus and it was a *nightmare* . . . but I made it." Very gradually, Lynn was able to build enough confidence to try her hand at shopping; "although I felt uncomfortable . . . you don't *enjoy* shopping, you don't enjoy these kind of things, but she was with me and she helped me."

It is in recounting their experiences of "consumer affairs" that the respondents reveal most about the effect of the disorder on their everyday lives:

> Non-phobics take a lot for granted. I did too when I was non-phobic. You take it for granted that you just go out and get on a bus and you go. I mean I could never take for granted that I'm going to lift my shopping bag and go and get some shopping. I cannae do it.
>
> (Carron)

"Shopping" provides a recurring, even unifying theme to their narratives, cropping up whether they are discussing, for example, their first panic attack, social restrictions on their lives, or in Maggie's case, issues connected with treatment and measurement of the extent of their recovery:

> So I gradually started going into [nearest large town] with my husband. And I'm no saying it was easy, sometimes I was sitting away down on the floor in the back [of the car] . . . things like that. But then gradually it did get better and I was staying longer in the shops.

Maggie can be seen to measure the extent of her recovery by her ability to stay in shops for increasing amounts of time. Even as her tolerance builds and her defenses grow stronger, the smallest details of her grocery requirements continue to be of tremendous significance; the replenishment of the larder, even the bread-bin, will never again be taken for granted:

> I can go the shopping an' that now, and I go down the street every day for the wee . . . I do a big shop once a week, and then I have to go down through the week if I need fresh bread or milk or whatever. And I can do that.

Sharing accounts of their problems with shopping often forms a focus for the self-help groups:

> Just the knowledge that other people suffer the way you do is so . . . helpful. When I'm in the supermarket and I start having a panic attack, and I think "oh oh," and then I think, "M will have had these bad turns too", and it just makes me feel so much better.
>
> (Fiona)

This is one of the reasons why attendance at the self-help group can be so very constructive – the sufferer learns that they are not alone in the world.[17] The other members know exactly how difficult it is to place yourself anywhere near shopping spaces, and will give you credit for your painful efforts:

We can give support, and understand . . . if you do manage to do such a simple thing . . . We can rejoice with them. But if you don't know what it's like and what it's cost that person, to pluck up the courage to do it [laughs], you know if you tell someone that isn't a sufferer, they think, you know, "well, big deal."

(Ann)

Sufferers' attempts to develop spatial strategies which enable them to cope on a day-to-day basis, and to regain some control over the geography of their lives, were also communicated around the theme of shopping. Both Carron and Maggie were put in contact with health care professionals who helped them to cultivate a tolerance of consuming places. By coming to their homes and, after careful preparation, taking them out, then into a shop, then a shopping center, they gradually and gently increased the time spent there on each occasion. Having prior knowledge of exactly how and when they would leave, a degree of control over the proceedings, made the experience (barely) tolerable. Forewarned, and tentatively forearmed, sufferers can just about manage to contain the rising tide of terror until it is time to make their escape. A sympathetic GP explained to Maggie that if she was

in a shop and I could feel a panic coming on, just to tighten up the muscles in my hands, he said "nobody'll see you, just let go, or bend your knees a little and walk about," it's things like that that help.

(Maggie)

These methods soothe because they remind the sufferer of the fact of her embodiment, of the location of the *limits* of her body. If she can place her boundaries before the panic takes hold, she may be able to hold on to some sense of herself, and prevent their dissolution.

However, it must be stressed that for many agoraphobics, *talking* about the issue is all that they can do; actually *going* shopping, *at all*, is simply not an option. When the women I interviewed move on to discuss their experiences of gradually regaining entry to the forbidding, *consuming* realm of shopping spaces, it is clearly after having spent *years* in the attempt. Only when they determine to set out on the road to "recovery" can they begin to think about being a consumer.

To enter the mall without fear and trembling one must become *sure of oneself* – of the self that *you* are – rather than those myriad others that are offered as alternatives. One must also feel secure in oneself, at ease in the body's bounds. But the shopping mall epitomizes those architectures of alienation that undermine security, seeking to play upon the feminine imagination *as consumer* and, at the same time, realize the misogynist *imagery of the woman as that which is consumed* by/for others. The woman who dares to enter spaces of consumption is forced to accept a subject position structured by these two poles, to abandon hope of being herself.

Inside the new churches of consumer capital the feminine self is sacrificed according to a patriarchal logic which (in Kierkegaard's words) regards "[a] woman who is happy without *self-abandonment*, that is, without giving all of her self, no matter what she gives it to, [as] altogether unfeminine" (1989: 81, emphasis added).

But perhaps hope is not entirely lost. As the respondents in this study show, though they may never become *carefree* consumers, neither must they remain confined within the four walls of their personal domestic realm. It is possible for a path to be forged between these poles, for the agoraphobic to re-constitute herself as a bounded yet free-flowing individual. In part this might depend upon coming to recognize the paradoxical nature of the relationship between anxiety, freedom, and selfhood.

This paradox is at the heart of Kierkegaard's philosophy. To be aware of oneself is to be aware of the self's possibilities, of its freedom to be otherwise. It is this freedom that makes us autonomous (human) rather than automatons. Through self-reflexivity we become aware of our-selves as selves, as a synthesis of the finite (a bounded and embodied subject) and the infinite (freedom), of "actuality" and the "potentiality." But this synthesis is difficult to achieve, for freedom can be a terrifying prospect and looking upon it we are subject to that "feminine" weakness "anxiety."

Never having the potential to be a self in her own right "woman" seems destined to remain in anxiety's purgatory. But Kierekgaard's misogynistic exegesis of the self entirely ignores the feminine predicament and in so doing he misrecognizes both the etiology of and the potential cure for such existential anxiety. Kierkegaard forgets that sensitivity to the self also entails sensitivity to the self's surroundings. *Sensitivity* to the self's possibilities also "brings home" the manner in which the external world threatens to intrude upon and call that self into question. In other words anxiety is not simply "*the dizziness of freedom*" (Kierkegaard 1980: 61, emphasis added). Anxiety can also be a mark of the self's recognition of those external forces which threaten to subvert its autonomy, to restrict or undermine its hard-fought freedoms. The struggle to maintain a conception of one's *self*-identity is made harder for a woman by her recognition that, in a masculine economy, her surroundings selectively seek to isolate and/or dissipate her identity, that they constantly call her to deny her-self. Indeed the feminine sensitivity to her surroundings of which Kierkegaard makes so much might itself be a product of this recognition of an environment that treats her as consumer and/or seeks to consume her.

If this is true, then there lies the potential for a reflexive recognition of the self, despite the manner in which the masculine economy mediates and distorts the feminine dialectic between freedom and anxiety. In part at least this might come from an understanding that the same phenomena that previously seemed to call her being into question can also serve to enhance her feeling of embodied identity. Susan Bordo writes, "[b]eing outside, which when I was agoraphobic had left me feeling substanceless, a medium through which body, breath and world would rush, squeezing my heart and dotting my vision, now gave me definition, body, focused my gaze" (Bordo *et al.* 1998: 83). The feelings associated with panic can begin to be translated as excitement. Like the child who spins in circles, manufacturing dizziness for the delightful disorientation it creates, the agoraphobic can learn that temporary loss of one's "normal" perspective can be liberating. To open oneself up to excitement, to learn to endure and even enjoy the *potentiality* of panic without giving oneself over to it completely, is the phenomenal freedom to which the agoraphobic aspires.

However, this process of *re-definition* is slow and often arduous. It is usually only achievable via a process of *acclimatization* to threatening space, and the patience to persevere through almost imperceptible improvements. Very gradually, her feelings of isolation and abandonment may become transformed and even re-placed by a sense of freedom and independence. Public space that challenged her boundaries can begin to be experienced positively, and need not entail a descent into the void. Bordo explains how, when overcoming her agoraphobia, she began to enjoy her "freedom," the "charge of leaving home, knowing that your body has been cut loose from the cycling habits of the domestic domain and is now moving unrooted across time and space, always to something new, alert to the defining gaze of strangers" (Bordo *et al.* 1998: 81). Similarly, Maggie describes her elation after having successfully negotiated a trip to hospital to visit her mother: "Once I got back in [her home town] on that bus, I felt like shouting in the square 'I've done it!' You know you just feel so good." Anxiety, despite, or perhaps because of, its association with the abyss, can be intensely life-affirming, rather than simply soul-destroying.

Acknowledgments

Thanks to Liz Bondi, Mick Smith, Charles Withers, and the editors of this collection for helpful comments and advice. I dedicate this chapter to Rionach, a truly great spirit.

Notes

1 Søren Kierkegaard's *Fear and Trembling: Dialectical Lyric* was first published in 1843 under the pseudonym Johanes de Silentio. Kierkegaard was a prominent and influential nineteenth-century philosopher. I suggest that his development of an existentialist analysis of human experience and emotion is particularly helpful for approaching and understanding the nature of agoraphobic life-worlds.
2 Rather they merely indicate that her role is to mediate between the world and *man*-kind; "only through Eve could Adam be seduced by [the possibilities offered by] the serpent" (Kierkegaard 1980: 66).
3 An article written by Susan Bordo and her two sisters concerning her own and their mother's experience of agoraphobia provides a recent and notable exception (Bordo *et al.* 1998). On the subject of "anxiety" more generally, there has been increased interest recently, as anxiety is seen by some as a defining feature of

contemporary life. See, for example, Giddens (1997), Kroker *et al.* (1989), on "panic postmodernism," and Dunant and Porter (1996). Linda McDowell also notes that "anxiety is a central theme in a great deal of current work" (McDowell 1996: 30).

4 Eight women from three self-help groups have participated in semi-structured interviews that have been taped and transcribed. They are referred to in the text by pseudonyms. I have also interviewed one man who described himself as an "ex-sufferer," and is now involved in organizing self-help groups and producing resource material for sufferers, and a woman who established a community-based "mobility initiative." She had found that, contrary to her expectations, many of her clients who experienced difficulties negotiating public spaces and transport were not physically disabled, but rather suffering from agoraphobia. She was able to provide some insights into the effects of the disorder from a non-phobic perspective.

5 "[*The Concept of Anxiety* and *The Sickness Unto Death*] are aptly enough called Kierkegaard's psychological works" (Hannay 1982: 157).

6 Danielle Quinodoz writes of the "inseparable alternation of claustrophobia and agoraphobia" (1997: 53). For Quinodoz, "it is clear that the problem of claustrophobic and agoraphobic patients in relating to their surroundings also reflects the difficulties they have in structuring their psychic space" (1997: 53). See also Kathleen Kirby (1996) on her experience of "post traumatic vertigo."

7 The definitions I employ are those set out in the most recent edition of the *Diagnostic and Statistical Manual of Mental Disorders* (DSM IV), produced by the American Psychiatric Association (1996).

8 See Sibley (1997), for a discussion of what he terms "geographies of exclusion."

9 In her oft-quoted essay "Notes toward a politics of location" (1986), Adrienne Rich refers to the body as "the geography closest in."

10 See Davidson (2000a, b), where I attempted to develop the characterization of agoraphobia as a disorder of the boundaries, and the panic attack as a boundary crisis that dissolves the barrier between "inner self" and "outer space."

11 In his introduction to Kierkegaard's *The Concept of Anxiety*, Reidar Thomte writes that "[f]ear is a threat to the periphery of one's existence and can be studied as an effect among other effects. Anxiety is a threat to the foundation and center of one's existence. It is ontological and can be understood only as a threat to *Dasein*" (xvii). Anxiety then, on this view at least, disrupts the very essence of our "*being in the world.*"

12 It can, though, be difficult to encourage interviewees to talk specifically about their embodiment at any length, and there is not much in the way of advice to be gleaned from existing literature. Emily Martin has, though, perhaps gone some way towards offering a framework for this kind of research (Martin 1989).

13 See Langman (1994), and Gabriel and Lang (1995: ch. 5).

14 Mathews *et al.* report a study which found "joining a line in a store" to be the most commonly reported anxiety-provoking situation amongst agoraphobics (96 percent) (1981: 4).

15 See for example, Campbell (1997), Langman (1994), and Miller (1997).

16 Although two of the women were now able to manage part-time employment outside the home (one as a care assistant in a residential home for the elderly, the other as a cleaner in the village hotel), there was a tendency among the women to refer to themselves as "housewives." Lynn, unable to do things for her children outside the home, complained of not being able to do her "so called *job* properly."

17 All of the respondents had positive experiences of self-help groups, but it is acknowledged that this is not always the case. As Ann explains, some people "only come for one meeting, because it might not be for them." Others "just think 'ah, this is a waste of time,' because they're not cured."

References

American Psychiatric Association (1996) *Diagnostic and Statistical Manual of Mental Disorders*, 4th edn, Washington, DC: American Psychiatric Association.

Battersby, C. (1998) *The Phenomenal Woman: Feminist Metaphysics and Patterns of Identity*, Cambridge: Polity Press.

Bordo, S. (1995) *Unbearable Weight: Feminism, Western Culture and the Body*, Berkeley, Los Angeles, and London: University of California Press.

Bordo, S., Klein, B., and Silverman, M. K. (1998) "Missing kitchens," in H. J. Nast and S. Pile (eds) *Places Through the Body*, London: Routledge: 72–92.

Burgin, V. (1996) *In/Different Spaces: Place and Memory in Visual Culture*, Berkeley, Los Angeles, and London: University of California Press.

Caillois, R. (1984) "Mimicry and legendary psychasthenia," *October 31* (Winter): 17–32.

Campbell, C. (1997) "Shopping, pleasure and the sex war," in P. Falk and C. Campbell (eds) *The Shopping Experience*, London: Sage Publications: 166–76.

Chambless, D. L. and Goldstein, A. J. (eds) (1982) *Agoraphobia: Multiple Perspectives on Theory and Treatment*, New York: John Wiley & Sons.

Clum, G. A. and Knowles, S. L. (1991) "Why do some people with panic disorder become avoidant?: A review," *Clinical Psychology Review* 11: 295–313.

Crawford, M. (1991) "The world in a shopping mall," in Michael Sorkin (ed.) *Variations on a Theme Park: The New American City and the End of Public Space*, New York: Hill & Wang.

Csordas, T. J. (ed.) (1994) *Embodiment and Experience: The Existential Ground of Culture and Self*, Cambridge: Cambridge University Press.

Davidson, J. (2000a) "'The world was getting smaller': women, agoraphobia and bodily boundaries," *Area* 32, 1: 31–40.

—— (2000b) "A phenomenology of fear: Merleau-Ponty and agoraphobic life-worlds," *Sociology of Health and Illness* 22, 5: 640–60.

Dunant, S. and Porter, R. (eds) (1996) *The Age of Anxiety*, London: Virago.

Featherstone, M. (1996) *Consumer Culture and Postmodernism*, London: Sage Publications.

Gabriel, Y. and Lang, T. (1995) *The Unmanageable Consumer: Contemporary Consumption and its Fragmentations*, London: Sage Publications.

Giddens, A. (1997) *Modernity and Self-Identity*, Cambridge: Polity Press.

Goss, J. (1992) "Modernity and post-modernity in the retail landscape," in K. Anderson and F. Gale (eds) *Inventing Places: Studies in Cultural Geography*, Cheshire: Longman.

Grosz, E. (1994) *Volatile Bodies: Towards a Corporeal Feminism*, Bloomingdale and Indianapolis: Indiana University Press.

Hannay, A. (1982) *Kierkegaard*, London: Routledge & Kegan Paul.

Kierkegaard, S. (1980) *The Concept of Anxiety: A Simple Psychologically Orienting Deliberation on the Dogmatic Issue of Hereditary Sin*, trans. Reidar Thomte in collaboration with Albert B. Anderson, Princeton, NJ and Chichester: Princeton University Press.

—— (1985) *Fear and Trembling: Dialectical Lyric*, trans. Alastair Hannay, London: Penguin Books.

—— (1989) *The Sickness Unto Death: A Christian Psychological Exposition for Edification and Awakening*, trans. Alastair Hannay, London: Penguin Books.

Kirby, K. M. (1996) *Indifferent Boundaries: Spatial Concepts of Human Subjectivity*, New York and London: The Guilford Press.

Kroker, A., Kroker, M., and Cook, D. (1989) *Panic Encyclopedia: The Definitive Guide to the Postmodern Scene*, London: Macmillan.

Langman, L. (1994) "Neon cages: shopping for subjectivity," in Rob Shields (ed.) *Lifestyle Shopping: The Subject of Consumption*, London and New York: Routledge: 40–82.

Lupton, D. (1998) "Going with the flow: some central discourses in conceptualizing and articulating the embodiment of emotional states," in S. Nettleton and J. Watson (eds) *The Body in Everyday Life*, London and New York: Routledge: 82–99.

McDowell, L. (1996) "Spatializing feminism: geographic perspectives," in N. Duncan (ed.) *BodySpace*, London and New York: Routledge: 28–44.

McNally, R. J. (1994) *Panic Disorder: A Critical Analysis*, New York and London: The Guilford Press.

Marks, I. M. (1987) *Fears, Phobias and Rituals*, New York and Oxford: Oxford University Press.

Martin, E. (1989) *The Woman in the Body*, Boston: Beacon Press.

Mathews, A. M., Gelder, M. G., and Johnston, D. W. (1981) *Agoraphobia: Nature and Treatment*, London and New York: Tavistock Publications.

Merleau-Ponty, M. (1962) *Phenomenology of Perception*, trans. Colin Smith, London: Routledge & Kegan Paul.

Miller, D. (1997) "Could shopping ever really matter," in P. Falk and C. Campbell (eds) *The Shopping Experience*, London: Sage Publications: 31–55.

Quinodoz, D. (1997) *Emotional Vertigo: Between Anxiety and Pleasure*, trans. Arnold Pomerans, London and New York: Routledge.

Rich, A. (1986) *Blood, Bread and Poetry: Selected Prose 1979–1985*, New York: Norton.

Sibley, D. (1997) *Geographies of Exclusion*, London and New York: Routledge.

13 Material bodies precariously positioned

Women embodying chronic illness in the workplace

Pamela Moss and Isabel Dyck

By way of introduction

Empirical themes in the disability and chronic illness literature in health geography prominently include issues around marginalization – in employment (Kitchin *et al.* 1998), in accessibility (e.g. Imrie and Wells 1993; Imrie 1996), and in daily life (Dyck 1995). Documenting responses to processes of exclusion and marginalization by persons with disabilities has been fruitful in creating a *spatial* understanding of disability. For example, persons with disabilities may appropriate certain place-specific exclusionary practices in order to re-define what it is to be disabled (see e.g. Dorn 1998). Also, in the production of formal and scientific knowledge – an exclusionary practice in the academy – geographers are writing about their personal experience of disability and disabling illness as a way forward to empowerment (e.g. Chouinard and Grant 1995; Chouinard 1997; Golledge 1997; Moss 1999). Accounting for the ways persons with disabilities are positioned within society has identified several of the mechanisms through which marginalization takes place (e.g. Gleeson 1999). Like other exclusionary processes, marginalization of persons with disabilities takes place in both public and private spaces at various spatial scales (see Sibley 1995; Butler and Bowlby 1997; see Parr and Philo (1995) and Radford and Park (1998) for examples in mental health). Social spaces created in and through these milieus of power are place-specific in that a singular configuration at any point in time is as unique in its configuration as it is similar to other social spaces – giving rise to the notion that the processes of marginalization are similar, but the outcomes are (or may be) different.

We too are interested in marginalization, but in a slightly different way. Most of these works (including our own) focus on the disabled body as a subject/object that is marginalized by systemic attitudes and practices, as an identity marginalized on account of a bodily impairment or disease process, as an end product. We prefer here to focus on the making of that end product, to intervene into the process of marginalization and look at the connections between bodies and environments. In this sense, we are interested in how women *embody* marginalization processes.

For us, *embodiment* refers to those *lived* spaces where bodies are located conceptually and corporeally, metaphorically and concretely, discursively and materially (following Grosz 1995; and Laws' 1997 interpretation of Grosz, pp. 48–52). This means *being* simultaneously part of bodily forms and their social constructions. With this definition, however, it is easy to forget that embodiment is an active process of *being*. Embodiment involves not only the body as a surface upon which society *inscribes* or "marks" a body so that it can be read in a culturally intelligible way, but also the activity of bodily *self-inscription* which can resist some cultural marks and create (perhaps) new ones, or what can be called "autonomous" (Grosz 1995: 36) representations.[1] But embodiment is not only about inscription and the discourses being inscribed. While living in and through spaces, bodies engage in material practices that produce and reproduce both the meanings of bodies, as for example, being "able" or "disabled," and the circumstances within which bodies exist, as for example, spaces being "accessible" or not. At the same time, meanings of spaces are produced and reproduced through both material practices and discourse, and, like inscriptions, are also resisted, contested, or refused. If we think in terms of this casting of embodiment, women's experiences of the workplace as possibly or potentially "abled," both materially and through various representations of an "ill" body, are very much a part of their identities and subjectivities. As such, women with chronic illness can either challenge or reinforce their own marginalization and the marginalization of other women with chronic illness. Acting on the experience of embodiment – through what Philo (1996: 38) calls *embodied* knowledge – women with chronic illness could draw on their "distinctive ways" through which they intersect, connect, and interact with their environments shaping their "sense of [them]selves in time, space, period and place." For example, an ideal result for women with chronic illness speaking out against discriminatory hiring policies would be the establishment of non-discriminatory hiring policies. Yet, these women also must be aware that heightening awareness to such a "malady" as chronic illness could provide fodder for the production of newer, even further marginalizing policies, as for example, closer scrutiny by employers of possible employees' medical histories and biomedical diagnoses.

Our intent in this chapter is to map women's embodiments of marginalization through an exploration of the precarious states of employment of women diagnosed with chronic illness. Thus, we access *embodiment* by querying how women diagnosed with chronic illness take on an "ill" or "disabled" identity; how these women structure and restructure their social and material spaces in order to accommodate the uncertainty and unpredictability of the physiology of the disease process; and how women negotiate their everyday lives while being marginalized, personally and systemically. We first elaborate a framework for specifically addressing the instability of employment and workplace environments for women with chronic illness. We then present the employment struggles of four women who have been diagnosed with chronic illness, either rheumatoid arthritis (RA) or myalgic encephalomyelitis (ME), popularly known as chronic fatigue syndrome. We show how these women were able to structure and restructure their working environments in order to accommodate the disabling progression of the illness. We link these stories by pulling out more general themes relating to chronic illness, body, and the workplace as sites of struggle.

Destabilization of material bodies and sites of struggle

Examining the daily lives of women diagnosed with chronic illness struggling with employment and working environments provides an excellent opportunity to pursue our interest in embodiment and marginalization. First, being diagnosed with chronic illness brings uncertainty and variability into a woman's life. She can no longer take for granted the proper functioning of her body that she could before onset of symptoms. In addition, the disease category itself is unstable. Several chronic illness diagnoses are inexact because they are "diagnoses of exclusion" – ruling out a series of other diseases through a host of biomedical procedures. This unsteady state of change is precisely the type of terrain through which specific practices can marginalize women. Because both the disease category and the feelings of illness themselves are unstable, women *precariously* forge "ill" or "disabled" identities.

Second, the material aspects of these women's bodies are in flux. Because the progression of chronic illness is unpredictable, prognosis for recovery is also unpredictable. Fluctuating transitory symptoms leave the women with chronic illness little leeway for planning activities or creating routines. This ongoing, but intermittent, destabilization of the material body invariably complicates women's daily lives, from getting out of bed to securing an income, from shopping for food to preparing a meal, from coping with family commitments to dealing with insurance adjusters. But in each case, the materiality (in terms of both economy and body) of their existence comes to the fore around, for example, issues of financial soundness, health maintenance and recovery, and support from social relationships. Because of the indecisive course of illness, women *precariously* structure their social environments in ways that accommodate the uncertainty of disease progression.

Third, the social organization of employment and workplace environments are predominately based on assumption(s) of the "working body" as an "able body." From the tasks comprising a job description to the manner and place in which they are carried out, ability is uncritically, unequivocally assumed. The tribulations in negotiating social and material spaces by women diagnosed with chronic illness in employment and workplace environments demonstrate the embedded continuity of social life and how disruptions can shift one's positioning in the labor force. In other words, new experiences, such as onset of chronic illness, rupture the flow of daily life socially – employment included – and signal a move toward a new set of experiences, repositioning women *vis-à-vis* previous constants in their lives. This repositioning may have considerable consequences materially, as for example, reduced hours resulting in reduced income, legal battles with insurance companies over disability claims, or unexpected dismissals for not being able to perform work tasks. In this sense, the workplace is a *site of struggle* whereby women with chronic illness are forced to contest definitions of "sick," sick leave, and illness in terms of an "ill" body as well as what constitutes disability or a "disabled" body. Because of the unstable state of their bodies and the momentarily fixed (indefinite) diagnosis, women *precariously* secure incomes through employment.

Women with chronic illness who are active in the labor force experience chronic illness, their bodies, and the workplace environment simultaneously. Because each is a site of struggle (in terms of both oppression and resistance), women with chronic illness are marginalized and excluded while being able to, at the same time, at least to some extent, resist oppression and thwart marginalization. The women embody chronic illness through their expectations of what it is to be "ill" as well as those of their employers, supervisors, and co-workers. In their attempts to negotiate the uncertainty, indeterminacy, and unpredictability of their illness, body, and workplace environment, they engage in specific material practices that reconfigure each as a site of struggle. These sites of struggle exist together, intermingled in the woman's ordinary, everyday goings-on. These integrated experiences are forever being woven and re-woven into the fabric of a woman's identity, an unevenly textured tapestry where threads are worn in some places, slightly ripped in other places, and newly meshed in still others. And each time we look we see yet another mélange, the same ingredients with a different configuration. In this sense there is no end product; there is only a series of interim stages of identity formation, (re)structuring of environments, and employment and workplace accommodation.

Material bodies precariously positioned

This chapter is based on research with women diagnosed with rheumatoid arthritis (RA) and myalgic encephalomyelitis (ME) living in the Vancouver and Victoria regions of British Columbia, Canada. The bulk of the project included in-depth interviews with forty-nine women, twenty-four of whom were diagnosed with RA, twenty-five with ME. All but one of the interviews (at the woman's request) were recorded and transcribed verbatim. RA is a progressive degenerative rheumatic autoimmune disease affecting bones and soft tissue. As the disease progresses, mobility becomes restricted as joints fuse causing permanent damage. During disease activity, major symptoms include fatigue, joint swelling, pain, and stiffness. ME is a disease of the central nervous system with no known origin. Primary symptoms include debilitating fatigue, pain, and cognitive impairment. Other ongoing symptoms include noise- and photo-sensitivity, anxiety, sore throat, nausea, imbalance, dizziness, muscle weakness, migraine-like headaches, sleep disturbance, forgetfulness, and blurred vision (Komaroff and Fagioli 1996; Schaefer 1995). Because the disease processes differ physiologically, the diseases affect the body differently: RA irreparably ravages joints whereas the damage from ME is not (seemingly) permanent. Yet comparing the two diseases is useful in that not only do both affect dexterity and mobility and both have as central symptoms pain and fatigue, but the disease progression is uncertain and unpredictable, forcing the women into precarious situations with regard to chronic illness, body, and workplace environments.

We include only four women's stories in this chapter for four reasons. First, because of the rich detail and voluminous amounts of material qualitative methods such as in-depth interviews produce, we cannot presume to report all of our "findings" in one short chapter. This chapter reports on only one of the many analytical themes we are pursuing – embodiment of chronic illness in the workplace.[2] Second, because of the process through which we build theory, a continual (re)thinking of abstract constructs and concrete information, we cannot presume to have a definitive framework created prior to analyzing any information. This chapter is but one piece of our overall research program that seeks to understand and explain in part women's daily lives. Third, because we are interested in the dynamics of the workplace with an employer, we only draw on the experiences of those women working for a company or organization. At the time of interview, eight women were employed in paying jobs and one was active in a part-time job without pay.[3] Our choice of four adequately represents the spectrum of accommodation strategies for women dealing with employers.

But these four women's stories are not unusual, atypical, or aberrant with regard to the other employed women in the study. In fact, they represent the range of ways these women embodied chronic illness in their working environments. Differences in diagnosis, disease progression, and recovery among these four specific women show the scope of embodied practices we encountered in the study by the women with chronic illness and their employers. We chose these particular four women to illustrate the topics we highlighted for discussion in the previous section: chronic illness, body, and workplace environments as sites of struggle. All the women are trained professionals with advanced education living in middle-income housing types. Despite this, their incomes vary widely. (For a brief overview of the women's socio-demographic and illness information see Table 13.1). After presenting the four vignettes, we draw out for discussion overlapping issues emerging from these women's sites of struggle.

Hiding behind success

Julia, in her early 40s, was employed in a high-pressure, prestigious job when she came down with ME symptoms. Her initial response was to pare down

Table 13.1 Socio-economic profiles of the four women with chronic illness

	Julia	Inge	Carolyn	Sandra
Age at time of interview	40	49	45	Late 30s
Year ill	1991 with ME	1983 with RA	1955 with RA	1995 with ME
Year diagnosed	1991	1993	1955	1995
Occupation	Previously producer; now retail sales	Nurse	Administrator/ activist	Health care provider
Education and training	Trade school	College, nursing	BA in psychology; experience in counseling	Training for dental hygienist
Individual income	No data[a]	$20,000/year	$9,000/year	$14,950/year
Source	Employment insurance; part-time retail jobs	Job	Social assistant; CPP[b]	Job
Household composition	Self	Self, husband, 2 sons	Self	Self, husband, son, daughter
Household income	Same as individual	$65,000/year	Same as individual	No data[a]
Tenure	Rent	Own	Rent	Own
Dwelling type	1-bedroom apartment	3-story, 4-bedroom house	3-bedroom ranch	2-bedroom bungalow

Notes
a "No data" means that the information was not reported.
b CPP (Canada Pension Plan) is disability income.

her non-employment activities so that she could keep her job. Strategies she used to maintain her employment centered on preventing disclosure of illness to anyone other than her direct supervisor and on restructuring the way in which she used her energy, particularly with regard to moving around the building.

> I pretty much just went to work and went home, 'cause I didn't want to lose that link with normal life – which was the job. I was afraid of, um, getting devoured by it [ME]. So I – that's why I thought the best thing is let all the other things slide and just go to work . . . My boss was well aware of what I had. And I probably worked not at all the same, not the same capacity. But she was very good, and very – I was very fortunate!

But I did not want to go on disability leave. So she kind of, you know, we took it into consideration. You start working in a different way. You've gotta get smarter, not run around so much. You get more methodical, more organized . . . You know, I wouldn't do that same kind of running around – I would save things up and just do one trip. And I probably didn't move as quickly . . . I was moving at a lot slower pace, but it was so important to me to keep my job.

By negotiating both her social space, in not letting anyone but her employer know of her illness, and her material space, in altering her manner and working "smarter," Julia was able to embody her illness in such a way as to protect herself from failure – she hid her illness behind her success.

Julia's motivation to hide her illness stemmed from wanting to keep a link to "normal life." For Julia, it made no sense to be employed and open about her illness when she would not get the respect she needed to do her job. She was frightened about giving in to an illness of cognitive impairment. In addition, she had seen "what happened to other people with disability leaves . . . One other woman in particular – she had breast cancer – and I didn't feel that she had been treated compassionately." What is somewhat unique in Julia's case is that nearly all of her support came from her supervisor.

I would miss the odd day, and my boss was good about [it]. I think what turned out, it was easier to keep me on board – even at my pace – with what I knew, rather than get somebody else new in, train that new person, and then have that person leave them. I was very committed to my job. I was good at it. I was very loyal to the boss. I mean, you know how that is when you're working with people, you want to have people that are on your team. Well, we were a team. And it was worth it more, I think, for her to keep me – even at my reduced . . . So I was very fortunate!

She and her boss even hired an assistant which lessened the burden of routine tasks, such as writing letters and running errands. This arrangement, nego- tiated in the first six months of the illness, remained intact for five years, two of which were worse than the other three. Throughout the time, Julia continued to improve. Yet, in what appeared to be an ironic twist of fate, just after she proclaimed she was fully recovered, Julia was among ten employees laid off through a corporate downsizing strategy.

Flexible identity; flexible work environment

Onset of disease for Inge, 49 years old, was just after the birth of her son fifteen years ago; a diagnosis of RA, however, was only in 1993. Like many women, Inge thought that her body was finally giving into the years of abuse she had bestowed on it – pushing beyond her body's limits in order to meet the inexorable goals she set for herself as a mother, wife, and nurse. Once diagnosed, however, she "began a new life":

> I decided what I really needed to ask myself was "what do I need this illness for?" If indeed there is any emotional, social, economic reason that I need that illness. So that was a question that I spent a lot of time thinking about. What were my gains? Were there any gains from being ill? . . . So that was the beginning of looking at what are my priorities. What's the most important to me? Because I can't live the way I used to. And that [way of thinking] was very beneficial.

Rather than blanketing her multiple identities with a singular notion of "ill," Inge reconstituted her identity as an "ill" mother, "ill" wife, and "ill" nurse. By re-sorting her priorities, by re-thinking what it was to be ill, by taking on a new way to live her life, Inge created a space through which her "ill" identities could emerge; a new space for her embodiment.

One such literal space for Inge was employment. Not being able to draw blood from patients prompted her initial visit to a rheumatologist. In contrasting her motivation to remain employed with her increasing need to ask for assistance in carrying out routine tasks, Inge clearly shows the interdependence between her material body and the material conditions of her everyday life.

> I couldn't stand to go with medical leave. I could leave work for any other reason but not because my body wouldn't work for me. That was too big. Too big. I probably could do it now. You know, because I think that I've established a new image for myself, a new self, one that I didn't have before. You know. That I feel like I no longer need – at that time it was a terrible drive to [pause]. I had to be completing things and accomplishing things. And I had to be involved. And I didn't have to be necessarily the cheeriest or the brightest, but a tremendous self-pressure to accomplish, and to succeed, and I think I don't need that so much now. I think I've nourished other areas of myself so that it's all right to sit back. And I'll ask somebody else to go ahead and do the work. That was hard. That was hard.

Once Inge became more flexible with her expectations of her body, her co-workers adapted more readily to her needs by offering their assistance without her asking. She also felt the "freedom to know that I wasn't going to lose my job if I had to take some time away." Relief from the worry of financial security permitted her the "freedom" to begin restructuring – re-embodying – her working life while living with RA.

Volunteer work for "worth" and identity

Carolyn, 45 years old, recounted her personal history primarily in terms of accessibility to the built environment. RA developed when she was about 2 years old. Extensive damage and progressive steroid therapy resulted in brittle bones and after having broken her leg three times by age 12, she chose to use a wheelchair for mobility.

Carolyn's lifelong struggle to be financially independent – from her parents and the state – has not been successful. Systemic discrimination against her, in terms of her illness, the deterioration of her body, and her restricted mobility, set up (invisible) barriers which prevented her from achieving in the workplace what non-disabled persons achieve with a similar set of qualifications. After attending university in the early 1970s, Carolyn was unable to secure permanent employment as a medical social worker. She was turned down, interview after interview, many of which were laced with subtle phrases and gestures of exclusion and overt acts of discrimination. She was concerned that her degree was not in social work, but a degree in the field (at that time) didn't seem to pose much of a problem for hospital administrators; what posed a problem clearly was Carolyn's difference.

> And he said, "Actually I prefer people that don't have social work degrees. So come on in and we'll do an interview." And I was really hopeful. And then when I got there he just kept asking me about how I would get around. And I kept looking at him, like what, was he imagining that as a problem? And I would say, "What do you mean how would I get around. Do you mean like from floor to floor?" I said, "There's an elevator. I would use the elevator. There's not a problem in me getting places." "But how would you get around?" He just kept sort of asking that question over and over again.

After two decades of searching, Carolyn has pretty much given up the idea of permanent full-time employment. She was only ever employed in part-time positions, which were often not associated with counseling, nor were they enough to cover living expenses.

A little over ten years ago Carolyn become involved with an advocacy group for rights for persons with disabilities. Several members encouraged her to take on the task of running the group, managing the office, and overseeing the (somewhat meager) finances. She accepted and has since been active on a daily basis. Carolyn finds the work satisfying and is pleased with some of the successes she and her group have been responsible for, as for example, low entry buses and a personal care service program. However, her poverty prevents her from being too supportive of the volunteer work sector.

> If you have the self-sufficiency then whatever your [material] circum-
> stances are become irrelevant because you can pay to get what you need.
> And people look at you as somebody who has money and they are more
> willing to respond to you as a paying customer. When you don't have
> money, now you are a charitable object. So everything that gets done for
> you, you have to be grateful for and grovel and be appreciative of them.
> Don't complain or bite the hand that feeds you come into play.

Socially, then, her work environment is enveloped in a cloud of disrespect
because of her unpaid status as a worker. She feels that her contributions are
not valued, particularly by the government employees with whom she works
who have similar educational backgrounds and less experience in the field.

Balancing support

Sandra, in her late thirties, did not take time off from the clinic where she
was employed as a health care provider, with the exception of a couple
of days here and there. Neurologists initially diagnosed multiple sclerosis
(MS) because of the breakdown in her central nervous system. After further
observations physicians diagnosed ME. Treatment for ME usually begins
with lifestyle changes. For Sandra, this meant slowing down.

> There's no question I'd have to slow down. And in some ways it was
> a blessing because you have to slow down. So you have to stop, and
> you have to take more time doing things instead of whipping around
> and doing a hundred things and doing it all at once.

In her working environment, this translated into fewer hours – going
from full time to three-quarters time. Reduction of hours did not lead to a
reduction in take-home pay, as it would in many cases; she received an hourly
wage raise to compensate for lost pay.

Such support in her work environment did not end there. With the MS
diagnosis, the physician with whom she worked had asked her to change
to him so he could monitor her condition daily. With the ME diagnosis,
the physician was still as supportive, and continues to monitor her illness.
Her supervisor, who also is a close friend, is able to observe Sandra and step
in when necessary. For example, when enduring "brain fog" (an extreme
form of "cloudy thinking" and arguably the most scary and debilitating
ME symptom), she may not be able to undertake simple, routine tasks such
as taking blood pressure or pulling files. The supervisor intercedes discreetly
and picks up where Sandra left off. Sandra feels comforted by this arrangement, especially because she sees it as only an interim measure while she
struggles to recover.

Sandra's openness with her supervisor and co-workers is not however
extended to patients. She rarely discloses the ME diagnosis when asked

because she knows there is resistance to an acknowledgment that ME exists, let alone that it is a debilitating disease.

> Where I work, in the medical clinic, and with patients and stuff, there are some patients that know that I'm sick. They get very concerned, and some of them I've told, some. They say "What's wrong?", "How come you're walking funny?", "Did you hurt your knee?" "Yes, I did." You know, when I can't walk very well, or I just am "sick." But sometimes, and I don't know if this is right or wrong, but people will say, and I don't like that I do this, but people say well what is your disease, and I tell them, it's basically I've got MS, except I don't actually have a lesion on my brain. Because people don't – because they don't understand it, the chronic fatigue thing bothers me, because they think you're just tired, and you're depressed.

This claim to legitimacy, having a "standard" chronic illness, rather than one that is contested, assists her in structuring the social aspects of her working environment in a way that permits her to keep her support intact. She is able to embody her illness on her own terms. By not revealing her disease, she is not continually thrown into doubt. Such doubt would strain the support she receives and exacerbate her symptoms.

Discussion

From these four vignettes, common themes emerge around financial soundness, health maintenance and recovery, and social relationships in the workplace environment. All the women were concerned about an income in tandem with pursuing career goals. These pursuits were complicated by disabling illness, some women being more severely affected than others. Yet without supportive social relationships in the workplace environment, none would have been able to remain employed or engage in volunteer work.

These four vignettes also provide information to scrutinize more closely our interests in embodiment, identity, and (re)structuring workplace environments. Even in successes over their struggles with regard to chronic illness, body, and employment, these women are still precariously positioned in their workplace environments.

Embodiment

Not only did specific work tasks and material spaces shape these women's working environments, but the social relations within which they engaged also structured the spaces through which they moved. For example, Julia was successful in maintaining employment by hiding her illness in a variety of ways. She closed off her life outside her job and worked "smarter" by limiting the amount of energy she expended on moving through the spaces of her environment. Even though this was effective, it was only through the emotional (understanding) and practical support (taking up the "slack" and hiring an assistant) of her employer that Julia was able to restructure her working environment. She refused to take on a public "ill" identity, which she thought would enable her co-workers to question her capabilities, and chose to remain "hidden" behind her success. Even though hidden, Julia still embodied the processes marginalizing ill women in the workplace. Her active participation in *hiding*, though strategic in securing an income, building a career, and exacting respect, further supported the systemic discrimination and marginalization against women who are ill in the workplace. In stark contrast is Sandra whose embodiment is more of a collective effort embedded in a web of social relationships in the workplace environment. She was open about her illness from the onset of her symptoms with her boss, supervisor, and co-workers. She has been able to maintain her employment at the same income because of the supportive social relations within the workplace. Together the entire staff work against marginalization of ill workers. Yet, like Julia, Sandra "hides" her illness, not behind the mask of success, but behind a mask of legitimacy, behind another chronic illness, behind MS. This demonstrates how delicate the balance is between acceptance and rejection of an embodied chronic illness in workplace relationships.

Both Julia and Sandra flexibly adjusted social relationships within the workplace so that they could accomplish their work tasks without setting into motion the dreaded uncertainty of a chronic illness diagnosis, Julia with her co-workers and Sandra with patients. Though both women are diagnosed with the same illness and endure(d) the same symptoms, the outcomes of their *embodiment* in the workplace differ. Their diverse experiences of job and career set them up to forge different paths in their workplaces – even though the materiality of their body and the disease process are comparable. They invoke similar strategies of disclosure, but not in the sense of the end product, an ill body in the workplace. Rather, it is in the process of anchoring the destabilization of the material body, the illness, within different contexts that produces the variation in embodiment.

Unstable identities of material bodies

Because of the instability of disease progression, the fluctuation of points to anchor identity in a particular context, and the dependence on flexible working styles, the women remain precariously positioned in their workplace environments. Even though workplace environments can be structured to accommodate both the fluctuation and progression of illness, material conditions of employment are still not secure. Similarly, stabilizing the deterioration of the material body also does not guarantee employment. Together these feed into the instability of identities as part of the women's material bodies.

For Julia and Carolyn, able-bodied persons are the yardstick by which to measure success in employment. Both project singular identities defined in terms of being able-bodied or not. Julia rejected her difference whereas Carolyn embraced hers. Julia refused to "give in" to the physiological process of the disease and proceeded as if she were "normal," that is, not ill. Julia, enjoying recovered health after having endured years of hidden accommodation, is now retraining and employed in part-time retail positions. This interim stability of health does not mean she will forever be without ME or another chronic illness. Nor does having a job connect her to the "normal life" she so desperately held on to while ill. This singularity in her claims to identity is itself unstable. Carolyn, who identifies herself as a person with disabilities, compares herself to able-bodied persons when it comes to employment based on qualifications and experience. Her tenacity in holding a singular identity has benefited other persons with disabilities through her advocacy work. She has used the political axis of disability in terms of social change. However, as Carolyn has continually experienced, systemic and personal discrimination against her singular identity as a person with disabilities has prevented her from securing permanent full-time employment. In its singularity, her identity has both positive and negative results, something that produces instability in her everyday life.

In contrast to Julia and Carolyn, Inge and Sandra have redefined themselves by integrating illness into their multiple identities. Both Inge and Sandra changed their fundamental approaches to life, which resulted in material changes in their workplaces. Initially, both Inge and Sandra were afraid to take medical leave, even if their body could not handle the work, in part because they gain some of their ongoing identity from employment – just like Julia and Carolyn. Their flexibility in accomplishing workplace tasks highlights the multi-faceted means through which workplace accommodation can be achieved – mostly by the woman with chronic illness, but only as part of the web of relationships in the workplace with bosses, supervisors, and co-workers. They are simultaneously ill and employed and their workplaces are set up to handle fluctuations in the uncertain progression of the disabling illness. Given the changes each has made in approaching her illness and her daily life, taking sick leave would probably not be so difficult now. However, instability still looms and the precariousness of their positions in the workplace is still present. If either were to change jobs or if any of the social relationships in the workplace were to shift, they would then again enter an uncertain environment where accommodation – with regard to health maintenance and recovery – would have to be negotiated all over again.

(Re)structuring workplace environments

The apparent simplicity of the choices these women made in securing employment and in finding personal satisfaction in unpaid political work hides the complexity of the processes that (re)shape, (re)constitute, and (re)structure illness, body, and workplace. That Inge decided to "begin a new life" once diagnosed with RA minimizes the effort she put into struggling against being ill, against her body, against having to change her work habits. By saying the change was "hard" only begins to describe the path she actually forged, a transformation of her own set of values which preceded all the material changes she made. From her experience, we can begin to understand how the destabilization of the material body can spark a change in the interpretation of context, of the milieus within which we exist, of our everyday life. Inge successfully restructured her workplace environment not only by redefining her approach to coping with the illness generally, but also in re-delimiting the material borders of her body's ability (in asking assistance for routine tasks).

Carolyn's experiences, too, indicate a range of processes that have marginalized her in employment. Disclosure of disability doesn't really play a role in Carolyn's life; her disability from RA is visible through the use of a wheelchair. Systemic and personal discrimination consistently denied Carolyn a paid position in counseling given her qualifications, gained primarily through part-time and self-employed jobs. The satisfaction Carolyn has found in working for an advocacy group for rights of persons with disabilities appears to resolve the tension around not being able to secure full-time employment. However, her unpaid status devalues her work in the same system and (often) to the same people that have prevented her from pursuing a career because she is not completely able-bodied.

Inge and Carolyn have had varying success in sorting out arrangements for employment even though both continually contest what it is to be ill with RA, what it is to have an unstable material body, and what employment means to them. Their different employment experiences reveal the diverse ways women with chronic illness challenge definitions of illness and disability in the workplace and in employment and reclaim them as a site of struggle.

Concluding remarks

Our mapping of women's embodiment of chronic illness in the workplace contributes to the overall mapping of women's "health" geographies. We use inverted commas around health because ours is a map of illness, something which, although defined as an absence of health, remains in the domain of women's health geographies. For our mapping, we provided details of how women with chronic illness are excluded and marginalized as well as of how they struggle to restructure their workplace environments socially and materially. We showed how women variously embody chronic illness in their workplaces, and how they both challenge and reinforce meanings of their chronically ill bodies. And, through these examples, we demonstrated just how precarious employment actually is for women with chronic illness, in maintaining a job and health at the same time, as well as in securing and keeping a paying job. Together a delicate collage of webbed relations appears, both for these individual women, and for women with chronic illness more generally.

Our vignettes, although representative of the women's stories we collected, should not be taken as the only way, nor indeed the most promising way, to deal with chronic illness in workplace environments. Details of these women's lives presented here also seem to indicate that women with chronic illness are successfully, though precariously, employed. We do not want to leave the impression that all women with chronic illness successfully maintain their employment after onset of disease. Success in getting a job and maintaining employment while ill with chronic illness is not necessarily the typical pattern for women with chronic illness. In our study, just over half of the women with RA and about a quarter of the women with ME (two of whom took a considerable amount of time off from employment and studies and the rest of whom cut their hours back drastically during the period with the most intense symptoms) were employed after the onset of the destabilization of their material body. Because ME is less widely accepted as a legitimate disease than RA and work tasks are more negatively affected (at least initially), disclosure is more of an issue for women with ME. Although more women remained employed after an RA diagnosis than after an ME diagnosis, insurance claims for RA were processed more quickly and with less struggle than those for ME. Our vignettes, as they have been written, are vehicles for theoretical exposition through which we can make sense of the everyday lives of women with chronic illness. And, as we make sense of these women's lives, we may be able to provide information toward contributing to forging employment policies sensitive to the unpredictability of chronic illness, devising innovative ways to deal with employment while ill, and building a politics inclusive of women marginalized through illness and disability.

Acknowledgments

Thanks to the women who told us their stories. Pamela also thanks the Geography Department at the University of Vienna, Austria, for its support while writing this paper. We appreciate the funding for this project – by the Social Science and Humanities Council of Canada, #410–95–0267. We dedicate this paper to Lorna Duncan who taught us much about living with chronic illness.

Notes

1   We are aware of the difficulty, if not impossibility, of creating "autonomous" inscriptions, and by extension, "autonomous" knowledge (with regard to the body, see especially Ebert 1996: 233ff). Inventions, like reinventions, are still part of the milieu within which we already exist. For us, then, any appearance of "autonomy," novelty, or innovation in inscriptions or in inscribing needs critical scrutiny.

2   Other themes include negotiation of physical and social space while living with chronic illness, embodied ways of knowing and being, and disciplining environments through deviant bodies.

3   Three women were self-employed. One had been self-employed when developing chronic illness, and upon recovery went back to the same employment arrangements. Self-employment for the other two women was a direct result of accommodating their illness through lifestyle change.

References

Butler, R. E. and Bowlby, S. (1997) "Bodies and spaces: an exploration of disabled people's experiences of public space," *Environment and Planning D: Society and Space* 15: 411–33.

Chouinard, V. (1997) "Making space for disabling differences: challenging ableist geographies," *Environment and Planning D: Society and Space* 15: 379–87.

Chouinard, V. and Grant, A. (1995) "On not being anywhere near the 'project': revolutionary ways of putting ourselves in the picture," *Antipode* 27, 2: 137–66.

Dorn, M. (1998) "Beyond nomadism: the travel narratives of a 'cripple'," in H. J. Nast and S. Pile (eds) *Places through the Body*, New York: Routledge: 183–206.

Dyck, I. (1995) "Hidden geographies: the changing lifeworlds of women with multiple sclerosis," *Social Science and Medicine* 40: 307–20.

Ebert, T. (1996) *Ludic Feminism and After: Postmodernism, Desire, and Labor in Late Capitalism*, Ann Arbor: University of Michigan Press.

Gleeson, B. (1999) *Geographies of Disability*, New York: Routledge.

Golledge, R. G. (1997) "On reassembling one's life: overcoming disability in the academic environment," *Environment and Planning D: Society and Space* 15: 391–410.

Grosz, E. (1995) "Bodies and knowledges: feminism and the crisis of reason," in E. Grosz, *Space, Time, and Perversion: Essays on the Politics of Body*, New York: Routledge: 25–43.

Imrie, R. (1996) *Disability and the City: International Perspectives*, London: Paul Chapman Publishing.

Imrie, R. F. and Wells, P. E. (1993) "Creating a barrier-free environment," *Town and Country Planning* 61: 278–81.

Kitchin, R., Shirlow, P., and Shuttleworth, I. (1998) "On the margins: disabled people's experience of employment in Donegal, West Ireland," *Disability and Society* 13, 5: 785–806.

Komaroff, A. L. and Fagioli, L. (1996) "Medical assessment of fatigue and chronic fatigue syndrome," in M. A. Dematrack and S. E. Abbey (eds) *Chronic Fatigue Syndrome: An Integrative Approach to Evaluation and Treatment*, New York: Guilford: 154–80.

Laws, G. (1997) "Women's life courses, spatial mobility, and state policies," in J. P. Jones, III, H. Nast, and S. Roberts (eds) *Thresholds in Feminist Geography: Difference, Methodology, Representation*, Lanham, MA: Rowman & Littlefield: 47–64.

Moss, P. (1999) "A sojourn into the autobiographical: researching chronic illness," in H. Parr and R. Butler (eds) *Mind and Body Spaces: Geographies of Disability, Illness and Impairment*, London: Routledge: 155–66.

Parr, H. and Philo, C. (1995) "Mapping 'mad' identities," in S. Pile and N. Thrift (eds) *Mapping the Subject: Geographies of Cultural Transformation*, London: Routledge: 199–255.

Philo, C. (1996) "Staying in? Invited comments on 'Coming out': exposing social theory in medical geography," *Health and Place* 2: 35–40.

Radford, J. and Park, D. C. (1998) "From the case files: reconstructing a history of involuntary sterilisation," *Disability and Society* 13, 3: 317–42.

Schaefer, K. M. (1995) "Sleep disturbances and fatigue in women with fibromyalgia and chronic fatigue syndrome," *Journal of Obstetric, Gynecologic, and Neonatal Nursing* 24, 3: 229–33.

Sibley, D. (1995) *Geographies of Exclusion: Society and Difference in the West*, London: Routledge.

14 The beauty of health

Locating young women's health and appearance

Andrea Litva, Kay Peggs, and Graham Moon

Introduction

Transitions are integral to the lifecourse. Puberty, when the individual moves from childhood to adolescence, and retirement, when paid work ceases to be a social expectation, are perhaps the two most notable transitions. One hallmark of lifecourse transitions is often a changing attitude to matters concerning health and bodily appearance. There may be resignation about increasing ill-health or enhanced concern with personal appearance; alternatively health may be taken for granted or the outward appearance of the body may cease to be a matter of great interest. Transitions are also often inherently spatialized. Not only do people's life concerns change, so too may their locations; they can literally "change place." These re-locations shift the contexts in which health and bodies are constructed. They expose well-learned behavior to new stimuli and threaten established understandings.

This chapter is concerned with the transition from adolescence to adulthood and with the spatiality of that particular transition. By this we mean to signal a concern with the way in which the transition from adolescence to adulthood may entail, often for the first time, leaving the parental home and, perhaps, moving away to a more or less distant location. We explore these themes through a grounded study of young women making the transition from home to university. The purpose of the chapter is the explication of the intersection of place with notions of beauty and of health, and the temporality of that intersection in so far as the young women in the study contrast their current views and actions with those they held before they moved to university.

The structure of the chapter is straightforward. In the next section we outline the theoretical context in which we will place our analysis. Attention then turns to our empirical study. We discuss briefly the structure and organization of the research before presenting and analyzing illustrative dialogue concerning place and health, and health and beauty. Our conclusions return us to more theoretical issues and provide a context for reflection on the extent to which young women's constructions of health and beauty shift and change as they undergo a key transition in their life and location.

Place, health, and the body

As the study of the body rose to prominence in social science and began to impact upon medical sociology, Dorn and Laws (1994) and Moon (1995) lamented its absence as a research theme in health geography. This neglect is no longer now so marked. The plethora of studies elsewhere in geography provides copious lessons for the study of the healthy body (see for example, Rodaway 1994; Bell and Valentine 1995; Longhurst 1995; Duncan 1996; Pile 1996). Within health geography the study of the chronically sick body and that of the disabled body have emerged as key areas of interest (Dyck 1995; Moss and Dyck 1996); for an exception to this trend see Longhurst (1994). As Parr (1998) notes, a number of geographical studies of the body have also focused on the cultural politics of gender. In this section we will locate the present study within this emerging research thematic. First, however, we address the general theoretical context for our study.

We all forge our identities within places. Pierre Bourdieu argues that three main factors underpin this process: social location, habitus, and taste (Bourdieu 1984). Social location concerns the material circumstances which contextualize individuals' daily lives and provide the circumstances for the development of their bodies (Shilling 1993: 129). Habitus refers to the internalization, as natural, of the ideas and attitudes of an individual's social peers (Frank 1991). Taste pertains to the ways in which individuals adopt lifestyles which are rooted in the material constraints of their circumstances. The way individuals discipline and handle their bodies reflects the complex interplay of each of these factors over time and space; people react within constraints with what Anthony Giddens (1991: 82) has termed "high modernity." However, we are not passive entities who merely absorb external influences. We contribute to and promote the social influences that affect us. Since we are constantly "on stage" (Goffman 1969) we seek to mirror desired body images. The mirroring body wants to reflect what is around it, but strives only to mirror images it has already internalized (Frank 1991).

The notion of "body regimes" is a particularly potent element in this process of identity formation (Featherstone 1991). Bodily control and body management are needed if we are to acquire the desired body image. Chris Shilling's discussion of the body as a *project* is useful here since it emphasizes that the body is unfinished at birth and "can be monitored and shaped by concerned individuals and social systems" (Shilling 1993: 200). In this way the body can be seen as plastic. It can be molded by individuals, who are expected to assume responsibility for the way they look, and transformed by lifestyle choices. Bodies can be seen as physical capital, since we can distinguish between those that assume responsibility and treat themselves as projects and those that do not (Bourdieu 1984). Body health and appearance thus reflect self-surveillance. Featherstone (1991) suggests that this indicates two basic body categories: the inner and the outer body. The inner body refers to concerns with the health and optimum functioning of the body whereas the outer body refers to appearance as well as the movement and control of the body within social space. A new "performing self" has emerged which places greater emphasis on the outer body but sees that body as crucially enabled by inner body health with dual maintenance of both bodies as a "virtuous leisure-time activity" which will secure lifestyle rewards resulting from an enhanced appearance (Hepworth and Featherstone 1982).

Dietary management is seen as crucial in the production of these "disciplined bodies" (Turner 1991). It provides one important way in which we can reorientate our general theoretical contentions about the body, health, and appearance to a more specific discussion of the relevance of these themes to young women. The images of young women in the media have created what Mirzoeff (1998: 183) terms an "impossible standard against which real people have judged their own bodies." For young women the epitome of bodily appearance has become the slender and toned body (Lloyd 1996). The "tyranny of slenderness" (Chernin 1983) haunts women, and young women in particular are encouraged to develop their bodies as objects of perception for others and held responsible for the various "defects" of their bodies (Bordo 1998). We can summarize these ideas with reference to the work of Elizabeth Grosz (1990, 1994). She sees women's bodies as sites inscribed by social expectations. Yet simultaneously she notes they also embody the potential for resistance; expectation can be confounded and women can and do resist what they believe may be expected of them in terms of body appearance and health and body-related behavior.

Both Grosz and Judith Butler (1990) also remind us that this inscription/resistance is largely understood in terms of relations between men and women. This cannot however always be taken to be the case even outside the specific case of lesbian relations. Heterosexual woman–woman relations can be significant, particularly in situations of transition where ties of friendship and influence may be changing. This brings us to the theoretical base to the present study. Following Cresswell (1996, 1999), our perspective in this chapter centers on the idea that bodies move in and between places, drawing meaning from their location. *Contra* Cresswell, we substitute transition for transgression: social location and tastes are framed within places and dislocated by changing places. We are interested less in the emergence of behavior that transgresses social expectations yet we share with Cresswell a concern for the way in which reactions and responses to social expectations shift and change according to location – in our case as young women grow older and move place. This position links back to existing studies in health geography: thus Dyck (1995) relates how women with multiple sclerosis make different use of home and neighborhood space after leaving the paid labor force. It also resonates with the conclusion to Katz and Monk (1993) where they note changes over women's lifecourses in the role of social and spatial mobility and the scale of women's social worlds. The study which follows explores how these ideas apply to young women's ideas of health and body appearance following their transition from parental home to a university setting.

Young women's perspectives on health and appearance

This research is located within an interpretative paradigm concerned with the understanding and analysis of meanings within specific contexts (Eyles 1988). We explore young women's perceptions of the relationship between appearance and health in one particular place: a university setting in southern England. We do not seek to create generalizable statements about the worlds of the women who were interviewed; rather we highlight "commonalities" in the positions that were revealed. We recognize that realities are multiple and flexible and therefore it is understood, *a priori*, that there is no way to distinguish between "cause" and "effect" in this type of study (Baxter and Eyles 1997). Instead, the emphasis is upon the credibility of the accounts. Credibility is understood as the degree to which the description of human experience is accurate enough to enable those who have the experience to recognize it, and those outside of the experience to relate to it or understand it (Lincoln and Guba 1985; Eyles 1988; McDowell 1992). Hence, our goal is to represent, as well as possible, the views of the young women who were interviewed; to enable them to recognize their experiences and to enable other young women, as well as our audience, to understand the reconstruction.

The selection of a university as the site for the research was both theoretically and practically driven. On a theoretical level, we recognized that there was a gap within qualitative health geography with regard to young, healthy women's perceptions of appearance and health. We also singled out the post-school transition to university as a key moment when existing life influences would be subject to (new) external stressors resulting from changing residence. In practical terms we needed a site that would provide a sample of young women fulfilling these criteria (young university students) but that was also readily accessible. This conditioned our choice of our own university. Our target population comprised young women between the ages of 18 and 24 years. The first author attended lectures from several different departments and at the end was allowed to ask for women volunteers to talk about their health. In total forty-eight women volunteered and seventeen were interviewed before saturation of emergent themes occurred. The women interviewed were spread evenly across the target age banding and all were attending three-year undergraduate courses. Both the volunteer and the interviewed students were all white and all were in full-time study. In order to exercise a degree of control over awareness of health issues, all interviewees were drawn from courses with a substantial input of health studies (sociology, social policy, and nursing).

We used in-depth interviews to focus on the interviewees' meanings and to locate them within their particular place-in-the-world (Blumer 1969). The concept of place-in-the-world incorporates the intersection of physical, emotional, and social space and contributes to the constructions of each person's "reality" or "truth." Prior to interviewing we put together a topic list of themes that we wanted to explore in the interviews. These included the meaning of health to participants, their health-related behavior, the impact of the university environment, and issues of stress. These themes were influenced by previous work on lay perceptions of health (Litva and Eyles 1994) where interviews with young women had revealed a relationship between health and appearance. The topic list ensured that the interview focused on the information we wanted to explore. The topics were introduced as they emerged in the conversation or at natural breaks. This allowed the interview to progress in a "conversation-like" manner. A grounded theory approach (Glaser and Strauss 1967) was used so that, as new themes emerged from the interviews, they were followed up in subsequent interviews. This enabled us to ascertain whether the new themes were specific to individuals or represented part of a collective reality. Interviewing continued until no new themes emerged. All the interviews were conducted by the first author, took place on campus, and were tape-recorded and then transcribed verbatim. Several transcripts were randomly selected and coded by two of the authors and a third, unconnected researcher in order to develop a list of categories for analysis. The transcripts were then coded and analyzed using NUD*IST, arguably the leading computer package for the coding of textual (and visual) research material and the automatic output of commonly coded themes.

Place and health: health status, being at university, and the transition to university

Each interview began with the question, "How would you describe your health right now?" The majority of the interviewees perceived their health to be poor or not as "good" as it could be. They often implied that they had been healthier at other times in their lives and that their health declined in response to being at university and the student way of life.

> Kirstie:[1] Mm, I don't know. I think it's difficult to be completely healthy because if you live in this sort of environment and you're under quite a lot of stress as well, because I mean, that takes it away quite a lot but . . . I don't know.
>
> (aged 22, studying sociology)

> Camilla: Um I think student life verges towards the unhealthy. I'm more healthy when I'm not doing term time. When it's more holidays I'm more healthy than I am when I'm actually here [university].
>
> (aged 21, studying social policy)

> Sally: I would say I'm more healthy than unhealthy. Not particularly healthy at the moment but that's probably because, like I said, I'm

a bit stressed out. In the summer, say, when I didn't have much hassles – I'd be a lot healthier.

(aged 20, studying nursing)

The stresses and strains of student life are coupled with lifestyle changes accompanying the transition to university. Moving place and fitting into a new milieu often involves changing habits; for younger university students this can be a prolonged process as they shuttle between a former home and college as terms begin and end.

Many of the interviewees also spoke of having "abused" their bodies in different ways since they came to the university. They see the beginning of their university life as the time when their physical health began to decline. It marked the beginning of a new phase in their lives when they were entirely responsible for themselves and did not have to worry about parental reactions to their behavior. Consequently many began smoking, drinking alcohol a great deal, not getting enough rest, and not eating properly.

Jo: I really feel like I've just abused my body since I've been at university.

I: Oh really?

Jo: Yeah because I did a two-year course before I came here. It was just like my third year away at University sort of thing. And I don't know . . . all I've really done is drink lager and smoke and just eat junk food and like, compared to what I used to be like, and I think it's maybe it makes me feel older.

(aged 22, studying social policy)

Michaela: From the first year onwards it's like . . . well in my first year I was out practically every night at the union [student pub], everyone was always drinking. You do things like go to McDonalds or eat pizza or like I say, cheese toasties . . . but yes, at the university, I think you just wander around and follow the crowd half the time and set a routine.

(aged 24, studying social policy)

The women associated the changes in their habits with a change in lifestyle and this was explained by their desire to fit in their new locale, using their bodies as mirrors to reflect what was around them (Frank 1991). For some these changes appear to be transient, marking the move from one lifestyle and place to another.

Liz: I am fitter than I was about two years ago. I went quite downhill when I started at uni. Because it was a complete . . . you know, you can go out to all hours. You can go and get absolutely rat-arsed without coming home and your mother going "Oh bloody hell. Have you been out on the piss again?" It's the freedom thing. And I suppose when I was at school, I did do sport because I wanted to and I was good at it.

(aged 21, studying nursing)

Several of the interviewees referred to the difficulty of maintaining a "healthy" diet while being a student. The theme of "routine" emerges in several women's discussions about diet. Michaela explains the importance of having a routine in order to be able to maintain a "good" diet. She sees the time and freedom associated with being at university as something that can sabotage the ability to have a routine and, by implication, the discipline required to eat healthily. Dietary management is crucial in the production of "disciplined bodies" (Turner 1991). Michaela sees many of her friends who, because of the circumstances created by the social spaces they inhabit, rely upon junk foods which are quick to make and eat.

> *Michaela*:   I think you've got to have a routine, especially when you're at university because you have got so much time and so much freedom. I see some of the junk some of my friends eat – it's absolutely untrue. I've always had proper meals and I've always tried to eat regularly. Not just binge and have fifty pizzas and then not have anything for the rest of the week. It's disgusting.
>
> (aged 24, studying social policy)

Jo and Michaela associate their poor diets with the responsibility of having to cook for themselves. Their comments suggest that the move from the parental home to university was accompanied, for them, by no longer being able to depend upon their parents to take care of their physical needs. This left them free to focus upon their social needs. University marks the transfer of the care of their inner body from parents to themselves, the transition to individual responsibility for body management and body discipline. In this sense their lives are receptive to what Michel Foucault (1998: 238) termed "oppositions," in this case between family space and social space. These views were reflected by other women who also stated that, when they were "back home" in "family space," they ate better because their parents were effectively able to take over the management of their inner body.

> *Jo*:   Probably not eating the right foods. Like, because when you are at home, you know, your mum always cooks you, like really healthy stuff. So you feel more healthy. But when you come to university, you're cooking for yourself. You don't really know what you're doing in the kitchen or I don't anyway. I don't know about anybody else. So I just ... like, "Oh well, I'm full but I feel awful" sort of thing.
>
> (aged 22, studying social policy)

Michaela: My health . . . it's deteriorated since I've come to the university I think. I don't get my mum cooking my meals for me or whatever. I have to cook for myself, buy my own food and stuff like that.

(aged 20, studying social policy)

In a society that associates older age with ill-health (Featherstone and Wernick 1995) it is not surprising that these young women do not perceive themselves as having any of the physical restraints or problems associated with advancing age. Consequently they tend to take both their physical body and their health for granted. The majority of the interviewees expect their lifestyles to radically change once again when they leave the social space of university. They see many of their behaviors as restricted to the university environment and that, once they move from this particular environment to another, their lifestyles should "improve." They explain that the damaging effect of anything they may be doing now is unlikely to have any major impact on their long-term health and therefore they do not worry.

Hayley: Occasionally now I think, "I'm at university." I've got three years, short term. I just think, you know, I can sort it out later. I'm going to do it. I'm going to do the three [years] and perhaps when I'm in a steady job I'll sit down and I'll think about, right, I've got to start eating healthy and I've got to sort myself out.

(aged 19, studying sociology)

Olivia: Yes, I think I've too much going on to think about . . . I think, feeling healthy is the last thing I'll think about at the moment . . . I think I am more concerned with worrying about my dissertation and other things.

(aged 20, studying social policy)

Health is not in the forefront of these young women's minds. What is, however, is how others see them. This impacts upon how they perceive themselves and their ability to cope with their new setting. Women are more likely than men to be trapped in narcissistic body management and presentation since they have been more exposed to the discourse of health and the glorification of the slim body (Warde 1997: 91). In the next section we explore the relationship between appearance and health, and the use of the body as a resource for coping with the socio-spatial worlds.

Beauty and health

To suggest that these women are not maintaining and managing their bodies because of their lifestyle is inaccurate; they manage their bodies very carefully. For many of these women creating and maintaining a healthy inner body is secondary to the task of creating and maintaining an attractive outer body. As Wendy Chapkiss (1986: 14) writes, "The body beautiful is women's responsibility and authority. She will be valued and rewarded on the basis of how close she comes to embodying the ideal." Our respondents were well aware that they are constantly judged by their appearance. How others perceive them affected how they perceived themselves. In order to feel good about themselves they, to different degrees, inscribed social values upon their bodies. Having a body that met some of the social criteria for beauty allowed them to feel good about themselves. As we shall see, if they felt that their bodies did not fit these criteria, they used what are often thought to be "health behaviors" in order to address their "deficiency." In this way their bodies became a resource for coping and managing uncertainty.

The interviewees had common and general notions of what a healthy person would look like. These conformed to a version of the "Martini people" (Hepworth and Featherstone 1982). They referred to healthiness as clear skin, shiny hair, nice teeth, being average weight, not too skinny or too fat, and "fit" or toned, rested and happy.

> *Rowena*: I don't know. Normal. Average weight. Clear skin and shiny hair.
>
> (aged 21, studying nursing)

> *Amy*: It sounds daft but an even proportioned body, although I'm not sure how that does equate with health, but . . . because it is nature isn't it, you know, how you're built and whatever, so, you know, clear skin, good hair, healthy looking hair.
>
> (aged 19, studying sociology)

> *Sarah*: I don't really know. Happy, again I think and laughing, because I think that's attractive. I suppose you'd have to say a good figure wouldn't you really. Nice teeth. Nice hair. I don't really know because everyone's different aren't they – you like them for who they are not what they look like really.
>
> (aged 20, studying social policy)

Far from bodies having natural shapes and sizes they represent highly skilled and socially differentiated achievements which are far from natural (Shilling 1993). The seeming contradiction between the body as plastic and malleable yet natural in shape and size provides evidence of competing pressures about the body. The unhealthy body is perceived to be at a physical extreme, either too fat or too thin in addition to being unhappy or irritable. Our respondents recognized these pressures and had very clear negotiating strategies which equated extreme body-molding activities with ill-health. At the same time they also tended to follow a popular lay equation of extreme body size with ill-health.

Jo: No I think it's a lot up here [in the mind] as well. It's like you hear about these women who can use really really crash course diets, you know, like models and stuff, but models aren't healthily thin at all, in the least bit and they starve themselves to have a set kind of look . . . I don't regard that as being in good health.

(aged 22, studying social policy)

Hayley: I think in people's mind, if you see a large person you think, you automatically think, oh they obviously don't eat properly. Obviously it's not a direct relation.

(aged 19, studying sociology)

The interviewees felt that there is a "look" of health since women with particular "desired" features are "looking" healthy while women with other "undesired" features, such as being overweight, tend to "look" unhealthy. Therefore what health "looks" like and actual bodily health are not necessarily analogous. Having "the look" (Featherstone 1991) is what is important. Amy's discussion sheds light on this, revealing an awareness that biological healthiness cannot be seen. Amy suggests that people cannot "see" that a person who is fat may be eating "properly" and in good health. Instead, the fatness is portrayed as an "unhealthy" body as it is not socially acceptable.

Amy: Because how do you . . . I suppose, how do you see health? You can't sort of . . . I mean a fat person might be healthy though, you know, it's not just because of being large that they're unhealthy. But I think generally people would make that relationship between being fat equals unhealthy.

I: You can't see health?

Amy: No. Well, maybe you can in that, I don't know, if you look at somebody's skin, if it's quite clear, you could sort of say that they're healthy or well my skin, if it's a bit spotty it's usually because I've got a bit run down so it's probably not going to be healthy.

(aged 19, studying sociology)

Behaviors such as eating a balanced diet and getting regular exercise are often viewed as laudable in a society where individuals are largely perceived to be responsible for their health (Lupton 1995). However, where such behaviors are not on view, judgment about the moral character of an individual can only be made by viewing the outer body. This leads to a focus, not on behaviors, but on being a "picture" of health, that is a beautiful body. The following quotes demonstrate that the women interviewed are aware of this double standard but are unlikely or unwilling to resist it.

Lisa: There was this girl last year and she was a very nice student, she was slim, but didn't do anything, she ate pizza all day. She didn't have any meals and I just think, she wasn't healthy. Didn't have a healthy lifestyle at all. Didn't make an effort with anything. She'd drink, she smoked, she used to get up late. She just didn't bother with herself at all but she still looked very good.

I: Do you think health and looking good are separate?

Lisa: I think they should be. I don't think they often are. Because health is for you isn't it. I suppose looking good is for yourself as well, but you should be able to be healthy and not worry about what you look like, or you should be able to think, oh that's okay but if you were naturally thin, you should really be healthy as well ... do you see what I mean?

(aged 19, studying social policy)

Nicole: I suppose you do. It's like these models, I mean maybe they don't have, I mean I don't know what they eat so I can't really say but maybe they don't ... they're probably not having enough protein and carbohydrates or whatever and not having enough calories in a day which your body actually does need to perform efficiently and maybe they're not eating properly, I mean some people aren't naturally born very slim but I think a lot of them are. Especially it's affecting teenagers and things through magazines.

(aged 19, studying nursing)

Consequently it is the outer, social body that is central in these young women's place-in-the-world. Their outer body is a form of physical capital upon which they are evaluated; physical capital influences their relationships with others. Thus, it is the resource that is most useful for coping with their day-to-day lives. As the following interviewees' words illustrate, biological health is not the reason that they manage their bodies with diet and exercise. The reason that they practice these and other lifestyle behaviors is primarily because they are perceived to affect how they will look.

Amy: Yes. I think, I mean exercise makes us healthier as well but it makes you happier in that you are achieving these looks that you want to maybe as well. I think those factors are just as important. You know, when I exercise, like when I was going to aerobics, it was not for the fun of going to aerobics, and I'm not keeping in mind, ooh I'm going to be slim or whatever, or I'm going to be really healthy. And I feel bad if I don't go and my friends are going to aerobics. It's almost sort of, bit like a competition, it's like mmm, you're going to be flabby and I'm not going to be flabby.

(aged 19, studying sociology)

Emma: I'm more concerned with how I look than how healthy I am, yes.

I: So you do this exercise more for fitness or for how you look?

Emma: More for, to just keep the weight down, like, visually so I haven't got ... you know, a minute on the lips, a lifetime on the hips kind of thing. But I don't do the exercise to be healthy. I'm doing exercise to look a bit better when it comes to summertime.

(aged 19, studying sociology)

Despite an awareness that they are often doing things which might not be good for the inner body, the women explained why it was important for them to lose weight or be fitter. They explain that when they *feel* that they are attractive it gives them confidence that is noticed by others. Hence feeling attractive to others enabled the interviewees to feel happy, valued, and good about themselves. This reinforces their focus of etching social expectations upon their physical bodies. The pursuit of an idealized body weight or shape becomes attached to concern about diet (Bordo 1998).

I: So there seems to be some sort of, you think, mental and physical connection?

Liz: Yes between health and positive feeling and stuff and I think it kind of reciprocates on itself. If you're feeling low and depressed, like binge-eating, if you're feeling low and depressed, you don't give a shit what you look like, you don't care about exercise, you just want to eat loads of stuff, and then you feel guilty so you throw it all up or whatever and then you look crap although you think you look great and it goes down and down and down whereas ... I mean it might be a bit psychological but I think if you feel better you project a more comfortable image towards other people.

(aged 21, studying nursing)

Melanie: Well I'm not really worried about other people, well I am, but I'm worried about ... it's more about making myself feel better really. It gives you a bit more confidence if you think that you look better but on the other hand I think, well, will I ever think that. Will I ever think I look better? Probably not.

(aged 19, studying sociology)

The following response from Olivia emphasizes how she perceives her health to be about looking good, feeling good, and liking herself. The connection here is between a healthy mind associated with confidence and happiness and having "the look" in the outer body.

Olivia: I am sure a lot of people, if they look better, they'll feel better, you know if they've sort of lost a lot of weight or whatever, then they feel much better with themselves. Full of more confidence. Go out and do things.

I: Are they healthier then?

Olivia: Well yes because if they've lost a lot of weight they are going to
be healthier and be happier in their minds won't they?

(aged 20, studying social policy)

Yet Emma's words, while illustrating how health and looking good are
closely connected, also show how it is unlikely that women can achieve
absolute health because they are never entirely happy with their lifestyles or
with the way they look.

I: You don't know any healthy people?

Emma: Not 100 percent healthy because like you say, I don't know
anyone who is perfectly happy with their lifestyle, who's perfectly
happy with the way they look, the way they do things. Everyone
always whinges about something in their life don't they so . . .

(aged 19, studying sociology)

Within these women's places-in-the-world they speak of many pressures.
There are pressures related to performing well at university but there are the
more central pressures of how they appear to others, particularly the opposite
sex, and the larger issue of societal expectations. We hear from these women
that they are very aware of these pressures and recognize that they are
unrealistic, yet they do not feel that they can, or want to, resist them.

Nicole: I feel pressure on myself to be sort of like better and like he
went to this warehouse because he is sponsored by this company and
he went to this warehouse to pick up some kit and brought me some
back and I felt like . . . and he said, "oh are you going to wear this?
Are you going to wear these trainers?" And bla bla bla and I just felt
this little dig as if to say, "Don't you think you should start toning
up a bit?" and I do sort of have this slight complex about sort of
like, my bum and stuff like this.

(aged 19, studying nursing)

Nicole has internalized a "fragmented body image" (Balsamo 1998) where
certain "flawed" parts need "fixing." The "gaze" of her male partner emphasizes this fragmentation. However, as Sarah Bartely suggests, the "panoptical
male consumer [who] resides within the consciousness of most women"
(quoted in Lloyd 1996: 91) means that most women discipline their physical
bodies with the male gaze in mind. The "tyranny of slenderness" (Chernin
1983) is aimed at purely physical transformation. The pressure can lead to
anxiety in a world where individuals are increasingly preoccupied with
promoting a particular self (Smart 1999). This is summed up by Olivia:

Olivia: You've got the health benefits, you've got the one side of it, it's
the benefit, you're healthy, but then, why do women exercise? Yes

it's because of their health, it's also to get ... you know so many women are on diets, it's also to get skinnier, why do they want to be skinnier? Because people perceive them as being fat or whatever and they probably think, well if I'm skinny, that bloke I fancy, he might like me if I'm a bit thinner. Women think like that. I'm sure they do. If their boyfriends or something say, oh well you're a bit fat, they think "oh, I'll go on a diet because he won't fancy me anymore" you know ... I'm sure of it. I mean you've got this one side which says it's good for your health but then, the other side, I mean – and there may be a lot of women who think they're dieting or doing exercise or whatever for themselves – but I'm sure that a lot of it is because of how society perceives us and expects us women to be.

(aged 20, studying social policy)

So these young women display gendered notions of health and beauty which locate the responsibility for their body image firmly in themselves. They expect to discipline their bodies, though not to a "pathological" level. Although they recognized that the appearance of their outer bodies does not necessarily portray a healthy inner body their main concern was portraying a healthy "image" in a society where "unprecedented value is placed on the youthful, trim and sensual body" (Shilling 1993: 3).

Amy: I think it's sort of you have to accept the way things are, I mean, I can't stand alone against society so, look, you've got to change. This is little me. I'm not going to make a difference so therefore I play the game. I go along with it.

(aged 19, studying sociology)

Conclusion

The young women in our study speak of their past as a time when they ate better and did more exercise. Some of this is due to the fact that while in the family home, there were others to take care of their bodily needs by, for example, cooking proper meals for them. This meant they did not have the responsibility of taking care of their physical body and so were able to focus more upon the needs of the social body. This is perhaps the crucial distinction between their recollection of their views prior to leaving school and their perspectives as university students – which might otherwise be expected to be similar. When they come to university, the interviewees are put into a situation where there is a high level of instability and they quickly develop resources to cope with this. In addition, they are also suddenly made responsible for their own physical well-being. For many it is a time of struggle and negotiation. It is a time when they relinquish the needs of the physical body in order to learn to cope with independence and freedom. This involves doing things that can make them "look better" and thus feel better about themselves and give them the confidence boost required to cope with unfamiliar situations. In this way the "health" needs of the physical body are manipulated or negated in order to develop and create a social body that is useful for negotiating their position with regard to others in their changed place in the world.

The change in lifestyle, resulting from a move to a new place, a university environment, had meant that these women felt unable to care for their bodies in the ways they had previously. Much of their current behavior reflects a student lifestyle which is popularly characterized by drinking and fast food – though interestingly clothes, another key aspect of this lifestyle, featured little in the interviews. In this sense the lifestyle decisions these young women were making were inextricably linked to a milieu which differed from the "healthy" and routinized space they associated with their former location. These lifestyle changes were seen as only temporary and in most cases a purposeful reaction designed to facilitate a smooth transition from their family space to the social space of the university. It appears that they also regard these changes in health-related behavior as transitory with regard to the future. Upon leaving university, they intend to adopt a "healthier" lifestyle. Thus the attitudes and viewpoints which we have been able to identify represent mobile meanings and reinscriptions concerning the body, in which transition across time and space draws on locational context.

Lifestyle, identity, and behavior are crucially constrained by context. Our study has shown how this conclusion can be applied to young women at a transitional stage in their lives. Their "presenting selves" seek an image that guarantees acceptance. The physical capital that these young women have in terms of youth is, in their own view, in need of enhancement by a "healthy" and "beautiful" appearance. The women know this amounts to the appearance of their outer bodies and may have little to do with the care of their inner bodies. They move in an environment dominated by younger people where they are constantly on display and they live in a consumer culture that encourages the display of bodies. Their notions of health and beauty are framed in place and changed by transition between places.

Note

1 All names have been changed to hide identities. "I" denotes the interviewer.

References

Balsamo, A. (1998) "On the cutting edge: cosmetic surgery and the technological production of the gendered body," in N. Mirzoeff (ed.) *The Visual Culture Reader*, London: Sage: 223–33.

Baxter, J. and Eyles, J. (1997) "Evaluating qualitative research in social geography: establishing 'rigour' in interview analysis," *Transactions of the Institute of British Geographers* 22: 505–25.

Bell, D. and Valentine, G. (1995) *Mapping Desire: Geographies of Sexualities*, London: Routledge.

Blumer, H. (1969) *Symbolic Interactionism*, New York: Prentice-Hall.

Bordo, S. (1998) "Reading the slender body," in N. Mirzoeff (ed.) *The Visual Culture Reader*, London: Sage: 214–22.

Bourdieu, P. (1984) *Distinction: A Social Critique of the Judgement of Taste*, London: Routledge.

Butler, J. (1990) *Gender Trouble: Feminism and the Subversion of Identity*, London: Routledge.

Chapkiss, W. (1986) *Beauty Secrets: Women and the Politics of Appearance*, Boston: South End Press.

Chernin, K. (1983) *Womansize: The Tyranny of Slenderness*, London: The Women's Press.

Cresswell, T. (1996) *In Place/Out of Place: Geography, Ideology and Transgression*, Minneapolis: University of Minnesota Press.

—— (1999) "Embodiment, power and the politics of mobility: the case of female tramps and hobos," *Transactions of the Institute of British Geographers* 24: 175–92.

Dorn, M. and Laws, G. (1994) "Social theory, body politics and medical geography," *Professional Geographer* 46: 106–10.

Duncan, N. (1996) *BodySpace: Destabilising Geographies of Gender and Sexuality*, London: Routledge.

Dyck, I. (1995) "Hidden geographies: the changing lifeworlds of women with multiple sclerosis," *Social Science and Medicine* 40: 307–20.

Eyles, J. (1988) "Interpreting the geographical world," in J. Eyles and D. Smith (eds) *Qualitative Methods in Human Geography*, Cambridge: Polity Press.

Featherstone, M. (1991) "The body in consumer culture," in M. Featherstone, M. Hepworth, and B. Turner (eds) *The Body: Social Processes and Cultural Theory*, London: Sage.

Featherstone, M. and Wernick, A. (1995) *Images of Ageing*, London: Routledge

Foucault, M. (1998) "Other spaces," in N. Mirzoeff (ed.) *The Visual Culture Reader*, London: Sage: 237–44.

Frank, A. (1991) "For a sociology of the body: an analytical review," in M. Featherstone, M. Hepworth, and B. Turner (eds) *The Body: Social Processes and Cultural Theory*, London: Sage.

Giddens, A. (1991) *Modernity and Self-Identity: Self and Society in the Late Modern Age*, Cambridge: Polity Press.

Glaser, B. and Strauss, A. (1967) *The Discovery of Grounded Theory*, Chicago: Aldine.

Goffman, E. (1969) *The Presentation of Self in Everyday Life*, Harmondsworth: Penguin.

Grosz, E. (1990) "Inscriptions and body-maps: representations and the corporeal," in T. Threadgold and A. Cranny-Francis (eds) *Feminine/Masculine and Representation*, London: Allen & Unwin.

—— (1994) *Volatile Bodies: Towards a Corporeal Feminism*, Bloomington: Indiana University Press.

Hepworth, M. and Featherstone, M. (1982) *Surviving Middle Age*, Oxford: Blackwell.

Katz, C. and Monk, J. (1993) *Full Circles: Geographies of Women over the Life Course*, London: Routledge.

Lincoln, Y. and Guba, E. (1985) *Naturalistic Inquiry*, Beverley Hills, CA: Sage.

Litva, A. and Eyles, J. (1994) "Health or healthy: why people are not sick in a southern Ontario town," *Social Science and Medicine* 39: 1083–91.

Lloyd, M. (1996) "Feminism, aerobics and the politics of the body," *Body and Society* 2: 79–98.

Longhurst, R. (1994) "The geography closest in: the body and the politics of pregnability," *Australian Geographical Studies* 32: 214–23.

—— (1995) "The body and geography," *Gender, Place and Culture* 2: 97–105.

Lupton, D. (1995) *The Imperative of Health: Public Health and the Regulated Body*, London: Sage.

McDowell, L. (1992) "Doing gender: feminism, feminists and research methods in human geography," *Transactions of the Institute of British Geographers* 17: 399–416.

Mirzoeff, N. (ed.) (1998) *The Visual Culture Reader*, London: Sage.

Moon, G. (1995) "(Re)placing research on health and health care," *Health and Place* 1: 1–4.

Moss, P. and Dyck, I. (1996) "Inquiry into environment and body: women, work, and chronic illness," *Environment and Planning D: Society and Space* 14: 737–53.

Parr, H. (1998) "Mental health, ethnography and the body," *Area* 30: 28–37.

Pile, S. (1996) *The Body and the City*, London: Routledge.

Rodaway, P. (1994) *Sensuous Geographies: Body, Sense and Place*, London: Routledge.

Shilling, C. (1993) *The Body and Social Theory*, London: Sage.

Smart, B. (1999) *Facing Modernity: Ambivalence, Reflexivity and Morality*, London: Sage.

Turner, B. (1991) "The discourse of diet," in M. Featherstone, M. Hepworth, and B. Turner (eds) *The Body: Social Processes and Cultural Theory*, London: Sage.

Warde, A. (1997) *Consumption, Food and Taste: Culinary Antinomies and Commodity Culture*, London: Sage.

15 Women in their place

Gender and perceptions of neighborhoods and health in the West of Scotland

Anne Ellaway and Sally Macintyre

Introduction

It has recently been argued that much health research has incorporated one of two types of gender bias (Ruiz and Verbrugge 1997). The first type of bias is the assumed equality or similarity of men and women. This is reflected in the way in which results from studies of men are extrapolated in an unquestioning way on to women. This is particularly the case for diseases which are often assumed (sometimes wrongly) to be more prevalent in men, such as heart disease; clinical trials and epidemiological studies of heart disease have commonly been undertaken in male-only samples, and the results then generalized to the total population. However this type of bias also applies to studies which include both men and women but which then treat gender as a control variable, a form of noise in the system, to be controlled away in multivariate analysis so that the supposedly true effect of a risk factor or treatment can be more correctly assessed.

The second type of bias is the assumption that men and women are fundamentally different. The basis of these differences is often unquestioned and this assumption may be expressed either in the use of different outcome measures for men and women (for example the safe number of units of alcohol per week), or in the use of single-sex samples with implicit comparisons being made with the unstudied gender (for example the physical and mental symptoms experienced by women around the time of the menopause are often studied but rarely compared systematically with the prevalence of similar symptoms among men of a similar age).

Both these types of bias are discernible in the study of gender, place, and health. Many area-based studies of health or risk factors associated with health have studied only men. Examples include the analysis of the relationship between median household income and the zipcode of residents in the US MRFIT study (Davey Smith *et al.* 1996), international comparisons of mortality by social class (Kunst and Mackenbach 1994), and the British Regional Heart Study (Shaper *et al.* 1981). Although there may be good reasons for using only men in these studies, the results are often seen as generalizable to both sexes. Other recent epidemiological studies of the relationship between area level income inequality and mortality have combined both sexes (Kennedy *et al.* 1996; Lynch *et al.* 1998). Again, there may be good reasons, in terms of data available, to combine both sexes, but the result is that one is unable to examine whether the effects of income inequality are greater for either men or women, and the impression given is that there are no gender differences in this regard.

On the other hand many studies of place and health assume, though without clearly demonstrating, that there are or inevitably will be gender differences and that therefore it is appropriate to study only one gender. Thus at a session on health and place at the fourth International Congress of Behavioral Medicine in Baltimore in 1996, Felicia Leclere presented an analysis which included males only, justifying this on the basis that "it is well-known that" men are more sensitive to the effects of the environment than women (Leclere and Rodgers 1996). In contrast, other writers have suggested, again often without providing empirical evidence, that women are more sensitive to the local physical and social environment (Payne 1991). The assumption that women are more sensitive to the local environment is often based on a further assumption that women spend more time at home or on domestic tasks which require local services. However, this assumption is often presented without any supporting empirical evidence from particular times, cultures, or places. What may well have been true in middle-class suburbs in Western societies in the 1950s, may not be true, nor may it ever have been true, of other sub-cultures, places, or cultures. In this chapter we will first explore the evidence for gender differences in perceptions of risk and relationships with health and then draw upon data collected in the West of Scotland to examine empirically whether there are gender differences in perceptions of the local environment and health.

Evidence for gender differences

Although much research on area variations in health does not focus directly on gender differences, it has recently been observed that both socio-economic and area variations in health may be more marked for men than for women (Macintyre 1997; Macintyre forthcoming). For example, there are stronger associations among men than among women between area-based deprivation and life expectancy in England (Raleigh and Kiri 1997) and area deprivation and mortality in Scotland (Macintyre forthcoming). This raises questions about potential differences between men and women in the social meanings of place, and in exposure or vulnerability to social and physical environments.

A substantial body of work shows that women tend to view the world as a more risky place than do men. Women tend to perceive greater risk from a wide range of events such as nuclear power, technological disasters, airplane and car accidents (Karpowicz-Lazreg and Mullet 1993; Flynn *et al.* 1994), and risks in the domestic arena such as fire in the home (Savage 1993). In the employment sphere, women in the same position in the same organization as men are more likely to report a poorer physical working environment (Emslie *et al.* 1999), even after "actual" differences in physical conditions have been measured by outside observers (Sternberg and Wall 1995).

Various explanations have been proposed to account for the gender difference in risk perception. Candidate explanations include women feeling more personally threatened by environmental problems than men, women tending to be more involved in local activities than men and therefore more knowledgeable about environmental issues, and women being more concerned than men with nurturing and maintaining life and less concerned than men with jobs and economic growth (Blocker and Eckberg 1989; Stern and Kalof 1993).

If there are gender differences in perceptions of the environment, how might these relate to health? We have previously reported that residents of socially contrasting neighborhoods in an urban area varied systematically in their perceptions of features of their local social and physical environment (such as area amenities, problems, crime, neighborliness, area reputation, and satisfaction) and that these varying perceptions were associated with self-reported health (Sooman and Macintyre 1995). A study of African-American mothers found that perceptions of features of their residential environment such as police protection, personal safety, cleanliness, and quietness were associated with very low birthweight in their infants after controlling for maternal health behaviors such as alcohol use and cigarette smoking (Collins *et al.* 1998).

Molinari (1998) examined men's and women's perceptions of the social and physical quality of their community and found that for women, it was their perceptions of the *social* quality of their local community (including problems such as unemployment, access to health care, youth violence, and the quality of public education) that were associated with their self-assessed health, whereas for men, it was their perceptions of the *physical* quality of their local community (such as the quality of indoor and outdoor air, drinking water, and waste disposal) that were associated with their self-assessed health (Molinari 1998).

In this chapter we use data from the West of Scotland to examine: first, whether there are gender differences in perceptions of the local, neighborhood environment; second, whether these might relate to employment and domestic roles; and third, whether perceptions of the environment relate to self-reported health, and if so whether this relationship differs between men and women. This is a very preliminary analysis of data collected in a particular time and place, but it is offered as a contribution towards the development of an empirical body of evidence about gender, health, and place.

Study design and methods

To examine these relationships, we draw here upon the locality component of the "Twenty-07 study: health in the community" based in the West of

Scotland in the United Kingdom (Macintyre *et al.* 1989). The Twenty-07 study, which began in 1987, is following three cohorts (aged 15, 35, and 55 when first interviewed in 1987) of individuals over a twenty-year period. The aim of the study is to explore the social processes producing social patterning in health, in particular by gender, age, socio-economic status, ethnicity, family composition, and area of residence. The study area encompasses a large, socially heterogeneous region centered around Glasgow and draws in areas formerly dominated by heavy industry (such as shipbuilding and steel-making) and some semi-rural agricultural communities.

One component of the study involves two socially contrasting localities in Glasgow city. These two localities (each comprising two neighborhoods) are the north-west (comprising the neighborhoods of the West End and Garscadden) and the south-west (comprising the neighborhoods of Mosspark and Greater Pollok). In the north-west of the city, the West End exists as a spatial representation of the social class divisions of Victorian times, the area being built for the middle classes of that time, physically separate from the heavy industry elsewhere in the city. The area consists of nineteenth-century sandstone villas and tenements, the latter frequently having retail premises on their ground floors at easily accessible road junctions. Today, addresses in this neighborhood are still among the most desirable in Glasgow.

Garscadden, also in the north-west, is a planned, mainly public housing extension to the city. The high-status council estates which predominate here were built between the two world wars with high rents and purpose-built community facilities (e.g. shopping parades) aimed at attracting the more affluent working classes. Today, many of the houses have been bought by their tenants. The West End is in the eastern part, and Garscadden the western part, of the north-west locality; they are spatially contiguous and some local services and amenities are equally available to both neighborhoods.

In the south-west of the city, Mosspark is, like Garscadden, an area of high-status interwar development. However, it also includes some low-rent council flats more typical of Glasgow and, being further from the city center than Garscadden and adjacent to a more deprived rather than more affluent area, it might be considered less socially advantaged.

Greater Pollok is the poorest of the four neighborhoods and the most remote from the city center. It is one of Glasgow's four postwar peripheral public housing "schemes." Unlike many of their interwar predecessors, these schemes lacked many basic local amenities (e.g. shops, schools, health centers, social centers) for decades after their construction. Because of the postwar housing shortage, properties were built to standards previously thought to be unacceptably low. Greater Pollok is at the other end of a spectrum of "desirability" from the West End. Mosspark and Greater Pollok are adjacent and some amenities and services are accessible to both.

The four neighborhoods thus differ in history, built environment, local amenities, and socio-demographic characteristics. The West End is the most socio-residentially advantaged and Greater Pollok the most disadvantaged. As one might expect, health also differs between these neighborhoods, with those living in the most affluent neighborhood reporting lower levels of limiting long-term illness, and having lower standardized mortality ratios at or around the 1991 census, compared with the most deprived neighborhood. Men reported slightly more limiting long-term illness compared with women in each neighborhood.

Data from respondents in the locality sample have been gathered on three occasions so far, with face-to-face interviews in 1987 and 1992, and a postal survey in 1997. Here we use data from 1997 on those respondents (265 men and 340 women) who were still resident within these localities. The numbers of respondents in each neighborhood were 178 in the West End (78 men, 100 women), 147 in Garscadden (60 men, 87 women), 41 in Mosspark (21 men, 20 women), and 239 in Greater Pollok (106 men, 133 women).

Measures of assessment of neighborhood

Respondents were asked a range of structured questions about how they perceived their local area. These included both general questions and more specific questions about particular characteristics of their local neighborhood. The focus of the questions ranged from respondents' perceptions of the provision of services and amenities to questions relating to the quality and safety of the local environment. Here we report on the responses to two suites of questions by gender.

Local problems

To measure respondents' perceptions of local problems, they were asked about eleven types of socio-environmental problem in their neighborhood. Respondents were invited to reply using a three-point scale ("not a problem," "minor problem," "serious problem"), with an option for "don't know." Table 15.1 shows the proportion of men and women reporting their perceptions of these items as a "serious" problem. Women were more likely to see most of these items as a "major" problem than were men, with the exception of perceptions of assaults and muggings and problems with dogs. Women's more negative assessments of local problems reported in Table 15.1 do not support an interpretation that women are in general more positive about their local neighborhood environment than are men.

To construct a variable indicating overall assessment of local problems, responses to each of the individual problems were summed (the scores can range from 13 to 39). Women had a significantly higher mean score than did males ($p < 0.05$); there was no significant difference by age although those in the 45-year-old cohort had the highest mean score; neighborhoods differed significantly in local problems score ($p < 0.001$) with those living in the most deprived neighborhood having the highest score; and there was a clear social

Table 15.1   Proportion of women and men reporting a "serious" problem with various aspects of the neighborhood

	Women %	Men %	Sig.
Lack of recreational facilities	34.9	25.3	**
Lack of safe places for children to play	30.6	23.8	*
Speeding traffic	21.6	16.9	
Litter and rubbish	18.3	13.4	
Burglaries	17.6	16.4	
Uneven or dangerous pavements	14.0	9.0	*
Vandalism	13.9	12.0	
Disturbance by children or youngsters	12.6	12.5	
Nuisance from dogs	12.3	13.6	
Reputation of neighborhood	8.1	4.4	*
Smells and fumes	5.6	2.2	*
Assaults and muggings	4.5	7.3	
Discarded needles and syringes	2.2	0.7	

Notes
* p' < 0.05
** p < 0.01

class gradient (p < 0.001) (according to the respondents' own social class using the Registrar General's classification of occupation (OPCS 1980)) with those in higher social classes reporting fewer local problems (see Table 15.2). The significant gender difference remained after adjustment for age, and after adjustment for age and area of residence (representing respondents' physical location but not their perceptions about aspects of their environment), but disappeared after adjustment for age and the respondent's own social class.

Perceptions of neighborhood cohesion

Recent debates within the field of health inequalities have highlighted the potential role that social cohesion might play as a determinant of health (Wilkinson 1996), although social cohesion has rarely been measured directly. We included a scale measuring perceived neighborhood cohesion (Buckner 1988). This was developed in the United States as a measure of psychological sense of community, attraction to neighborhood, and the extent of social interaction, within geographically bounded neighborhoods. It has been found to be associated with home ownership and years of residence in an area; there are conflicting findings on the presence of children in the home and the relationship between neighborhood cohesion and income. We used the version of the scale as validated in Canada (Robinson and Wilkinson 1995). It contains seventeen statements about the neighborhood, respondents being invited to describe their agreement or disagreement with each on a five-point Likert scale (ranging from "strongly agree" to "strongly disagree"). The items include statements such as: "If I need advice about

Table 15.2 Mean local problems and neighborhood cohesion scores: means by
gender, cohort, social class, and neighborhood of residence

	Local problems score (mean)	Neighborhood cohesion score (mean)
Gender	*	ns
Women	21.4	57.8
Men	22.3	59.2
Cohort	ns	**
25-year-olds	21.6	52.5
45-year-olds	22.3	58.3
65-year-olds	21.8	62.4
Social class	**	ns
I/II/III non-manual	20.1	58.4
III manual	22.1	58.6
IV/V	24.8	58.8
Neighborhood of residence	**	**
West End	19.1	60.1
Garscadden	21.7	59.0
Mosspark	20.1	60.1
Greater Pollok	24.5	56.6

Notes
* p < 0.05
** p < 0.001
ns not significant

something I could go to someone in my neighborhood," "I believe my
neighbors would help in an emergency," and "I visit with my neighbors in
their homes." The total scores can range from 17 to 85, with higher scores
representing higher perceived neighborhood cohesion.

There was no significant difference between men and women in total
neighborhood cohesion score although men were slightly more negative
in their assessment. There was a significant difference by age (p < 0.001) with
older respondents having a more positive assessment of neighborhood
cohesion. There was no significant difference by social class, but there was
by neighborhood (p < 0.001), with respondents in the most deprived area
having the most negative assessment (see Table 15.2). The lack of gender
difference persisted after adjustment for age, social class, and area of
residence (there were no significant interactions).

Whilst there was no overall gender difference in the total score, there were
differences between the proportions of men and women "strongly agreeing"
with some of the individual items of the scale (Table 15.3). For every item,
including the two (5 and 15) which were phrased in a negative way, a higher
proportion of women compared with men reported that they "strongly
agreed" with the statement (the only exception was item 6 where a slightly
higher proportion of men reported "strongly agreeing" with this item).
It may be that this pattern of responses reflects a tendency on women's part
to be more likely to agree with such Likert type scales.

Table 15.3 Proportion of women and men reporting "strongly agree" with individual component statements of the neighborhood cohesion scale

	Women %	Men %	Sig.
1 Overall, I am very attracted to living in this neighborhood	26.7	22.1	
2 I feel like I belong to this neighborhood	23.1	20.4	
3 I visit with my neighbors in their homes	8.6	5.0	
4 The friendships and associations I have with other people in my neighborhood mean a lot to me	13.9	2.3	
5 Given the opportunity, I would like to move out of this neighborhood	8.3	5.7	
6 If the people in my neighborhood were planning something, I'd think of it as something "we" were doing rather than "they" were doing	4.8	5.0	
7 If I need advice about something I could go to someone in my neighborhood	10.7	5.7	*
8 I think I agree with most people in my neighborhood about what is important in life	5.9	3.8	
9 I believe my neighbors would help in an emergency	38.6	27.9	**
10 I feel loyal to the people in my neighborhood	15.0	11.9	
11 I borrow things and exchange favors with my neighbors	8.0	5.4	
12 I would be willing to work together with others on something to improve my neighborhood	19.5	14.5	
13 I plan to remain a resident of this neighborhood for a number of years	22.7	19.1	
14 I like to think of myself as similar to the people who live in this neighborhood	13.9	9.6	
15 I rarely have neighbors over to my house to visit	10.7	8.8	
16 I regularly stop and talk with people in my neighborhood	22.8	16.4	*
17 Living in this neighborhood gives me a sense of community	10.9	6.9	*

Notes
* $p < 0.05$
** $p < 0.01$

We examined whether gender differences in perceptions of place were more marked in some neighborhoods than in others (Table 15.4). For the local problems score, there was a larger gender difference in the most deprived area (Greater Pollok) than in the other neighborhoods, although this gender difference was not significant even there ($p < 0.09$), whereas for the neighborhood cohesion score the gender difference was only significant in the most affluent area (the West End, $p < 0.05$).

Table 15.4 Mean local problems and neighborhood cohesion scores: means (adjusted for age) for men and women, by neighborhood

	West End	Garscadden	Mosspark	Pollok
Local problems				
Gender difference *				
Women	19.2	22.1	20.6	25.3
Men	18.7	21.0	19.9	23.9
Area difference**				
All respondents	19.0	21.6	20.3	24.7
Neighborhood cohesion score				
Gender difference[ns]				
Women	62.5	58.9	58.9	57.2
Men	59.3	56.9	61.0	56.9
Area difference**				
All respondents	61.1	58.1	60.0	56.9

Notes
* p < 0.01
** p < 0.001
ns not significant

Explanations for gender differences in perceptions

Theorizing about gender differences in perceptions of place has tended to be based on assumptions that men and women are differentially exposed to their local neighborhoods, for example because women are less likely to go out to work, or because they spend more time at home, or have more localized social networks. How true are any of these assumptions in our study?

Employment status

We combined those respondents who reported being in one of the following categories as "not working" – disabled/permanently sick, retired, "caring for home", or unemployed – and compared them with those currently reporting themselves as "working." In our sample, a slightly higher proportion of women (48.2 percent) reported that they were "working" compared with men (46.8 percent) which is not what stereotypes would suggest. Overall, those respondents who were "working" had a more positive view of their neighborhood on the local problems score compared with those "not working" (p < 0.001); this significant difference persisted after adjustment for age and when men and women were examined separately. Women still had a more negative view of their areas than men, whether or not they were "working" (although this did not reach statistical significance), but with women who were "not working" having the most negative view of all (Table 15.5). Thus "working" men had the most positive and "non-working" women the most negative views of local problems. This suggests that

Table 15.5 Mean assessment of local problems and perceived neighborhood cohesion scores, by gender and employment status

	"Working" mean	n	"Not working" mean	n
Local problems				
Women	21.4	147	23.0	148
Men	20.2	114	22.1	122
All respondents	33.4	261	35.4	270
Perceived neighborhood cohesion				
Women	57.5	149	61.8	154
Men	56.2	115	59.9	126
All respondents	56.9	264	60.9	280

Note
Totals differ as a result of missing cases on some of the variables.

employment outside the home may explain some, but not all, of the gender difference in the measure (there was still a significant gender difference in local problems score after controlling for age and employment status ($p < 0.01$)).

A rather different pattern emerged with the neighborhood cohesion score in relation to employment outside the home; in this case it was those respondents who were "not working" who had the most positive view of neighborhood cohesion ($p < 0.001$) although this significant difference disappeared after controlling for age. When we examined this separately for men and women, it was women who were "not working" who had the most positive and men who "worked" who had the most negative assessment of neighborhood cohesion.

Presence of children in the home

It is sometimes assumed that mothers are particularly sensitive to their local neighborhood both because they interact with other, local mothers and because activities with children can be helped or hindered by features of the neighborhood (play spaces, transport, schools, etc.).

Women who had children (defined here as under 18 years of age) in their household had the most negative view of their local neighborhood according to both the local problems score and neighborhood cohesion score (although this was only statistically significant for the local problems score). There was little difference between men in these scores according to whether or not there were children present in the home (Table 15.6).

Interestingly, the presence of children in the home does not appear to affect the neighborhood differences in perceptions shown earlier (Table 15.4) as a higher proportion of respondents in West End have children under 18 in

Table 15.6 Mean local problems and neighborhood cohesion scores, by gender and presence of children

	Children in home mean	n	No children in home mean	n
Local problems				
Women	23.4	77	22.0	245
Men	21.4	53	21.4	202
All respondents	22.6	130	21.7	447
Perceived neighborhood cohesion				
Women	57.7	79	59.8	257
Men	58.4	54	57.8	207
All respondents	58.0	133	58.9	464

the home (West End 29 percent, Garscadden 21 percent, Mosspark 5 percent, Pollok 21 percent).

Relationships with health

Are there any associations between assessment of local problems, perceived neighborhood cohesion, and self-perceived health and, if so, are there different patterns for men and women? General linear modeling (GLM) was used for all the multivariate analysis (SPSS 1996) with separate models constructed sequentially for the variables of interest (local problems and neighborhood cohesion scores) which were adjusted for all the socio-demographic variables preceding them in the model (age, social class, and area of residence).

Health measures

Mental health: We used the General Health 12 questionnaire (GHQ12), a measure of minor psychiatric morbidity (Goldberg and Williams 1988). It comprises a series of statements (examples include "Have you recently lost much sleep over worry," "felt constantly under strain," "been able to enjoy your normal day-to-day activities?") and the respondent has to choose the level of agreement on a four-point scale (scored from 0 to 3, so total scores can range from 0 to 36).

Number of symptoms in the previous month: Respondents were asked to ring all of the symptoms they had suffered within the previous month from a list of twenty common symptoms (scored 1 for "yes" and 0 for "no" so total scores could range from 0 to 20).

"Malaise" type symptoms: We extracted from the total symptoms score those commonly thought to reflect psychosocial "malaise" (headaches,

Table 15.7 Summary of associations by gender between health measures and overall assessment of area and perceived neighborhood cohesion

	Model 1 age	Model 2 age and social class	Model 3 age, social class, and area of residence	Model 4 Model 3 + local problems score		Model 5 Model 3 + neighborhood cohesion score	
	$R^2 \times 100$	$R^2 \times 100$	$R^2 \times 100$	$R^2 \times 100$	$R^2 \times 100$ change	$R^2 \times 100$	$R^2 \times 100$ change
GHQ12 score							
Men	1.4	6.1	6.9	10.8***	3.9	9.4**	2.5
women	2.5	4.3	5.5	7.8**	2.3	6.3 ns	0.8
Total n. symptoms score							
Men	0.7	6.0	6.4	11.4***	5.0	8.4*	2.0
Women	0.1	1.8	5.4	15.6***	10.2	9.5***	4.1
"Malaise" type symptoms							
Men	3.8	8.2	8.5	13.1***	4.6	10.3*	1.8
women	3.7	3.9	5.4	13.3***	7.9	8.2**	2.8
"Physical" type symptoms							
Men	0.8	4.9	5.7	9.2**	3.5	7.1 ns	1.4
Women	2.8	5.2	8.9	15.3***	6.4	11.7**	2.8

Notes
* $p < 0.05$
** $p < 0.01$
*** $p < 0.001$
ns not significant

difficulty sleeping, problems with nerves, always feeling tired, difficulty concentrating, and worrying over every little thing). Scores could range from 0 to 6.

"Physical" symptoms reported in the previous month: We then looked at number of symptoms reported in the previous month excluding "malaise" ones. This list of "physical" symptoms included symptoms categorized as "respiratory," such as colds and flu, hay fever, and persistent cough; those categorized as "musculoskeletal," such as painful joints and problems with a "bad back"; those categorized as "gastrointestinal," such as constipation and indigestion/stomach trouble; and those categorized as "other," such as faints or dizziness, palpitations or breathlessness, trouble with feet, ears, or eyes, or kidney or bladder trouble. Scores could range from 0 to 14.

We first examined if there were significant relationships between assessment of local problems and perceived neighborhood cohesion and any of these health measures after controlling for age, social class, and area of residence. We found that among men and women taken together both local problems scores and neighborhood cohesion scores were significantly associated with all of the health measures after controlling for these sociodemographic factors.

We then went on to explore these associations separately for men and women. Table 15.7 shows the results of the analyses and utilizes the $R^2 \times 100$ statistic which can be interpreted as the percentage of variance in the outcome measure which is "explained" statistically by the predictor variable (age, social class, area scores). This method of presentation allows us to explore, for each health outcome, the additional contribution that perceived local problems or neighborhood cohesion make to models with age, social class, and area of residence and whether these might be different for men and women.

The first column shows for each health variable the $R^2 \times 100$ of model 1 which just has age; the second column (model 2) shows the outcome of adding social class to model 1; the third column (model 3) shows the outcome of adding area of residence to the model 2. Column 4 (model 4) shows the outcome of adding local problems score, while column 5 reports the corresponding change in $R^2 \times 100$. Column 6 (model 5) shows the outcome of adding perceived neighborhood cohesion to model 3, while column 7 shows the corresponding change in $R^2 \times 100$.

GHQ12: After taking into account age, social class, and area of residence, the local problems score is significantly associated with GHQ12 score in both women and men. Neighborhood cohesion scores were significantly related to GHQ12 score in men but not in women.

Total symptoms: Local problems are strongly and significantly associated with the total number of symptoms score in the previous month in both men and women, but with a much greater change in $R^2 \times 100$ for women than for men. Neighborhood cohesion scores were much more strongly associated with the total symptoms in women than in men.

"Malaise" symptoms: Local problems score is strongly significantly associated with "malaise" symptoms in both men and women. Neighborhood cohesion was much more strongly associated with the "malaise" symptoms for men than for women.

"Physical" symptoms: Local problem and neighborhood cohesion scores were significantly associated with "physical" symptoms in the previous month in women; but among men, there was weaker association between local problems and "physical" symptoms and no significant relationship between neighborhood cohesion and the "physical" symptoms.

Thus after controlling for age, social class, and neighborhood, local problems predicted all four health measures, in the case of "physical" symptoms more strongly in women. Perceived neighborhood cohesion related to GHQ12 only in men, and to "physical" symptoms only in women. Two of the health measures (total symptoms reported in the previous month and "malaise" symptoms) were associated with neighborhood cohesion in both sexes, but the association was stronger among women.

In three of the four health measures, both local problems and neighborhood cohesion scores explained more of the remaining variance (after taking account of age, social class, and neighborhood) among women than among men. In contrast, for the GHQ12 score, the additional affect of adding local problems or neighborhood cohesion scores was greater for men than for women.

Discussion

We have found few reports of empirical studies examining potential differences between men and women in experiences or perceptions of the local neighborhood, or how these might be associated with health. This chapter uses empirical data from a study in urban Scotland to provide a preliminary and descriptive analysis of this topic. We found no significant gender difference in one measure of perceptions of the neighborhood (perceived neighborhood cohesion); for another (assessment of local problems), women had a significantly more negative view of the area. Thus whether or not one observes gender differences in perceptions of area may depend on the particular measure or domain of perception used.

Gender differences in these perceptions also seem to be related to domestic circumstances and to type of neighborhood. The most negative perceptions were in women with children, and in women who were not employed outside the home. This lends some support to the idea that women at home with children may be more exposed or sensitive to features of their local neighborhood than are men or women in employment. While, as expected, the most negative views about local problems in the neighborhood were found in the most deprived area among both men and women, the difference between men and women was also greater there. By contrast, gender differences in perceptions of neighborhood cohesion were only significant in the most affluent neighborhood. This suggests that some gender differences may differ between different area contexts.

In this analysis we used self-assessments of health and of the neighborhood. We therefore cannot assume that any observed associations between assessments of area and of health are causal. People in poor health (particularly poorer psychosocial health) may be more likely to be negative about their areas; or people with a generally pessimistic world-view may be more likely to report both their health and their area as being poor. Furthermore, the observed differences between men and women in the associations between perceptions of the area and health may be due to different reporting styles among men and women.

Nevertheless, we think it interesting that, as we have previously shown, perceptions of the area are associated with health, and that for some measures these associations are stronger in one gender compared with the other. For one mental health measure (GHQ12) the association seemed to be stronger for men than for women, while for "physical" symptoms the association was stronger for women than for men. Our data do not allow us to examine directly why this is and we would be interested to know whether the observation is found in other studies. In further analysis we plan to take a longitudinal approach and explore whether perceptions of the area in 1987 predict health in 1997, and whether perceptions of the area are associated with directly measured aspects of health (such as blood pressure, respiratory function, immune function, and cardiovascular reactivity) and whether there are gender differences in these associations. The observations reported here raise more questions about gendered experience and consequences of place than they answer. We hope they will stimulate further research in other places and using similar or different measures.

References

Blocker, T. and Eckberg, D. (1989) "Environmental issues as women's issues: general concerns and local hazards," *Social Science Quarterly* 70: 586–93.

Buckner, J. C. (1988) "The development of an instrument to measure neighborhood cohesion," *American Journal of Community Psychology* 16, 6: 771–91.

Collins, J. W., David, R. J., Symons, R., Handler, A., Wale, S., and Andes, S. (1998) "African-American mothers' perception of their residential environmental, stressful life events, and very low birthweight," *Epidemiology* 9, 3: 286–9.

Davey Smith, G., Neaton, J. D., Wentworth, D., Stamler, R., and Stamler, J. (1996) "Socioeconomic differentials in mortality risk among men screened for the Multiple Risk Factor Intervention Trial 1: white men," *American Journal of Public Health* 86, 4: 486–96.

Emslie, C., Hunt, K., and Macintyre, S. (1999) "'Gender' or 'job' differences? Reported working conditions amongst men and women in similar white-collar occupations," *Employment, Work and Society* 13, 4: 711–29.

Flynn, J., Slovic, P., and Mertz, C. (1994) "Gender, race, and perception of environmental health risks," *Risk Analysis* 14, 6: 1101–8.

Goldberg, D. and Williams, P. (1988) *A User's Guide to the General Health Questionnaire*, Windsor: NFER-Nelson.

Karpowicz-Lazreg, C. and Mullet, E. (1993) "Societal risk as perceived by the French public," *Risk Analysis* 13: 253–8.

Kennedy, B. P., Kawachi, I., and Prothrowstith, D. (1996) "Income-distribution and mortality – cross-sectional ecological study of the Robin Hood Index in the United States," *British Medical Journal* 312, 7037: 1004–7.

Kunst, A. and Mackenbach, J. (1994) "International variations in the size of mortality differences associated with occupational status," *International Journal of Epidemiology* 23, 4: 742–50.

Leclere, F. and Rodgers, R. (1996) "Socioeconomic status and mortality in the United States: individual and community correlates," The Fourth International Congress on Behavioral Medicine, Washington, DC, The Society of Behavioral Medicine.

Lynch, J., Kaplan, G., Pamuk, E., Cohen, R., Heck, K., Balfour, J., and Yen, I. (1998) "Income inequality and mortality in metropolitan areas of the United States," *American Journal of Public Health* 88, 7: 1074–80.

Macintyre, S. (1997) "What are spatial effects and how can we measure them?" in A. Dale (ed.) *CCSR Occasional Paper No. 12: Exploiting National Survey and Census Data: The Role of Locality and Spatial Effects*, Manchester: University of Manchester.

—— (forthcoming) "Gender differences in the relationship between wealth and health: what can these tell us about the mechanisms producing social inequalities in health?", in D. Lean and G. Walt (eds) *Poverty, Inequality and Health*, Oxford: Oxford University Press.

Macintyre, S., Annandale, E., Ecob, R., Ford, G., Hunt, K., Jamieson, B., McIver, S., West, P., and Wyke, S. (1989) "The West of Scotland Twenty-07 study: health in the community," in C. Martin and D. McQueen (eds), *Readings for a New Public Health*, Edinburgh: Edinburgh University Press.

Molinari, C. (1998) "The relationship of community quality to the health of women and men," *Social Science and Medicine* 47, 8: 1113–20.

OPCS (1980) *Classification of Occupations and Coding Index*, London: HMSO.

Payne, S. (1991) *Women, Health and Poverty: An Introduction*, London: Harvester Wheatsheaf.

Raleigh, S. and Kiri, V. (1997) "Life expectancy in England; variation and trends by gender, heath authority and level of deprivation," *Journal of Epidemiology* 51: 649–58.

Robinson, D. and Wilkinson, D. (1995) "Sense of community in a remote mining town – validating a neighborhood cohesion scale," *American Journal of Community Psychology* 23, 1: 137–48.

Ruiz, M. and Verbrugge, L. (1997) "A two way view of gender bias in medicine," *Journal of Epidemiology and Community Health* 51: 106–9.

Savage, I. (1993) "Demographic influences on risk perceptions," *Risk Analysis* 13: 413–20.

Shaper, A., Pocock, S., Walker, M., Cohen, N., Wale, C., and Thomson, A. (1981) "British regional heart study: cardiovascular risk factors in middle-aged men in 24 towns," *British Medical Journal* 283, 6285: 179–86.

Sooman, A. and Macintyre, S. (1995) "Health and perceptions of the local environment in socially contrasting neighborhoods in Glasgow," *Health and Place* 1: 15–26.

SPSS (1996) *SPSS Advanced Statistics 7.0*.

Stern, P. and Kalof, L. (1993) "Value orientations, gender and environmental concerns," *Environment and Behavior* 25: 322–48.

Sternberg, B. and Wall, S. (1995) "Why do women report 'sick building symptoms' more often than men?", *Social Science & Medicine* 40, 4: 491–502.

Wilkinson, R. (1996) *Unhealthy Societies: The Afflictions of Inequality*, London: Routledge.

Index